Gastro-Esophageal Reflux Disease

Pathogenesis, Diagnosis, Therapy

Edited by

DONALD O. CASTELL, M.D.

Chief, Gastroenterology Section
Professor of Medicine
Bowman Gray School of Medicine
Winston-Salem, North Carolina

WALLACE C. WU, M.B., B.S.

Associate Professor of Medicine
Bowman Gray School of Medicine
Winston-Salem, North Carolina

DAVID J. OTT, M.D.

Associate Professor of Radiology
Bowman Gray School of Medicine
Winston-Salem, North Carolina

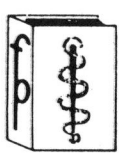

Futura Publishing Company, Inc.
Mount Kisco, New York
1985

Library of Congress Cataloging in Publication Data

Main entry under title:

Gastro-esophageal reflux disease.

    Includes bibliographies and index.
    1. Gastroesophageal reflux. I. Castell, Donald O.
II. Wu, Wallace C. III. Ott, David J. (David James),
1946-   . [DNLM: 1. Gastroesophageal reflux disease.
2. Gastroesophageal reflux disease. WI 250 G25691]
RC815.7.G36 1985   616.3'2   85-6789
ISBN 0-87993-239-2

Copyright © 1985
Futura Publishing Company, Inc.

Published by
Futura Publishing Company, Inc.
295 Main Street, P.O. Box 330
Mount Kisco, New York 10549

L.C. No.: 85-70526
ISBN No.: 0-87993-239-2

Contributors

Charles F. Barish, M.D.
 Fellow, Gastroenterology Section
 Bowman Gray School of Medicine
 Winston-Salem, North Carolina

Canan Avunduk Bonnice, M.D., Ph.D.
 Assistant Professor of Medicine
 University of Massachusetts Medical Center
 Worcester, Massachusetts

Donald O. Castell, M.D.
 Chief, Gastroenterology Section
 Professor of Medicine
 Bowman Gray School of Medicine
 Winston-Salem, North Carolina

Robert J. Cowan, M.D.
 Director of Nuclear Medicine
 Professor of Radiology
 Bowman Gray School of Medicine
 Winston-Salem, North Carolina

Tom R. DeMeester, M.D.
 Chairman, Department of Surgery
 Professor of Thoracic and Cardiovascular Surgery
 Creighton University
 Omaha, Nebraska

Wylie J. Dodds, M.D.
 Professor of Radiology and Medicine
 Medical College of Wisconsin
 Milwaukee, Wisconsin

Andre Dubois, M.D., Ph.D.
 Assistant Director of Digestive Disease Division
 Associate Professor of Medicine
 Uniformed Services University of the
     Health Sciences School of Medicine
 Bethesda, Maryland

Gregory L. Eastwood, M.D.
Director, Gastroenterology Division
Professor of Medicine
University of Massachusetts
Worcester, Massachusetts

Kim R. Geisinger, M.D.
Assistant Professor of Pathology
Bowman Gray School of Medicine
Winston-Salem, North Carolina

James F. Helm, M.D.
Assistant Professor of Medicine
Medical College of Wisconsin
Milwaukee, Wisconsin

Walter J. Hogan, M.D.
Professor of Medicine
Medical College of Wisconsin
Milwaukee, Wisconsin

Philip O. Katz, M.D.
Fellow, Gastroenterology Division
Bowman Gray School of Medicine
Winston-Salem, North Carolina

Roy C. Orlando, M.D.
Associate Professor of Medicine
University of North Carolina School of Medicine
Chapel Hill, North Carolina

David J. Ott, M.D.
Associate Professor of Radiology
Bowman Gray School of Medicine
Winston-Salem, North Carolina

William J. Ravich, M.D.
Assistant Professor of Medicine
Clinical Director, The Swallowing Center
The Johns Hopkins University School of Medicine
Baltimore, Maryland

Joel E. Richter, M.D.
    Assistant Professor of Medicine
    Bowman Gray School of Medicine
    Winston-Salem, North Carolina

Wallace C. Wu, M.B., B.S.
    Associate Professor of Medicine
    Bowman Gray School of Medicine
    Winston-Salem, North Carolina

Preface

Symptomatic gastroesophageal (GE) reflux manifested by heartburn or acid regurgitation is an extremely common problem in the United States. Although a great number of scientific publications have been written during the past decade concerning the mechanisms and manifestations of GE reflux, there has been little attempt to bring this information together in a treatise. The intent, therefore, of this book was to consolidate the available information on GE reflux. We have endeavored to cover in detail the pathogenesis, diagnosis, and therapy of GE reflux disease by reviewing both the older and newer literature. We sought to identify the most relevant aspects of GE reflux and its complications by inviting those individuals with special expertise and research experience in these areas to participate in this project. Because of the cooperation and enthusiasm of the many experts who prepared the chapters of this book, the final result is proudly presented as a statement of the current thinking on GE reflux disease. Newer concepts in the pathogenesis, diagnosis, and therapy of this common malady are balanced with older views that have been time-honored. We hope that this material will prove valuable to those physicians and clinical investigators having an interest in the problem of GE reflux disease. We apologize if the reader identifies some inconsistencies or disagreements within this text. We recognize the potential for their presence since it is a multi-author work, but we definitely prefer that each chapter author state his own concepts.

DONALD O. CASTELL, M.D.
WALLACE C. WU, M.D.
DAVID J. OTT, M.D.

Acknowledgment

The authors wish to recognize and thank Ms. Karen Chatman and Ms. Rebecca Southard for their expert editorial assistance in preparation of this book.

Contents

PATHOPHYSIOLOGY

DIAGNOSIS

THERAPY

PATHOPHYSIOLOGY

1

Introduction to Pathophysiology of Gastroesophageal Reflux

Donald O. Castell, M.D.

Chapter Contents

Gastroesophageal (GE) reflux and its major manifestations, heartburn and acid regurgitation, are an extremely common problem in our population. It has been shown that approximately 10% of Americans will suffer daily heartburn and that greater than one-third of us will experience it at less frequent intervals.[1] It is important to recognize that major objective manifestations of reflux, such as esophagi-

From Castell DO, Wu WC, Ott DJ (eds): *Gastroesophageal Reflux Disease: Pathogenesis, Diagnosis, Therapy.* Mount Kisco, NY, Futura Publishing Co., Inc., 1985.

tis, are not always present in a patient with chronic reflux. For this reason, it has become more convenient to use the term *GE reflux disease* to cover the whole spectrum of manifestations of chronic reflux, including the patient who has recurring heartburn without objective disease and the individual who presents with severe esophageal injury but with no symptoms until advanced disease develops. It is also important to recognize that patients with reflux symptoms who are seen by physicians only represent the tip of the iceberg. It has been estimated that the majority of individuals with reflux have only intermittent symptoms and are not seen by physicians. These individuals treat themselves with various over-the-counter antacid preparations. Those patients with more severe reflux symptoms or complications of chronic GE reflux disease are the ones that require decisions about appropriate management. These concepts are portrayed in Figure 1.

For a number of years, many investigators focused their attention on the lower esophageal sphincter (LES) as the crucial factor in the development of reflux disease. It now seems more reasonable to suggest that reflux disease is multifactorial in its pathogenesis, and to include a number of aspects that lead to important symptoms and/or esophageal structural abnormalities. The following should all be considered in evaluating the possible development of reflux disease:

1. Efficiency of the anti-reflux barrier at the EG junction.
2. Irritant effect of gastric juice.
    a. acid
    b. pepsin
    c. bile
3. Efficiency of the esophageal clearing mechanism.
    a. tissue resistance of the esophageal mucosa
    b. salivary flow and HCO_3^-
4. Efficiency of gastric emptying.
    a. effectiveness of intragastric volume

Anti-reflux Barrier

The LES still should be considered the *major* mechanism responsible for the prevention of reflux. Although many recent studies have indicated a poor correlation between sphincter pressures measured in the fasting state and reflux symptoms, there are ample data to indicate that the level of pressure is quite crucial to the development of reflux. Modern concepts on the anti-reflux barrier are discussed by Drs. Ott, Katz, and Wu in Chapter 3.

GERD ICEBERG

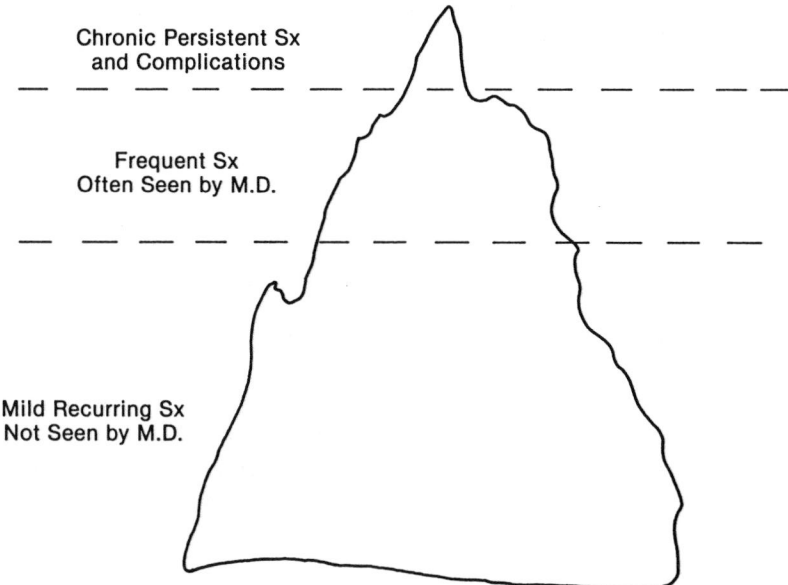

Figure 1: *The gastroesophageal reflux disease (GERD) iceberg illustrates the concept of the relative incidence of symptomatic reflux and its forms of presentation. It has been estimated that the majority of patients with reflux disease have symptoms that are only mildly troublesome and usually do not seek the help of a physician. The larger group of those reflux patients seen by the physician has more persistent symptoms without complications. It is only the tip of the iceberg that is represented by those chronic reflux sufferers, who have complications of their reflux disease. Sx = symptoms.*

The circular muscle at the LES has many unique features that enable it to behave as a sphincter. Yet, the mechanism by which this sphincter becomes incompetent due to weakening of this muscle remains unclear. Although the relationship to hiatus hernia has been emphasized for many years, there is little evidence to suggest that it has a primary role in the pathogenesis of reflux. An important consideration is the observation that LES pressure varies remarkably during the day. This is particularly related to the effects of foods and other agents that affect LES pressure, notably fat, alcohol, chocolate, and smoking.[2] Recent observations have indicated that patients with reflux will show transient relaxations in LES pressure, allowing important episodes of acid reflux to occur. The specific cause of these relaxations is unknown. Three different mechanical mechanisms of

GE reflux due to changes in pressure relationships between the stomach and LES have been proposed:[3]

1. Transient LES relaxation
2. Intra-abdominal pressure transient increases
3. Spontaneous free reflux.

Gastric Juice

Acid and pepsin have been shown to be very caustic to the esophageal mucosa. Bile, when present in high concentration in the stomach, also is a potentially strong irritant factor during episodes of GE reflux. This "alkaline reflux" has been shown to be extremely damaging to the esophageal mucosa.[4] There is also evidence to indicate the excessive acid secretion, as seen in patients with the Zollinger–Ellison syndrome, can result in severe esophageal injury.[5] This may relate as much to the greater intragastric volumes as to the actual levels of acid present. The ability of increased gastric volume to promote greater reflux has been shown in recent investigations.[6]

Esophageal Clearance

The importance of esophageal clearing in the production of GE reflux disease has been demonstrated primarily through studies of overnight pH recording.[7] These studies have indicated that patients with chronic reflux will demonstrate slower clearing of acid reflux episodes, creating a situation of double jeopardy produced by increased frequency of reflux and slower clearing. Thus, their esophageal acid exposure time becomes greatly prolonged. The importance of elevating the head of the patient's bed at night has been stressed as a simple measure to significantly improve some of this abnormal esophageal clearing by using the effect of gravity. Recent studies have shown that bicarbonate present in the saliva may function as a buffer for small volumes of acid present in the esophagus.[8] It has been stressed that normal, effective peristalsis is extremely important to clear most of the acid that occurs during reflux and that salivary bicarbonate may neutralize the remaining small amounts of material. It is now well documented that decreased peristaltic amplitudes and frequent episodes of abnormal peristalsis are seen in patients with reflux. It is not clear, however, which comes first. That is, does the abnormal esophageal motility produce the reflux disease or does the reflux disease produce the abnormal esophageal squeezing pressures? Esophageal clearing factors are discussed by Drs. Helm, Dodds, and Hogan in Chapter 2.

Gastric Emptying

There have been recent studies to indicate that many patients with chronic GE reflux disease will have delayed gastric emptying.[9] This factor may also contribute importantly to the production of reflux by allowing acid/pepsin mixtures to remain in the stomach for longer periods of time and also by allowing greater gastric volumes of fluid. It has been suggested that metoclopramide may be particularly effective in treating patients who demonstrate delayed gastric emptying as an important aspect of their reflux abnormality.[10] In Chapter 5, Dr. Dubois discusses gastric factors in relation to GE reflux.

GE Reflux and Abnormal Esophageal Contractions

Although it has generally been accepted that reflux occurs secondary to low LES pressure and possibly abnormal peristalsis, this concept has recently been questioned. New information on the abnormal esophageal pressures seen in patients with chronic reflux has suggested that the abnormal pressures may not occur first. This has generated some of the concepts shown in Figure 2. The popular concept of reflux disease is that an incompetent lower esophageal sphincter allows GE reflux that produces esophagitis. Indeed, low sphincter pressures do frequently accompany reflux. More recently, low peristaltic amplitude and abnormal esophageal clearing have also been shown in such patients. But did these pressure abnormalities produce the reflux disease or are they a result of it? Perhaps an episode of reflux may produce acute injury resulting in alterations in peristaltic amplitude and clearing and in decreased lower esophageal sphincter tone. These events may then allow continued reflux and decreased clearing of the damaging acid from the distal esophagus. This hypothesis is supported by recent animal studies. Induction of esophagitis by acid instillation into the mid-esophagus in both cats and baboons has been shown to result in significant decreases in lower esophageal sphincter pressure.[11,12] In addition, concomitant decreases in esophageal peristaltic amplitude were shown in the distal esophagus. These experiments suggest that in human reflux

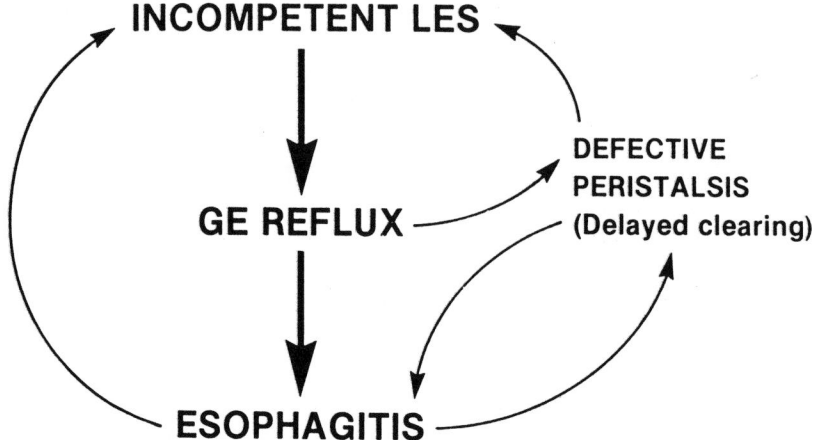

Figure 2: *Schematic representation of classical concept of pathogenesis of gastroesophageal (GE) reflux disease and various cyclic mechanisms of potential importance. LES = lower esophageal sphincter.*

disease, cyclic mechanisms may occur that allow perpetuation of this process once it has begun.

References

1. Nebel OT, Fornes MF, Castell DO: Symptomatic gastroesophageal reflux: Incidence and precipitating factors. *Am J Dig Dis* 1976; 21: 953–956.
2. Castell DO: The lower esophageal sphincter: Physiologic and clinical aspects. *Ann Intern Med* 1975; 83:390–401.
3. Dodds WJ, Dent J, Hogan WJ, Helm JF, Hauser R, Patel GK, Egide MS: Mechanisms of gastroesophageal reflux in patients with reflux esophagitis. *N Engl J Med* 1982; 307:1547–1552.
4. Pellegrini CA, DeMesster TR, Wernly JA, Johnson LF, Skinner DB: Alkaline gastroesophageal reflux. *Am J Surg* 1978; 135:177–183.
5. Richter JE, Pandol SJ, Castell DO, McCarthy DM: Gastroesophageal reflux disease in the Zollinger–Ellison syndrome. *Ann Intern Med* 1981; 19:37–43.
6. Ahtaridis G, Snape W, Cohen S: Lower esophageal sphincter pressure as an index of gastroesophageal acid reflux. *Dig Dis Sci* 1981; 26:993–998.
7. DeMeester TR, Johnson LF, Joseph GJ, Toscano MS, Hall AW, Skinner DB: Patterns of gastroesophageal reflux in health and disease. *Ann Surg* 1976; 184:459–470.
8. Helm JF, Dodds WJ, Hogan WJ, Soergel KH, Egide MS, Wood CM: Acid neutralizing capacity of human saliva. *Gastroenterology* 1982; 83: 69–74.

9. McCallum RW, Berkowitz DM, Lerner E: Gastric emptying in patients with gastroesophageal reflux. *Gastroenterology* 1981; 80:285–291.
10. McCallum RW, Ippolitti AF, Cooney C, Sturdevant R: A controlled trial of metoclopramide in symptomatic gastroesophageal reflux. *N Engl J Med* 1977; 296:354–357.
11. Eastwood GL, Castell DO, Higgs RH: Experimental esophagitis in cats impairs lower esophageal sphincter pressure. *Gastroenterology* 1975; 69:146–153.
12. Sinar DR, Fletcher JR, Cordova C, Eastwood GL, Castell DO: Acute acid-induced esophagitis impairs esophageal peristalsis in baboons. *Gastroenterology* 1981; 80:1286.

2

Esophageal Clearance

James F. Helm, M.D.,
Wylie J. Dodds, M.D., and
Walter J. Hogan, M.D.

Chapter Contents

From Castell DO, Wu WC, Ott DJ (eds): *Gastroesophageal Reflux Disease: Pathogenesis, Diagnosis, Therapy.* Mount Kisco, NY, Futura Publishing Co., Inc., 1985.

Gastroesophageal reflux is a common event in asymptomatic normal subjects, as well as in patients with reflux esophagitis.[1,2] In the event of gastroesophageal reflux, esophageal clearance is an important defense against the development of reflux esophagitis.[3] The efficacy of esophageal clearance determines the exposure of the esophageal mucosa to refluxed gastric fluid. The likelihood of mucosal injury and the severity of esophagitis are related to the potency of the refluxed fluid and the duration of its contact with the esophageal mucosa.[4-8]

Hydrochloric acid, pepsin, bile acids, and trypsin have been identified as constituents of gastric fluid with potential for causing esophageal injury.[3] Although the actual composition of fluid refluxed into the esophagus has never been studied comprehensively, pepsin and significant concentrations of bile acids have been found in esophageal aspirates from patients with gastroesophageal reflux disease.[9,10] Hydrochloric acid, pepsin, and bile acids in combination are particularly damaging to the esophageal mucosa.[8,11] Clearance of pepsin and bile acids from the esophagus has not been investigated. Esophageal acid clearance is more readily studied.

Esophageal acid clearance is the restoration of a normal intraluminal hydrogen ion concentration after acid gastroesophageal reflux. As the term has been commonly used, esophageal acid clearance has not been clearly distinguished from the emptying of an acid volume from the esophagus. This distinction is important, however, because a reduction in intra-esophageal acid volume alone would not decrease the hydrogen ion concentration of the acid remaining in the esophagus. Esophageal acid clearance and the emptying of an acid volume from the esophagus are related, but not equivalent events.

Measurement of Esophageal Emptying and Acid Clearance

Esophageal emptying of a fluid volume may be assessed qualitatively by observing the emptying of barium from the esophagus at fluoroscopy. For most clinical purposes, the barium swallow is an adequate measure of the emptying of liquids from the esophagus. However, radiation exposure limits fluoroscopic observation of esophageal emptying to brief periods.

Radionuclide imaging techniques provide a more quantitative measure of esophageal emptying than fluoroscopy, in addition to requiring negligible radiation exposure. In such studies a radiolabeled bolus is swallowed or injected into the esophagus through a catheter, while the scintillation count rate is recorded over the esophagus.[12-15] Most radionuclide studies of esophageal emptying have been semi-quantitative, because they used the absolute count rate or a percentage of the maximum count rate as a relative measure of the intra-esophageal bolus volume at a given time. Recently, a method has been devised to convert the count rate recorded from a radiolabeled bolus within the esophagus to the corresponding volume.[12] The accurate measurement of intra-esophageal bolus volume, however, is limited to the initial clearance of fluid volume. After near-complete emptying of a radiolabeled bolus, a small residual count rate persists over the esophagus despite repeated dry or wet swallows. The residual count rate is due to adherence of radionuclide to the esophageal mucosa. After near-complete esophageal emptying, the apparent fluid volume corresponding to the residual esophageal count rate is largely artifactual, and only an upper limit for the true residual volume. Thus, conclusions about the completeness of esophageal emptying based on the residual count rate may be subject to considerable error.

Esophageal acid clearance is monitored by a pH electrode stationed in the distal esophagus. The pH electrode records hydrogen ion concentration at a single site within the esophagus and cannot distinguish between large and small acid volumes. Usually the studies are conducted with the subject supine to eliminate any influence of gravity. Esophageal acid clearance may be studied after spontaneous or simulated acid gastroesophageal reflux. Acid reflux is commonly simulated by injection of a 15-ml bolus of 0.1N HCl (pH 1.2) through a catheter into the distal esophagus. After acid injection, swallowing is usually standardized by having the subject take a dry swallow every 30 seconds. Whether an acid reflux episode is spontaneous or simulated, the efficacy of acid clearance is commonly measured by the time required for the return of esophageal pH to a given value that should not cause mucosal injury. The values most commonly used for this purpose are pH 4 or 5. Some justification for the empiric choice of these values is provided by the observation that acid by itself at a pH greater than 2 does not cause esophageal injury in the cat, while pepsin is inactivated at pH values greater than 3.[4] The time required for esophageal acid clearance after spontaneous acid reflux has been shown to correlate with that after simulated acid reflux.[16]

Normal Esophageal Emptying

Peristalsis is the major mechanism for esophageal emptying in normal subjects. Studies of esophageal emptying show that a normal peristaltic contraction wave generally empties virtually all fluid volume from the esophagus.[12,17,18] In some instances, part of the fluid bolus escapes from the peristaltic wave at the level of the aortic arch, only to be cleared from the esophagus by the next peristaltic sequence.

The mechanism by which peristalsis empties the esophagus is shown by correlating the peristaltic stripping of a barium bolus from the esophagus with the manometrically-recorded peristaltic pressure complex (Figure 1).[19] During esophageal emptying, the barium bolus is propelled along the esophagus in advance of the peristaltic contraction wave. The peristaltic wave is seen radiographically as an aborally-propagated, lumen-obliterating contraction which imparts an inverted-V configuration to the tail of the barium bolus. The bolus tail is formed by approximation of opposing esophageal walls, and corresponds to the onset of the manometrically-recorded peristaltic pressure complex. Thus, esophageal emptying is dependent on the normal propagation of the lumen-obliterating leading edge of the peristaltic pressure complex, rather than on the contractile activity that follows. These observations suggest that esophageal emptying is not dependent on the specific amplitude or duration of the peristaltic pressure complex, as long as that pressure complex is sufficient to obliterate the esophageal lumen and strip all fluid from the esophagus. Furthermore, esophageal emptying will be unaffected by repetitive rises in the peristaltic pressure complex if the leading edge of the complex propagates normally.

Normal Esophageal Acid Clearance

Studies of spontaneous acid reflux in normal subjects show that in 90% of reflux episodes acid is cleared to pH 4 in less than five minutes.[1] Acid clearance may be delayed for as long as 30 minutes or more in the occasional event that a subject falls asleep before clearance of acid from the esophagus is complete. In studies of simulated acid reflux, a majority of normal subjects clear acid to pH 4 in less than five minutes with swallows taken at 30-second intervals.[20] However, the time required for acid clearance to pH 4 varies widely from one subject to another, and may be as long as 10–15 minutes.

Mechanism of Esophageal Acid Clearance

The importance of peristalsis as a mechanism for esophageal acid clearance is suggested by the observation that during acid clearance

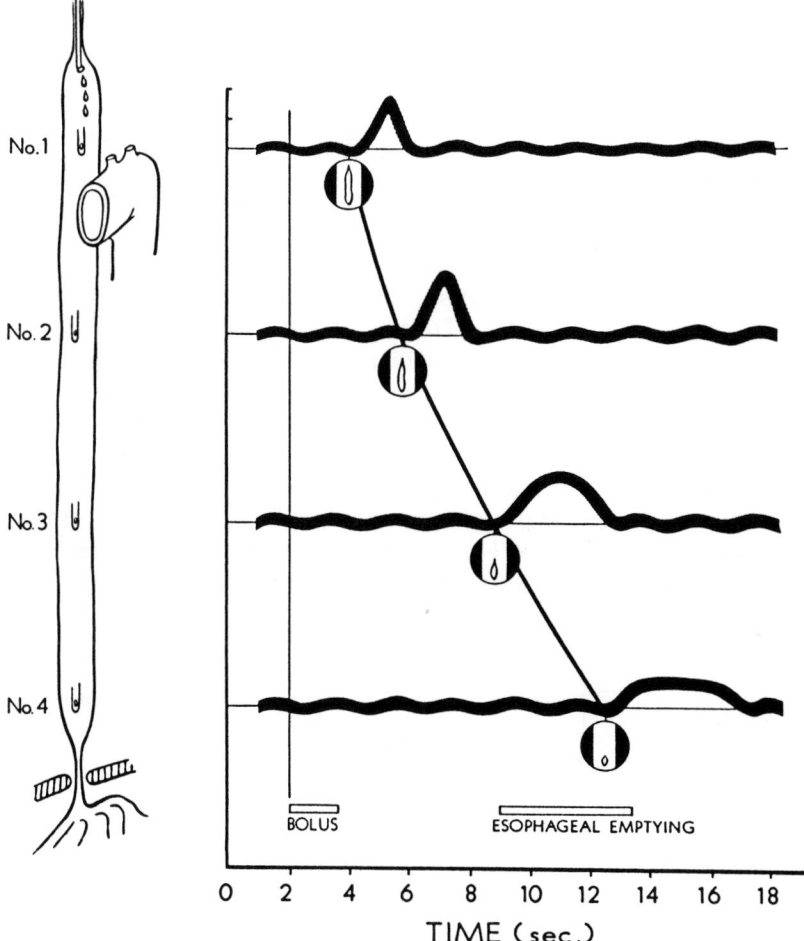

Figure 1: *Relation between passage of the barium bolus tail and mano-metrically-recorded pressure complexes in the cat. Injection of barium into the esophagus occurred during the interval marked* BOLUS. *Passage of the bolus tail is indicated by the solid line. The circular insets represent draw-ings of the cineradiographic appearance of the barium bolus as the bolus tail passed each manometric recording site. Barium passed into the stomach during the interval marked* ESOPHAGEAL EMPTYING. *The passage of the bolus tail past each recording site coincides with the onset of the peristaltic pressure complex at each site. (Modified from* J Clin Invest *1973; 52:1–13 with permission of The American Society for Clinical Investigation.)*

esophageal pH increases in a series of steps, each associated with a peristaltic sequence (Figure 2).[20] The step increase in esophageal pH does not occur when swallowing occasionally fails to initiate a peristaltic sequence. Between peristaltic sequences negligible change occurs in esophageal pH. Increasing the interval between swallows delays acid clearance.

Esophageal acid clearance has been commonly attributed to the progressive emptying of acid from the esophagus by peristaltic sequences. However, acid clearance cannot result from peristalsis alone, because a progressive reduction in intra-esophageal acid volume by itself would not change the pH of the remaining acid. Recent studies have shown that esophageal acid clearance occurs by a series of step increases in pH as a result of acid neutralization by saliva carried into the esophagus with each swallow.[20] Diversion of saliva from the esophagus by oral aspiration abolishes the discrete step increases in pH by which acid clearance occurs, despite repeated swallows (Figure 3). During saliva aspiration esophageal acid clearance is markedly delayed. The esophageal pH rises almost imperceptibly, perhaps due to acid neutralization by esophageal secretions or leakage of hydro-

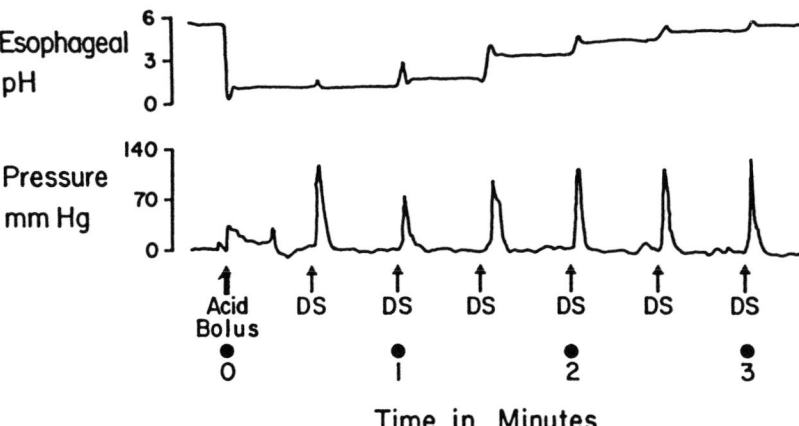

Figure 2: *Relation of esophageal acid clearance to peristalsis. Only peristaltic pressure complexes from the distal esophagus are shown. The initial pressure rise was due to the injection of a 15-ml bolus of 0.1N HCl. Dry swallows are indicated by DS. After injection of the acid bolus, esophageal pH returned to its original value in a series of step increases, each associated with a swallow-induced peristaltic sequence. (Reprinted by permission of Elsevier Science Publishing Co., Inc. from "Determinants of Esophageal Acid Clearance in Normal Subjects,"* Gastroenterology, *Vol No. 85, pp: 607–612 © 1983 by The American Gastroenterological Association.)*

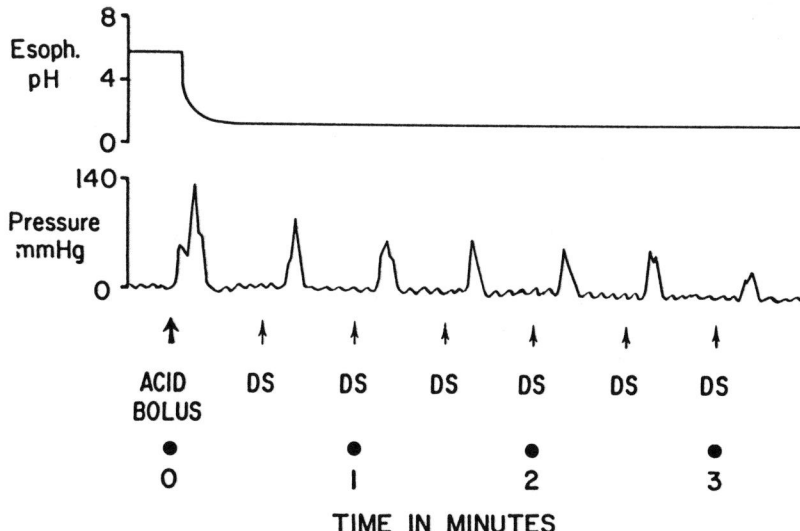

Figure 3: *Effect of oral aspiration of saliva on esophageal acid clearance. Only peristaltic pressure complexes from the distal esophagus are shown. Dry swallows are indicated by DS. Despite repeated swallow-induced peristaltic sequences, saliva aspiration effectively abolished esophageal acid clearance. (Modified from* N Engl J Med *1984; 310:284–288 with permission.)*

gen ions across the esophageal mucosa. Replacement of aspirated saliva with a bicarbonate solution reproduces the step increases in esophageal pH and restores acid clearance, while replacement with water alone does not improve acid clearance.

In the past, investigators proposed that if saliva had any role in esophageal acid clearance, its role was primarily one of lubrication or rinsing, rather than acid neutralization.[21] Neutralization of acid by saliva was believed to contribute little to esophageal acid clearance because of the finding that large volumes of saliva were needed to neutralize a 15-ml volume of 0.1N HCl. More recent studies, however, have shown that physiologic rates of saliva flow are capable of neutralizing small acid volumes of 1 ml or less within minutes.[22] These observations suggest that intra-esophageal acid must be reduced to a sufficiently small amount before neutralization of acid by swallowed saliva can be effective in clearing acid from the esophagus.

Esophageal acid clearance normally occurs as a two-step process.[12] First, virtually all acid volume is emptied from the esophagus by one or two peristaltic sequences, and then the minimal residual acid is neutralized by swallowed saliva. As shown in the example

of Figure 4, injection of a 15-ml acid bolus into the esophagus commonly elicits a secondary peristaltic sequence that reduces esophageal acid to a minimal residual that sustains a low pH. The residual
acid may enter an "unstirred" mucous layer that coats the esophageal
mucosa.[23] Despite nearly complete emptying of the acid volume by
the secondary peristaltic sequence, the esophageal pH does not begin
to rise until the first swallow, 30 seconds after bolus injection. Once
acid has been reduced to a minimal residual, acid neutralization by

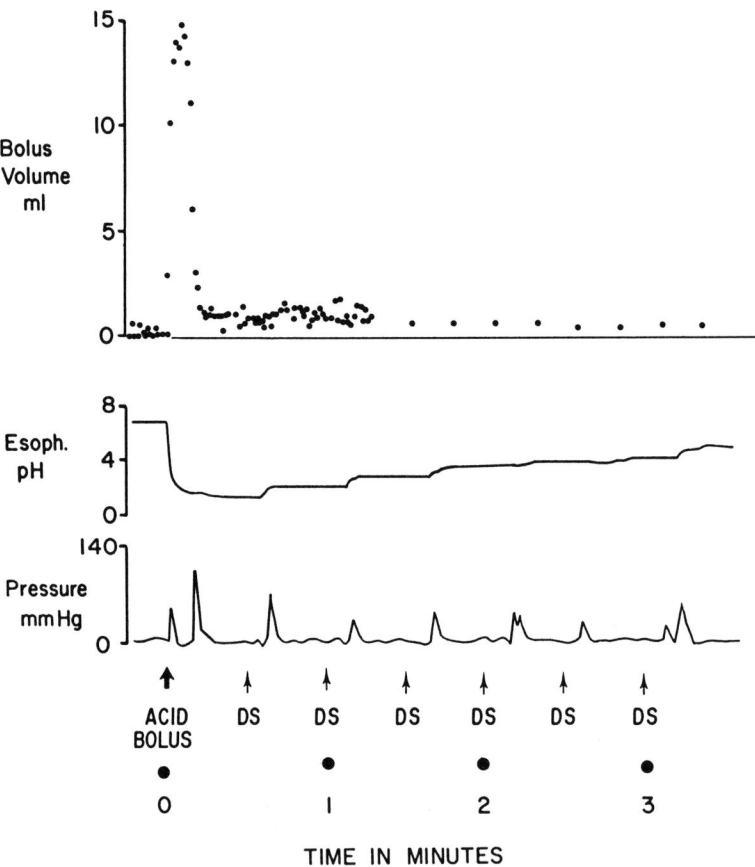

Figure 4: *Relations among esophageal acid clearance, motor activity, and
emptying of fluid volume. Esophageal emptying was monitored by radionuclide imaging. Only peristaltic pressure complexes from the distal esophagus are shown. Dry swallows are indicated by DS. Despite clearance of
the injected bolus volume to less than 1 ml by the second peristaltic
sequence, esophageal pH did not begin to rise until the first dry swallow, 30
seconds after bolus injection. (From N Engl J Med 1984; 310:284–288 with
permission.)*

swallowed saliva restores esophageal pH to normal in a series of step increases. The apparent residual acid volume that persists long after near-complete esophageal emptying is largely artifactual, resulting from adherence of radionuclide to the esophageal mucosa. When secondary peristalsis occasionally fails to reduce acid volume to a minimal residual, then acid clearance is delayed until after near-complete emptying of the acid by the first swallow-induced peristaltic sequence (Figure 5). The esophageal pH remains low and rises only

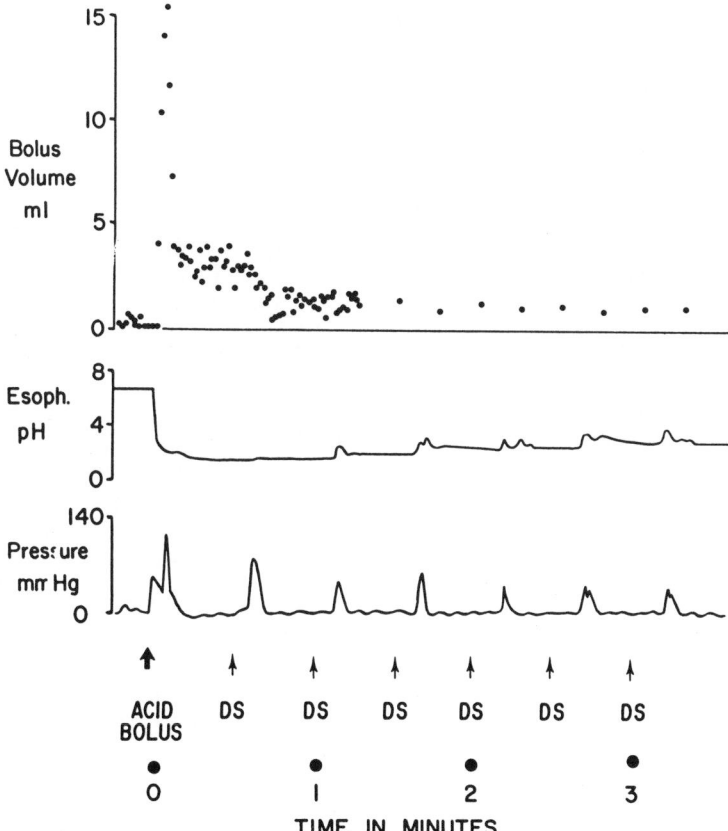

Figure 5: *Relations among esophageal acid clearance, motor activity, and emptying of fluid volume. Esophageal emptying was monitored by radionuclide imaging. Only peristaltic pressure complexes from the distal esophagus are shown. Dry swallows are indicated by DS. The secondary peristaltic sequence reduced the injected bolus volume from 15 to 4 ml, and 30 seconds later the remaining bolus volume was cleared to less than 1 ml by the first dry swallow. Esophagel pH, however, did not begin to rise until the second dry swallow, 30 seconds later. (From N Engl J Med 1984; 310:284–288 with permission.)*

with the second swallow, 60 seconds after acid injection. Thus, emptying of the esophageal acid must be virtually complete before swallowed saliva can begin to restore esophageal pH toward its normal resting value.

Non-critical Factors

Contrary to popular belief, peristaltic amplitude, gravity, and acid volume are not factors of critical importance for acid clearance in healthy subjects with normal peristalsis. Although peristalsis is important for acid clearance, knowledge of the amplitude of peristaltic contractions is of no value in predicting the time required for acid clearance in normal subjects.[20] The time required for esophageal acid clearance does not correlate with the amplitude of peristaltic contractions. How might one account for this apparent paradox? A plausible explanation is that the specific amplitude of normal peristaltic contractions is not a critical factor for acid clearance because any contraction amplitude within the broad range of normal is sufficient to obliterate the esophageal lumen and strip all fluid from the esophagus.

Gravity contributes little to esophageal acid clearance in the healthy subject with normal peristalsis. Studies of both spontaneous and simulated acid reflux episodes have shown only a slight tendency for improvement in acid clearance in the upright position.[20,21,24] A 15° head-down position has been reported to prolong acid clearance as compared with the supine position.[21] Gravity is of minimal importance for acid clearance in a healthy subject because a single peristaltic sequence can efficiently strip virtually all fluid from the esophagus.[12,17,25] For this same reason, esophageal acid clearance is not influenced by the acid volume in subjects with normal peristalsis. For injected acid boluses varying in size from 2 to 15 ml, the times required for acid clearance are comparable.[12]

Determinants of Acid Clearance Time

As discussed, esophageal acid clearance normally occurs as a two-step process consisting of esophageal emptying followed by acid neutralization. The time required for esophageal acid clearance is the sum of times required for each of the two sequential steps by which acid clearance occurs. Esophageal emptying, the first of these steps, is virtually complete after one or two peristaltic sequences and commonly requires as little as 10–15 seconds. Because of the rapidity with which esophageal emptying normally occurs, the time required for acid clearance is determined primarily by the rate of acid neutralization. Neutralization of acid, and hence the time required for acid clearance, is a function of salivation and the frequency with which saliva is carried into the esophagus by swallowing. Without altering the frequency of swallowing, stimulation of saliva flow by an oral lozenge markedly improves acid clearance, while oral aspiration of saliva virtually abolishes acid clearance.[20] By itself, doubling the natural swallowing frequency of about one per minute more than halves the time required for acid clearance.[20]

Peristalsis

Secondary peristalsis seldom occurs spontaneously, but is often elicited by acid gastroesophageal reflux as a result of esophageal distension and possibly acid pH.[1,26,27] Contrary to the common notion, however, primary peristalsis is the dominant esophageal motor activity during acid clearance.[1] This finding has two possible explanations. First, esophageal distension is usually a transient stimulus for secondary peristalsis, due to the virtually complete emptying of fluid volume from the esophagus by one or two peristaltic sequences. Thus, the major stimulus for secondary peristalsis is normally short-lived. Secondly, primary peristalsis has a high natural frequency of about one per minute already operative when acid reflux occurs.[1,28,29] Furthermore, the frequency of primary peristalsis shows a tendency to increase immediately after acid reflux.[1,26]

Circumstantial evidence links the frequency of spontaneous swallowing to the flow of saliva. An increase in saliva flow, such as occurs with stimulation by an oral lozenge, bethanechol, or intubation, is accompanied by a proportionate increase in the spontaneous frequency of swallowing.[30] During sleep, saliva flow virtually ceases[31] and peristalsis seldom occurs.[1] Abolition of saliva flow by atropine reduces, but does not eliminate spontaneous swallowing, indicating that the frequency of swallowing is not dependent on saliva flow alone.[30]

Saliva

All saliva is believed to be secreted in response to stimulation mediated by cholinergic nerves.[32–36] In an awake subject with minimal external stimulation, saliva flows continuously at a low rate of about 0.5 ml/min,[22] whereas, saliva flow ceases during sleep.[31] Abolition of saliva flow by atropine is cited as evidence for the mediation of saliva secretion by cholinergic nerves.[32,34,36]

In the mouth, saliva functions as a buffer to resist change in the relatively alkaline pH that is thought to be protective against dental caries. In the esophagus, however, swallowed saliva serves to neutralize refluxed acid and thereby restores esophageal pH to normal, rather than to buffer acid and resist a decrease in pH.[22] The ability of saliva to neutralize acid can be quantitated by titration of saliva against 0.1N HCl (pH 1.2) (Figure 6). In the titration of HCl, a strong acid, saliva acts as a weak base with the inflection point of the titration curve below pH 7. Titration of a strong acid to complete neutrality cannot be accomplished with a weak base, because excess uncombined base begins to accumulate as the titration proceeds beyond the point of inflection. However, titration to the point of inflection at

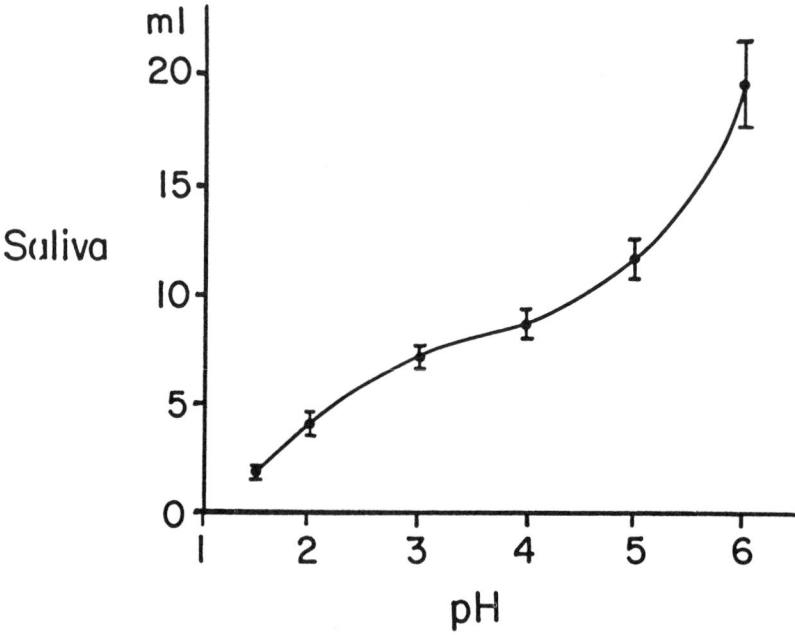

Figure 6: *Titration curve of resting saliva against 1 ml 0.1N HCl. Mean values obtained from 31 normal subjects. Vertical lines indicate ± 1 SE. (Reprinted by permission of Elsevier Science Publishing Co., Inc. from "Acid Neutralizing Capacity of Human Saliva,"* Gastroenterology, *Vol. No. 83, pp. 69–74. © 1982 by The American Gastroenterological Association.)*

about pH 4 does permit an estimation of the capacity for acid neutralization of saliva. With titration to pH 4, more than 99% of the acid has been neutralized without accumulation of excess base. With knowledge of the saliva volume required to titrate a known quantity of H^+ to pH 4, the capacity for acid neutralization of saliva can be determined as the quantity of H^+ neutralized per volume of saliva.

Just as salivary bicarbonate is the primary buffer in the mouth, bicarbonate is also primarily responsible for the ability of saliva to neutralize acid in the esophagus.[22] Bicarbonate accounts for an average of about 50% of the capacity for acid neutralization of resting saliva. The capacity of saliva for acid neutralization is directly related to the bicarbonate concentration. With stimulation of saliva by an oral lozenge, the capacity for acid neutralization increases as a result of a rise in bicarbonate concentration, while the contribution of the non-bicarbonate component to acid neutralization remains relatively constant. The non-bicarbonate component may be largely protein.

Abnormal Esophageal Acid Clearance

The duration of mucosal exposure to acid is an important factor in the development of reflux esophagitis. In patients with symptomatic reflux, the esophageal mucosa is usually exposed to acid for a greater percentage of time than in normal subjects.[37] Excessive exposure of the esophageal mucosa to acid may be the result of an increased frequency of gastroesophageal reflux, delayed esophageal acid clearance, or both.[24,38] An early study suggested that the time required for acid clearance in patients with symptomatic reflux is invariably greater than in normal subjects.[39] Subsequent studies, however, showed that the time required for acid clearance varies widely among patients with reflux symptoms, and that about half of such patients demonstrate normal acid clearance.[16,40] In theory, esophageal acid clearance may be prolonged by abnormal esophageal emptying or impaired salivation in patients with gastroesophageal reflux disease.

Abnormal Esophageal Emptying

Esophageal motor disorders are commonly associated with abnormal esophageal emptying. For example, when esophageal peristalsis is compromised as in the patient with scleroderma or diffuse esophageal spasm, barium or a radiolabeled fluid bolus is retained in the esophagus for long periods while the patient is recumbent.[13,18] The contribution of peristalsis to esophageal emptying is further illustrated by the abolition of peristalsis with the anti-cholinergic propantheline (Figure 7).[12] After propantheline, esophageal emptying in supine normal subjects is delayed and incomplete. In the absence of peristalsis, a 15-ml acid bolus injected into the esophagus will be retained for one to two minutes. Partial emptying of the bolus then occurs abruptly, and usually in association with a low-amplitude, non-peristaltic pressure transient. A residual of 2 to 8 ml persists after incomplete emptying. If peristalsis fails to reduce acid to a sufficiently small amount, swallowed saliva is incapable of neutralizing the residual acid and restoring esophageal pH to normal. However, acid clearance is abolished by propantheline not only because esophageal emptying is impaired, but also as a result of the elimination of saliva.

Esophageal emptying is impaired in patients with reflux symptoms who have esophageal motor dysfunction. In studies utilizing a radiolabeled bolus, reflux patients with non-specific esophageal motor abnormalities had incomplete emptying of the radiolabel from the esophagus despite repeated swallows.[13] In patients with normal peristalsis, emptying of the radiolabel from the esophagus was nearly complete after a single swallow, just as in healthy subjects with normal peristalsis. After repeated swallows, however, the residual esophageal count rate in patients with normal peristalsis was a little greater than in normal subjects, but still much less than in patients with esophageal motor abnormalities. In healthy subjects with normal peristalsis, the residual esophageal count rate is explained by adherence of radionuclide to the esophageal mucosa, rather than by incomplete emptying of the bolus.[12] Although the investigators discounted the possibility, adherence of radionuclide to the esophageal mucosa could be greater than normal in reflux patients with normal peristalsis, and one need not conclude that esophageal emptying is abnormal. Emptying of barium from the esophagus is normal in reflux patients with normal peristalsis.

Studies of esophageal motor function in patients with reflux esophagitis are conflicting and incomplete. Early studies using non-perfused manometry catheters suggested that up to 75% of patients with esophagitis manifest abnormal esophageal motor activity with deglutition, and that the severity of the esophagitis parallels the degree of the motor abnormality.[41,42] In a majority of the patients with motor abnormalities, peristalsis appeared to be ineffective or absent, and many had non-peristaltic, often-repetitive contractions.

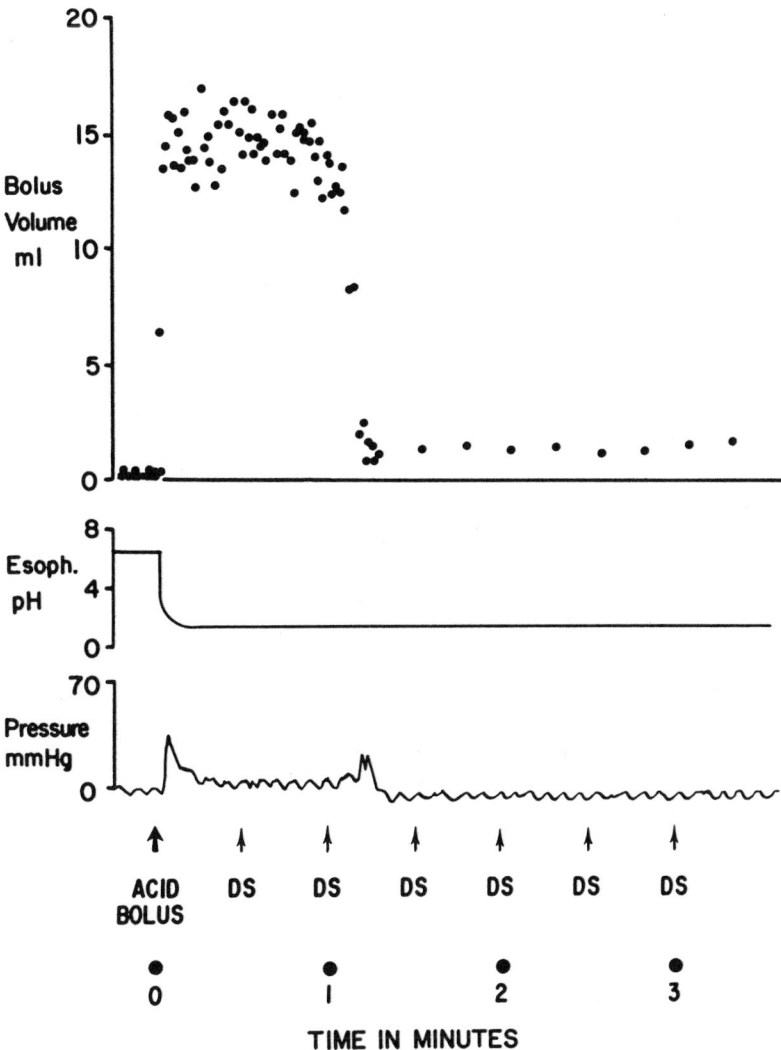

Figure 7: *Effect of the anti-cholinergic propantheline (30 mg i.v.) on esopha-geal emptying, acid clearance, and motor activity. Esophageal emptying was monitored by radionuclide imaging. Only pressures recorded from the distal esophagus are shown. Dry swallows are indicated by DS. With elimi-nation of peristalsis by propantheline, the injected 15-ml bolus was retained within the esophagus for about 1 minute. At that time, partial emptying of the esophagus occurred abruptly, in association with a non-peristaltic pres-sure transient. A residual of 2 ml persisted after incomplete esophageal emptying.*

Subsequent studies with perfused manometry catheters suggest that as few as 20% of esophagitis patients demonstrate abnormal primary peristalsis.[43-45] Furthermore, the severity of the esophagitis was unrelated to the degree of esophageal motor dysfunction in these more recent studies. Secondary peristalsis in patients with reflux esophagitis remains virtually uninvestigated.

Esophagitis itself has been suggested as a cause for the esophageal motor dysfunction found in some patients with esophagitis. Return of normal esophageal motor function after healing of esophagitis is cited as presumptive evidence that the motor abnormality is secondary to the esophagitis. Persistence of esophageal motor dysfunction after resolution of esophagitis suggests that the motor dysfunction either preceded the onset of esophagitis, or resulted from irreversible injury due to esophagitis. Animal studies indicate that acute esophagitis can cause marked motor abnormalities that resolve with healing of the esophagitis.[8,46] However, these motor abnormalities occur only with severe ulcerative esophagitis accompanied by transmural inflammation. Although not extensively studied in man, the return of normal esophageal motor function after healing of chronic esophagitis is probably uncommon.[44] We believe that the esophageal motor dysfunction found in some patients with reflux esophagitis is usually an antecedent condition that may contribute to the development of esophagitis in some instances. Nevertheless, esophagitis may be the cause of esophageal motor dysfunction in the occasional patient.

Impaired Salivation

Esophageal emptying is normal in some patients with delayed acid clearance. The small acid residual that coats the esophageal mucosa after the normal emptying of an acid volume from the esophagus may be just as capable of causing injury as a larger acid volume of the same pH. Impaired neutralization of this residual acid by swallowed saliva will delay acid clearance. Neutralization of residual acid may be impaired by reduced saliva flow accompanied by a decreased frequency of swallowing, or by a diminished capacity of saliva for acid neutralization.

A recent study suggested that as a group, patients with reflux esophagitis have a resting saliva flow that does not differ from that of normal subjects.[47] Nor does the bicarbonate concentration of saliva appear to differ between esophagitis patients and normal subjects. In this study, measurement of parotid saliva flow during stimulation with sublingual citric acid suggested that the secretory capacity of the salivary glands of esophagitis patients is comparable to that of normal subjects. Because reflux esophagitis is a disorder with multiple etiologic factors,[3] however, it still seems likely that impaired salivation may be a contributing factor in a subpopulation of patients with reflux esophagitis. We have recorded exceedingly low basal saliva flows in a few patients with reflux esophagitis. Esophagitis often accompanies scleroderma, a disorder in which saliva flow is commonly reduced and esophageal peristalsis is absent. Although saliva flow is decreased in Sjögren's syndrome, it is unknown whether or not patients with this disorder are prone to develop reflux esophagitis as a result.

Perfusion of the esophagus with acid has been reported to increase saliva flow in healthy young volunteers, but not in older normal subjects or esophagitis patients.[47] The increase in saliva flow with esophageal acid perfusion was attributed to stimulation of acid-sensitive mucosal receptors whose ability to respond to acid perfusion is lost with age. The investigators speculated that development of reflux esophagitis might be favored by an age-related loss of this apparent salivary response to acid gastroesophageal reflux. In contrast to these findings, studies in our laboratory have shown that esophageal acid perfusion unaccompanied by heartburn does not affect salivation, irrespective of age.[48] However, saliva flow does increase concurrent with the onset of heartburn induced by esophageal acid perfusion, in esophagitis patients as well as in healthy young volunteers. The increased saliva flow that normally accompanies heartburn may serve as a protective response to symptomatic acid reflux. When the increase in salivation that accompanies heartburn becomes clinically evident, some refer to this hypersalivation as waterbrash. We have encountered a few patients with symptomatic reflux esophagitis in whom profuse salivation was the dominant feature of the clinical presentation. Episodic hypersalivation is one of the more unusual presentations of reflux esophagitis, and one that could be misdiagnosed easily.

Nocturnal Acid Clearance

Overnight studies show that gastroesophageal reflux and esophageal acid clearance do not occur during electroencephalographically defined sleep in normal subjects (Figure 8).[1] During the night, transient lower esophageal sphincter relaxation and gastroesophageal reflux occur only during a transient arousal from sleep or when a

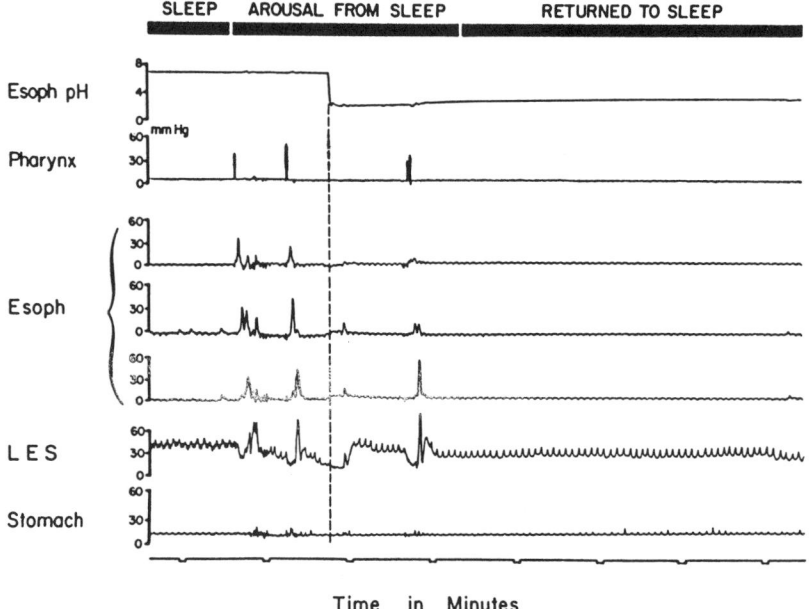

Figure 8: *Gastroesophageal reflux and partial clearance of acid from the esophagus during transient arousal from sleep. Following two spontaneous swallows that occurred after arousal from sleep, the lower esophageal sphincter relaxed transiently and acid gastroesophageal reflux occurred, as indicated by the vertical dashed line. One minute later a single primary peristaltic sequence, triggered by two closely-spaced swallows, led to only a slight increase in esophageal pH. The subject then returned to sleep and no further swallows or motor activity occurred until 20 minutes later when he had another arousal. During this 20-minute interval, the esophageal pH rose very slowly but remained less than 4. (Reprinted from J Clin Invest 1980; 65:256–267 with permission of The American Society for Clinical Investigation.)*

subject is fully awake, but not during sleep. If esophageal acid clearance is not completed before a subject resumes sleep, acid clearance is delayed until another arousal from sleep. Furthermore, if acid is injected into the esophagus during a period of sleep, clearance is markedly delayed in normal subjects and esophagitis patients alike.[49,50] Effective esophageal acid clearance does not occur during sleep, because peristalsis seldom occurs[1,28,51] and saliva flow virtually ceases during sleep.[40]

Extended periods of esophageal acid exposure have been observed during the night in normal subjects[1] as well as in esophagitis patients.[24,52] In some esophagitis patients, however, it may be possible that a high incidence of nocturnal gastroesophageal reflux, and perhaps impaired acid clearance, increase the chances of acid being present in the esophagus at the onset of sleep. Alternatively, some esophagitis patients with extremely low or absent lower esophageal sphincter pressures might experience free reflux during sleep. In either case, these patients would be more likely to experience periods of prolonged esophageal acid exposure during the night because effective acid clearance does not occur during sleep.

Therapeutic Implications

Esophageal acid clearance may be delayed by impaired esophageal emptying, an abnormality in the neutralization of acid by swallowed saliva, or both. In theory, treatment aimed at improving acid clearance should restore effective esophageal emptying or stimulate salivation.

Gravity is important for esophageal emptying in patients with esophageal motor dysfunction. In the absence of normal lumen-obliterating peristaltic contractions, barium is retained in the esophagus while the patient is recumbent but empties rapidly into the stomach when the patient assumes the upright position. Some patients with reflux esophagitis have esophageal motor abnormalities that compromise esophageal emptying in the recumbent position, and thereby prolong acid clearance.[13,16] Esophageal acid clearance is often improved in esophagitis patients by elevation of the head of the bed at night.[16,53,54] Presumably, elevation of the head of the bed aids in reducing intra-esophageal acid to a sufficiently small amount that swallowed saliva is capable of neutralizing. Elevation of the head of the bed would be expected to significantly improve acid clearance only in those patients lacking effective esophageal peristalsis, because a single peristaltic sequence can strip virtually all fluid volume from the esophagus.

Bethanechol has been shown to improve esophageal acid clearance in both normal subjects and in patients with reflux esophagitis.[20,38,54,55] This beneficial effect has been attributed to improvement in esophageal emptying as the result of a small increase in the amplitude of peristaltic contractions.[56,57] Strengthening of normal peristaltic contractions, however, would not appear to explain the improvement in acid clearance with bethanechol, because a wide range of contraction amplitudes obliterate the esophageal lumen and strip virtually all fluid from the esophagus in a single peristaltic sweep. Bethanechol has been shown to increase saliva flow and the ability of saliva to neutralize acid, similar to the effect of the oral lozenge.[22] Saliva stimulation, therefore, is the likely explanation for the improvement in acid clearance after bethanechol, because oral aspiration of saliva reverses the effect of bethanechol and markedly delays acid clearance in healthy subjects with normal peristalsis.[20] Only in reflux patients with ineffective esophageal emptying could the effect of bethanechol on esophageal motor function potentially make a significant contribution to acid clearance.

Improvement in esophageal acid clearance by oral saliva stimulation suggests a potential use for lozenges in the treatment of reflux symptoms. In a study of apparently healthy individuals selected for their use of antacid tablets, most were found to have symptomatic gastroesophageal reflux.[58] Although the antacid tablets had an acid-neutralizing capacity far below that considered useful for treatment of peptic ulcer disease, they were effective in relief of reflux symptoms. Oral saliva stimulation may be the mechanism for relief of reflux symptoms by antacid tablets. Indeed, we have encountered patients who report that they obtain relief from heartburn by sucking on candy or chewing on gum. The potential of oral saliva stimulation for relief of heartburn deserves further study.

References

1. Dent J, Dobbs WJ, Friedman RH, Sekiguchi T, Hogan WJ, Arndorfer RC, Petrie DJ: Mechanism of gastroesophageal reflux in recumbent asymptomatic human subjects. *J Clin Invest* 1980; 65:256−267.
2. Dodds WJ, Dent J, Hogan WJ, Helm JF, Hauser R, Patel GK, Egide MS: Mechanisms of gastroesophageal reflux in patients with reflux esophagitis. *N Engl J Med* 1982; 307:1547−1552.
3. Dodds WJ, Hogan WJ, Helm JF, Dent J: Pathogenesis of reflux esophagitis. *Gastroenterology* 1981; 81:376−394.
4. Goldberg HI, Dodds WJ, Gee S, Montgomery C, Zboralske FF: Role of acid and pepsin in acute experimental esophagitis. *Gastroenterology* 1969; 56:223−230.
5. Goldberg HI, Dodds WJ, Montgomery C, Baskin SA, Zboralske FF: Controlled production of acute esophagitis. *Invest Radiol* 1970; 5:254−256.
6. Dodds WJ, Goldberg HI, Montgomery C, Ludemann WB, Zboralske FF: Sequential gross, microscopic and roentgenographic features of acute feline esophagitis. *Invest Radiol* 1970; 5:209−219.
7. Harmon JW, Johnson LF, Maydonovitch CL: Effects of acid and bile salts on the rabbit esophageal mucosa. *Dig Dis Sci* 1981; 26:65−72.
8. Henderson RD, Mugashe FL, Jeejeebhoy KN, Szczpanski MM, Cullen J, Marryatt G, Boszko A: Synergism of acid and bile salts in the production of experimental esophagitis. *Can J Surg* 1973; 16:12−17.

9. Aylwin JA: The physiological basis of reflux oesophagitis in sliding hiatal diaphragmatic hernia. *Thorax* 1953; 8:38–45.
10. Mittal R, Reuben A, Magyar L, McCallum RW: Identification of bile acids in the esophagus during gastroesophageal reflux in man (abstract). *Gastroenterology* 1984; 86:1184.
11. Gillison EW, DeCastro VAM, Nyhus LM, Kusakari K: The significance of bile in reflux esophagitis. *Surg Gynecol Obstet* 1972; 134:419–424.
12. Helm JF, Dodds WJ, Pelc LR, Palmer DW, Hogan WJ, Teeter BC: Effect of esophageal emptying and saliva on clearance of acid from the esophagus. *N Engl J Med* 1984; 310:284–288.
13. Tolin RD, Malmud LS, Reilley J, Fisher R: Esophageal scintigraphy to quantitate esophageal transit (quantitation of esophageal transit). *Gastroenterology* 1979; 76:1402–1408.
14. Russell COH, Hill LD, Holmes ER III, Hull DA, Gannon R, Pope CE II: Radionuclide transit: A sensitive screening test for esophageal dysfunction. *Gastroenterology* 1981; 80:887–892.
15. Kazem I: A new scintigraphic technique for the study of the esophagus. *Am J Roentgenol Radium Ther Nucl Med* 1972; 115:681–688.
16. Stanciu C, Bennett JR: Oesophageal acid clearing: One factor in the production of reflux esophagitis. *Gut* 1974; 15:852–857.
17. Longhi EH, Jordan PH: Simultaneous cineradiographic and manometric analysis of incomplete emptying of the esophagus. *Am J Surg* 1971; 121:229–237.
18. Dodds WJ: Esophagus and esophagogastric region: Radiology. In: Margulis AR, Burhenne HJ, eds. *Alimentary Tract Radiology*. St. Louis: C.V. Mosby Co., 1983: 529–603.
19. Dodds WJ, Stewart ET, Hodges D, Zboralske FF: Movement of the feline esophagus associated with respiration and peristalsis. *J Clin Invest* 1973; 52:1–13.
20. Helm JF, Dodds WJ, Riedel DR, Teeter BC, Hogan WJ, Arndorfer RC: Determinants of esophageal acid clearance in normal subjects. *Gastroenterology* 1983; 85:607–612.
21. Kjellen G, Tibbling L: Influence of body position, dry and water swallows, smoking, and alcohol on esophageal acid clearing. *Scand J Gastroenterol* 1978; 13:283–288.
22. Helm JF, Dodds WJ, Hogan WJ, Soergel KH, Egide MS, Wood CM: Acid neutralizing capacity of human saliva. *Gastroenterology* 1982; 83:69–74.
23. Teeter BC, Helm JF, Dodds WJ, Linehan JH, Hogan WJ, Pelc LR, Egide MS: Computerized model of the mechanisms governing esophageal acid clearance (abstract). *Dig Dis Sci* 1982; 27:664.
24. DeMeester TR, Johnson LF, Guy JJ, Toscano MS, Hall AW, Skinner DB: Patterns of gastroesophageal reflux in health and disease. *Ann Surg* 1976; 184:459–470.
25. Fisher RS, Malud LS, Applegate G, Rock E, Lorber SH: Effect of bolus composition on esophageal transit: Concise communication. *J Nucl Med* 1982; 23:878–882.
26. Wallin L, Madsen T: 12-hour simultaneous registration of acid reflux and peristaltic activity in the oesophagus. *Scand J Gastroenterol* 1979; 14:561–566.
27. Corazziari E, Pozzessere C, Dani S, Anzini F, Torsoli A: Intraluminal pH and esophageal motility. *Gastroenterology* 1978; 75:275–277.

28. Lear CSC, Flanagan JB, Moorrees CFA: The frequency of deglutition in man. *Arch Oral Biol* 1965; 10:85–99.
29. Dodds WJ, Hogan WJ, Reid DP, Stewart ET, Arndorfer RC: A comparison between primary esophageal peristalsis following wet and dry swallows. *J Appl Physiol* 1973; 35:851–857.
30. Kapila YV, Dodds WJ, Helm JF, Hogan WJ: Relationship between swallow rate and salivary flow. *Dig Dis Sci* 1984; 29:528–533.
31. Schneyer LH, Pigman W, Hanahan L, Gilmore RW: Rate of flow of human parotid, sublingual, and submaxillary secretions during sleep. *J Dent Res* 1956; 35:109–114.
32. Kerr AC: *The Physiological Regulation of Salivary Secretions in Man.* New York: Pergamon Press, 1961.
33. Schneyer LH, Schneyer CA: Inorganic composition of saliva. In: Code CF, ed. *Handbook of Physiology. Sec. 6: Alimentary Canal, Vol. II.* Washington D.C.: American Physiological Society, 1967: 497–530.
34. Emmelin N: Nervous control of salivary glands. In: Code CF, ed. *Handbook of Physiology. Sec. 6: Alimentary Canal, Vol. II.* Washington D.C.: American Physiological Society, 1967: 595–632.
35. Jenkins GN: *The Physiology of the Mouth.* Philadelphia, Pa.: E.A. Davis Co., 1966.
36. Emmelin N: Interactions between sympathetic and parasympathetic nerves in control of the salivary glands. In: Brooks CM, Koizumi K, Sato A, eds. *Integrative Functions of the Autonomic Nervous System.* New York: University of Tokyo Press and Elsevier/North-Holland Inc., 1979: 5–23.
37. Stanciu C, Bennett JR: Correlation between a physiological test of gastroesophageal reflux and sphincter squeeze. *Proceedings of the Fourth International Symposium on Gastrointestinal Motility, Banff, Canada, September 6–8, 1973.* 1974; 131–138.
38. Johnson LF, DeMeester TR: Evaluation of elevation of the head of the bed, bethanechol, and antacid foam tablets on gastroesophageal reflux. *Dig Dis Sci* 1981; 26:673–680.
39. Booth DJ, Kemmerer WT, Skimmer DB: Acid clearing from the distal esophagus. *Arch Surg* 1968; 96:731–734.
40. Boesby S: Gastro-oesophageal sphincter pressure, motility and acid clearing. *Scand J Gastroenterol* 1977; 12:407–416.
41. Olsen AM, Schlegel JF: Motility disturbances caused by esophagitis. *J Thorac Cardiovasc Surg* 1965; 50:607–612.
42. Affolter H: Pressure characteristics of reflux esophagitis. *Helv Med Acta* 1966; 33:395–402.
43. Dodds WJ, Hogan WJ, Miller WN: Reflux esophagitis. *Dig Dis Sci* 1979; 21:49–67.
44. Russell COH, Pope CE, Gannon RM, Allen FD, Velasco N, Hill LD: Does surgery correct esophageal motor dysfunction in gastroesophageal reflux? *Ann Surg* 1981; 194:290–296.
45. Heddle R, Dent J, Toouli J, Lewis I: Esophageal peristaltic dysfunction in peptic esophagitis (abstract). *Gastroenterology* 1984; 86:1109.
46. Henderson RD, Mugashe F, Jeejeebhoy KN, Cullen J, Boszko A, Szczpanski M, Marryatt G: The motor defect of esophagitis. *Can J Surg* 1974; 17:112–116.
47. Sonnenberg A, Steinkamp U, Weise A, Berges W, Wienbeck M, Rohner HG, Peter P: Salivary secretion in reflux esophagitis. *Gastroenterology* 1982; 83:889–895.

HG, Peter P: Salivary secretion in reflux esophagitis. *Gastroenterology* 1982; 83:889–895.

48. Helm JF, Dodds WJ, Hogan WJ: Effect of esophageal acid perfusion on salivation in normal subjects and patients with reflux esophagitis (abstract). *Gastroenterology* 1983; 84:1185.
49. Orr WC, Robinson MG, Johnson LF: Acid clearance during sleep in the pathogenesis of reflux esophagitis. *Dig Dis Sci* 1981; 26:423–427.
50. Orr WC, Johnson LF, Robinson MG: Effect of sleep on swallowing, esophageal peristalsis, and acid clearance. *Gastroenterology* 1984; 86:814–819.
51. Lichter I, Muir RC: The pattern of swallowing during sleep. *Electroencephalogr Clin Neurophysiol* 1974; 38:427–432.
52. Lichter I: Measurement of gastro-oesophageal acid reflux: Its significance in hiatus hernia. *Br J Surg* 1974; 61:253–258.
53. Stanciu C, Bennett JR: Effects of posture on gastro-oesophageal reflux. *Digestion* 1977; 15:104–109.
54. Miller WN, Ganeshappa KP, Dodds WJ, Hogan WJ, Barreras RF, Arndorfer RC: Effect of bethanechol on gastroesophageal reflux. *Am J Dig Dis* 1977; 2:230–234.
55. Farrell RL, Roling GT, Castell DO: Cholinergic therapy and chronic heartburn. A controlled trial. *Ann Intern Med* 1974; 80:573–576.
56. Humphries TJ, Castell DO: Effect of oral bethanechol on parameters of esophageal peristalsis. *Dig Dis Sci* 1981; 26:129–132.
57. Phaosawasdi K, Malmud LS, Tolin RD, Stelzer F, Applegate G, Fisher RS: Cholinergic effects on esophageal transit and clearance. *Gastroenterology* 1981; 81:915–920.
58. Graham DY, Smith JL, Patterson DJ: Why do apparently healthy people use antacid tablets? *Am J Gastroenterol* 1983; 78:257–260.

3

Anti-reflux Barrier

David J. Ott, M.D.,
Philip O. Katz, M.D., and
Wallace C. Wu, M.B., B.S.

Chapter Contents

Elucidation of the anatomy and physiology of the esophagogastric region (EGR) has been attempted since the time of Hippocrates.[1] Considerable controversy, however, still persists over the morphologic and functional features of this rather short anatomic segment.[2] In particular, the exact nature of the anti-reflux barrier, and its relationship to normal and abnormal esophagogastric anatomy, remains confusing.

From Castell DO, Wu WC, Ott DJ (eds): *Gastroesophageal Reflux Disease: Pathogenesis, Diagnosis, Therapy.* Mount Kisco, NY, Futura Publishing Co., Inc., 1985.

Part of this confusion relates to different perceptions of the EGR formed by various disciplines. The anatomist studies structural relationships without functional correlation in cadaveric dissections. The manometrist interprets pressure variations in the lower esophageal sphincter (LES) under varying circumstances, but often in the absence of anatomic considerations. On the other hand, the radiologist visualizes the EGR maximally distended with barium, occurring only during relaxation of the LES. A combined approach to the study of the EGR appears needed to understand better the nature of the anti-reflux barrier.

In this chapter, we will review the anatomy and physiology of the EGR, and its role in preventing gastroesophageal reflux. Pertinent normal and abnormal radiographic anatomy will be reviewed, and comment will be made on the debated relationship between hiatal hernia and gastroesophageal reflux disease (GERD). The physiologic and manometric nature of the LES will be discussed, along with the role of the LES as the major candidate for the anti-reflux barrier.

Esophagogastric Anatomy

The terminology used to describe the anatomy of the EGR has been long and often contradictory. Several decades ago, considerable controversy focused on the nature of the lower termination of the esophagus. The concept that two saccular structures existed at the lower end of the esophagus was widely accepted at that time.[3] More recent evidence, however, has revised this idea, with the current view being that the esophagus terminates as a single sac.[4-8] Unfortunately, numerous and occasionally conflicting terms have been used to name this saccular structure or parts of it.

In the normal resting state, the lower esophageal sac straddles the diaphragmatic hiatus, with most of the structure lying above the hiatal level and a shorter portion located below the hiatus within the abdomen. The two most commonly accepted labels describing these components were the *phrenic ampulla* for the portion lying above the diaphragm and the *submerged segment* for the infrahiatal portion. In addition, the term *esophageal vestibule* became popular as a label for the whole lower esophageal sac.

The normal EGR has been shown to be mobile relative to the diaphragmatic hiatus, changing its relationship in response to swallowing, respiration, and positioning.[5,7,9-12] On deep inspiration, the diaphragmatic hiatus slides down the esophagus, while the esophageal vestibule moves orad during the longitudinal shortening associated with esophageal peristalsis. Under these circumstances, the esophagogastric junction will approximate the level of the diaphragmatic hiatus, thereby partially or completely obliterating the intra-abdominal portion of the esophagus.

Because of the changeable relationship between the diaphragmatic hiatus and the esophageal vestibule, its division into the phrenic ampulla and the submerged segment would seem somewhat factitious. In fact, it has been suggested that the term "phrenic ampulla" be discarded to simplify the terminology of the EGR.[1] The concept of the submerged segment, however, remains important since its disappearance radiographically is often associated with symptomatic gastroesophageal reflux, and its reconstruction during anti-reflux surgery is believed to be an important factor in preventing gastroesophageal reflux.[13-20]

The location of the anatomic junction between the esophagus and the stomach has also been surrounded by controversy. The major argument has focused on the use of the squamocolumnar mucosal union, or Z line, as a valid demarcator of the esophagogastric junction. However, recent anatomic and histologic evidence appear to refute the role of this mucosal transition as a reliable indicator of the junction.[1,5-7,12] Indeed, the upper level of the gastric sling fibers has become the most widely accepted criterion for localizing the esophagogastric junction. These muscle fibers lie within the gastric wall, demarcate the left lateral margin of the esophagogastric junction by straddling the cardiac incisura superiorly, and extend toward the lesser curvature of the stomach inferiorly. The squamocolumnar mucosal transition normally lies within a few centimeters above the upper level of the gastric sling fibers.

The existence of an anatomic sphincter in the EGR has been long debated. The presence of a structural sphincter near the lower end of the esophagus was widely accepted several decades ago.[21-23] This structure was called the *inferior esophageal sphincter*, and was localized to the junction between the tubular and vestibular portions of the esophagus. Both manometric and correlative radiologic investigations, however, have not verified such a structure. On the other hand, the presence of a physiologic sphincter characterized by a 2–4 cm high pressure zone in the EGR has been also acknowledged for nearly three decades.[8,24-26] This high pressure zone has been called the *lower esophageal sphincter*, or *LES*, and is believed to be the main candidate for the anti-reflux barrier. Attempts to identify the LES anatomically have been largely unsuccessful, although asymmetrical muscle thickening in the vicinity of the cardiac incisura has been shown recently.[27]

Because of this clearer understanding of the anatomy and function of the EGR, simplification of the terminology of this region is warranted (Figure 1). Basically, the esophagus consists of a cylindrical tube with a saccular termination. The cylindrical portion is defined as the *tubular esophagus*, while the saccular end is best labeled the *esophageal vestibule*. The tubulovestibular junction represents the union between these two esophageal segments. The upper level of the gastric sling fibers best demarcates the esophagogastric junction. Consequently, these respective junctions define the upper and lower boundaries of the esophageal vestibule. The squamocolumnar mucosal line lies near but slightly above the site of the gastric sling fibers. Two other pertinent terms that need to be mentioned are the *A level* and *B level*, popularized mainly in the radiologic literature.[8] The A level corresponds to the tubulovestibular junction and the B level to the *Z* line.

Esophagogastric Radiography

Proper radiographic evaluation of the EGR requires a thorough understanding of its morphology and function.[28,29] The upper margin of the manometric LES approximates the tubulovestibular junc-

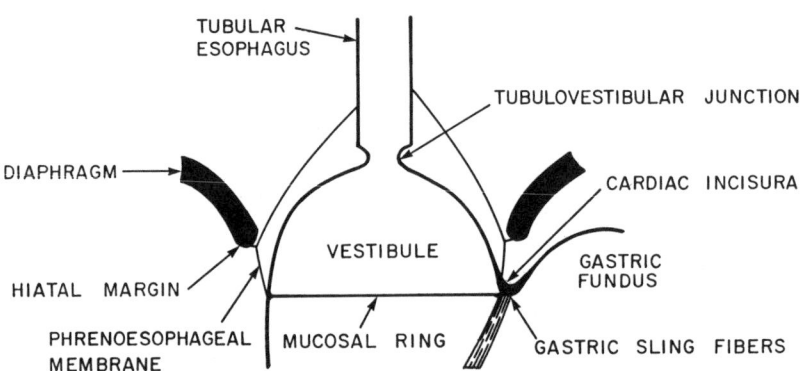

Figure 1: *Diagram of lower esophageal anatomy with simplification of terminology. Esophageal vestibule is defined by tubulovestibular junction superiorly and by upper margin of gastric sling fibers inferiorly. When present, mucosal ring approximates level of gastric sling fibers and, for practical purposes, demarcates the esophagogastric junction. (Modified with permission from* West J Med 1970; 112:33–51.)

tion, while its lower margin approaches the level of the gastric sling fibers.[8,9,24,26] Thus, the high pressure zone of the LES generally coincides in position to that of the esophageal vestibule, although their morphologic and functional interrelationship still remains unclear. During maximal radiographic distension of the EGR, the esophageal vestibule, corresponding to the relaxed LES segment, assumes a bulbous configuration in contrast to the cylindrical appearance of the tubular esophagus (Figure 2). Conversely, during the resting state, the tubular esophagus and esophageal vestibule are collapsed with the LES tightly closed because of its normal resting pressure.

The radiographic landmarks of the EGR are best appreciated following swallowing and subsequent relaxation of the LES. This permits maximal distension of the esophageal vestibule and its adjacent structures. The tubular esophagus terminates at the tubulovestibular junction as the vestibule begins and flares outward. Rarely, a smooth, changeable narrowing called the muscular ring, or A ring, may be seen at this upper vestibular border (Figure 3). With full distension, the esophageal vestibule assumes a bell-shaped configuration ending at the esophagogastric junction. Several ring-like narrowings may occur at the lower border of the esophageal vestibule. These include the lower esophageal mucosal ring, or B ring (Figure 4), and the annular peptic stricture. Radiographic differentiation among these various esophagogastric narrowings is usually not difficult.[2]

An axial hiatal hernia exists when the esophagogastric junction and a portion of adjacent stomach extend above the esophageal hiatus of the diaphragm. Unfortunately, a direct radiographic landmark for the upper margin of the diaphragmatic hiatus does not exist, thus requiring indirect signs.[5,11] Radiographic landmarks useful for delineating the esophagogastric junction include the lower esophageal mucosal ring (Figure 4), notch from the gastric sling fibers (Figure 3), orad level of the areae gastricae of the stomach (Figure 5), and termination site of esophageal peristalsis.[1,2,4–9,12,18,30–32] Hiatal hernia is diagnosed when these landmarks project above the estimated level of the esophageal hiatus, best recognized fluoroscopically as a transient narrowing of the EGR, the so-called "pinch-cock effect," as the patient sniffs or inspires deeply (Figure 6). Normally, however, the esophagogastric junction moves orad during respiration and primary esophageal peristalsis, approaching the level of the diaphragmatic hiatus. For this reason, some have argued that the esophagogastric landmarks must project at least 1–2 cm above the esophageal hiatus to be used as valid signs of hiatal herniation.[1,2,9,18]

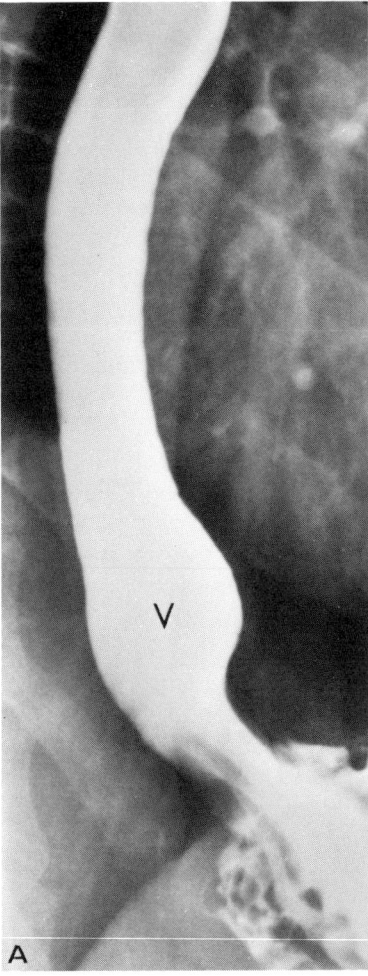
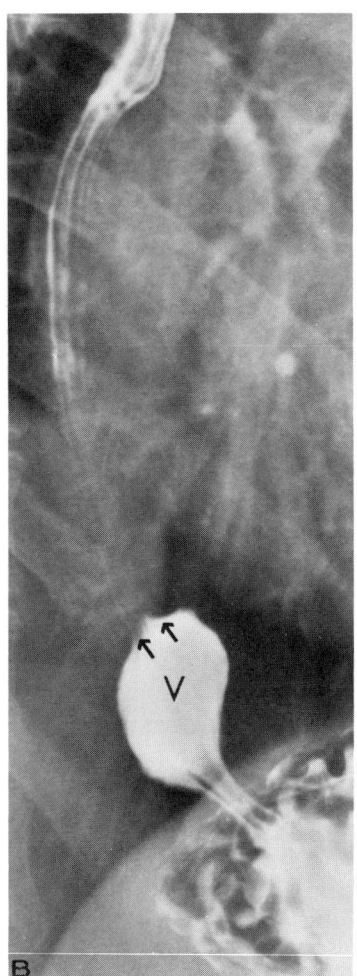

Figure 2: *Serial films of the esophagogastric region demonstrating its changeable appearance during various stages of swallowing.* **A.** *During maximal relaxation, the esophageal vestibule (V) is fully distended, and barium passes through the relaxed LES segment.* **B.** *When the primary peristaltic contraction reaches the tubulovestibular junction (arrows), the vestibule begins to collapse, and may be mistaken for hiatal hernia.* (Continued).

Hiatal Hernia and Reflux

In the past, the finding of hiatal hernia was often equated with the presence of reflux esophagitis. This misconception led to inappro-

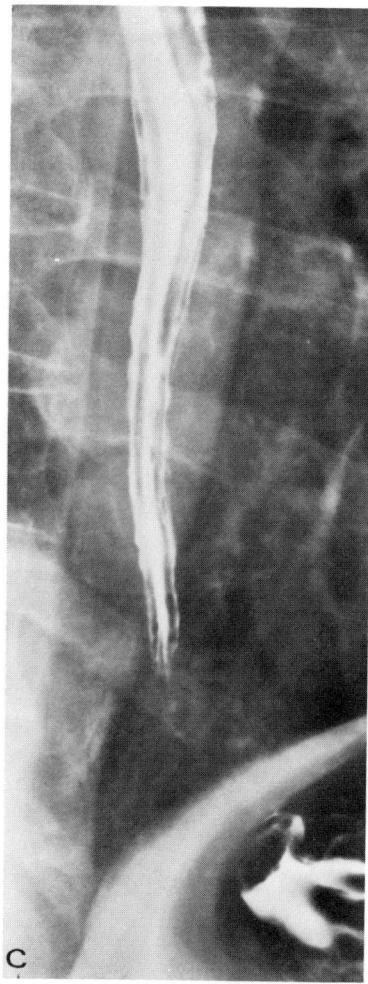

C

Figure 2C: *With complete collapse of the lower esophagus, the normal radiographic landmarks of the EGR are no longer apparent.*

priate surgical therapy directed at correction of the hiatal hernia rather than prevention of gastroesophageal reflux. Currently, the notion is that gastroesophageal reflux is caused primarily by LES dysfunction, with hiatal hernia being largely ignored in the pathogenesis of GERD.

A direct causal relationship between hiatal hernia and GERD has not been established.[18] Certainly, hiatal hernia is the most common diagnosis made during the radiographic examination of the upper gastrointestinal tract. The prevalence of hiatal herniation, however, is difficult to estimate due to differences in examining techniques and diagnostic criteria used. Although the reported radiographic inci-

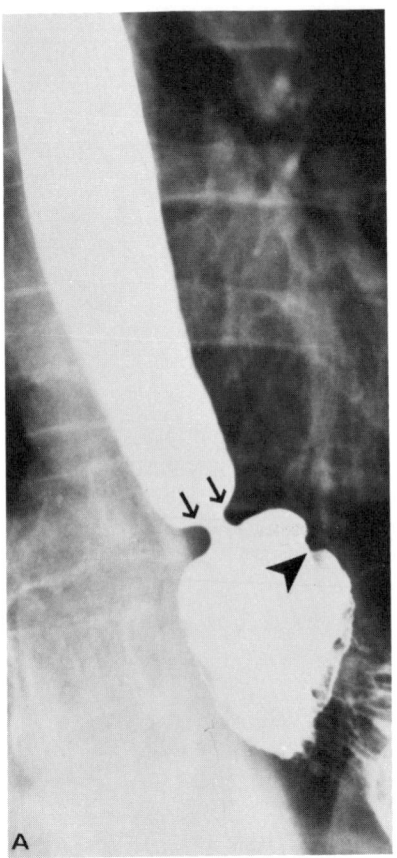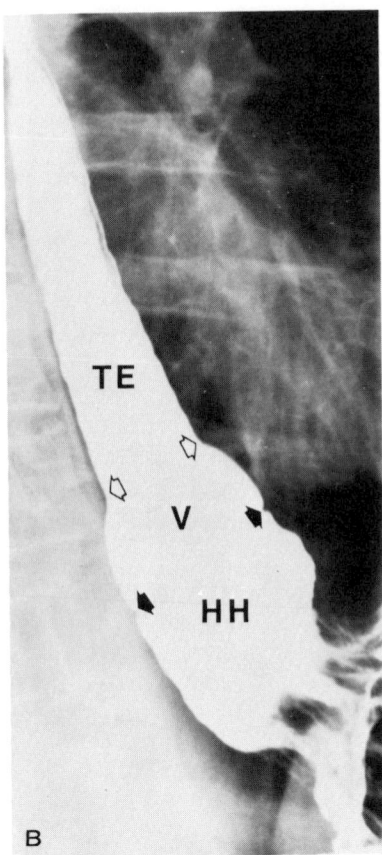

Figure 3: *Two views of the EGR taken moments apart.* **A.** *Changeable, smooth narrowing (arrows) of a muscular ring located at the tubulovestibular junction, well above the notching from the gastric sling fibers (arrowhead).* **B.** *Full distension of the EGR. The tubular esophagus (TE) has a cylindrical appearance, ending as the esophageal vestibule (V) flares outward at the tubulovestibular junction (open arrows). The lower end of the vestibule is demarcated by a widely patent mucosal ring (solid arrows). A sliding hiatal hernia (HH) lies below the vestibule (Reproduced with permission from Semin Roentgenol 1981; 16:168–182.)*

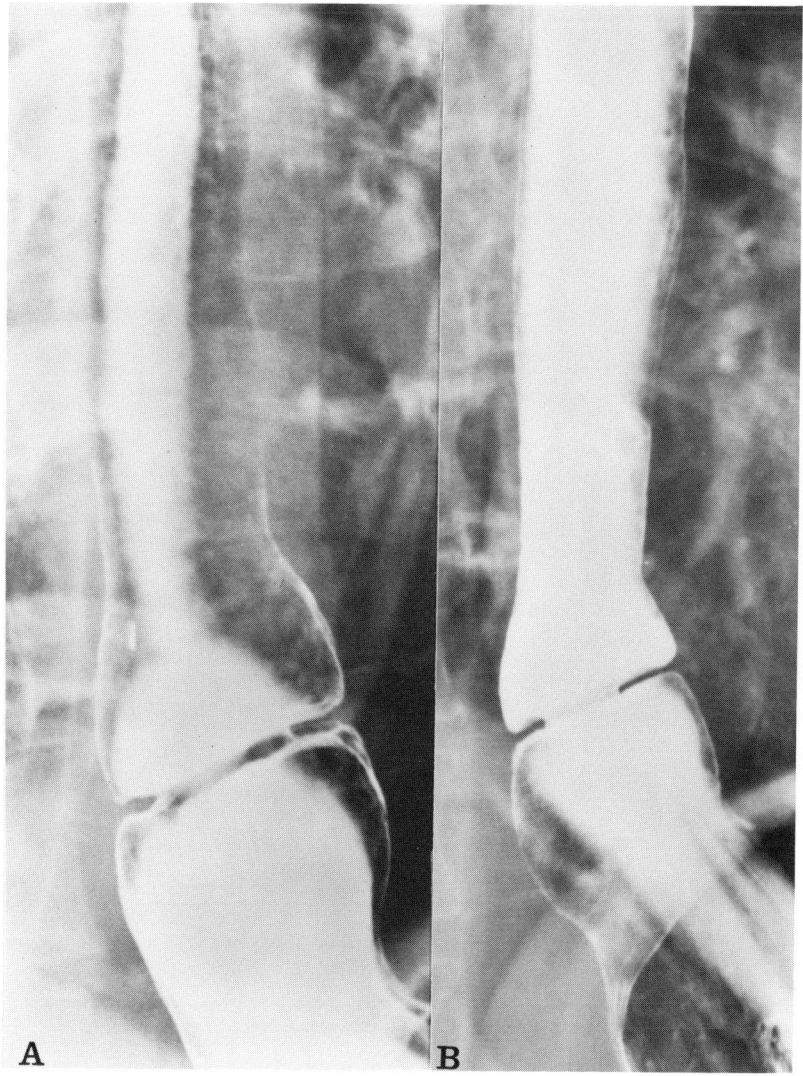

Figure 4: **A:** *Asymptomatic lower esophageal mucosal ring measuring 24 mm in caliber (with permission[2]).* **B.** *Lower esophageal mucosal ring measuring 12 mm in a patient with episodic dysphagia to solid food.*

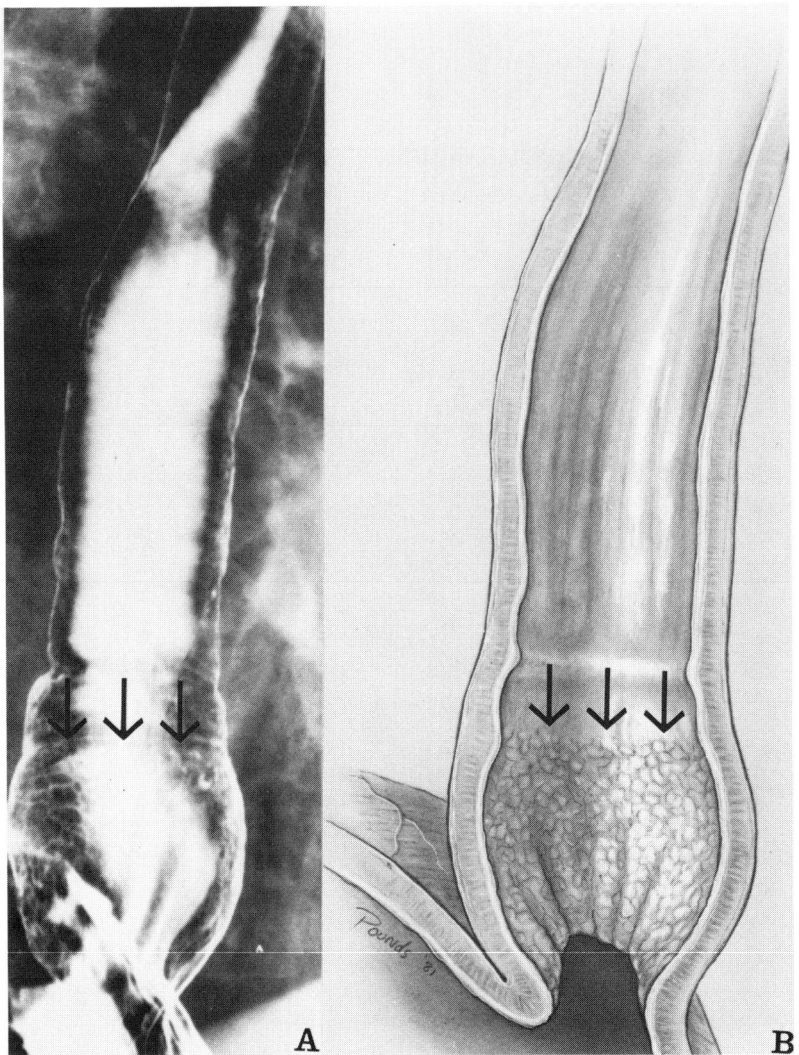

Figure 5: **A.** *Radiographic and* **B.** *Pictoral demonstration of the mucosal transition (arrows) between the stomach and esophagus. The reticulated pattern below the mucosal junction represents the areae gastricae of the stomach. The presence of area gastricae above the esophageal hiatus indicates hiatal herniation (Reproduced with permission from Elsevier Bio-medical,* Esophageal Function in Health and Disease, *1983: 211–235.)*

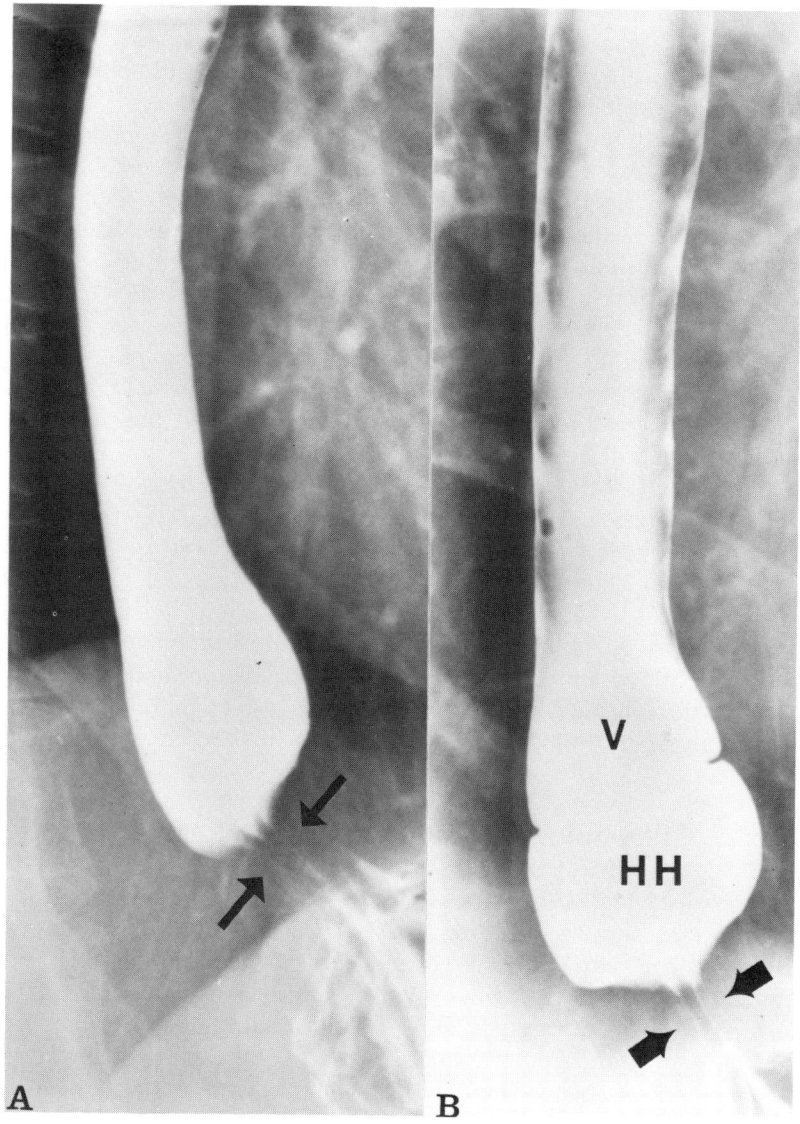

Figure 6: **A.** *Pinch-cock effect (arrows) on the normal EGR from compression of the esophageal hiatus with deep inspiration.* **B.** *Similar effect (arrows) in a patient with hiatal hernia (HH) (V = vestibule) and a widely patent lower esophageal mucosal ring (Reproduced with permission from* AJR *1984; 142:281–287.)*

dence of hiatal hernia has varied considerably, recent publications would indicate a 40–60% occurrence in adults.[17,18,33–38] Hiatal hernia is presumably an acquired condition, being uncommon in childhood, and increasing frequently with advancing age.[33]

Most individuals with hiatal hernia do not have endoscopic evidence of reflux esophagitis.[39,40] On the other hand, approximately 90% of those with GERD can be shown to have a concomitant hiatal hernia if appropriate radiographic techniques are used.[16–18] Although a normal esophagogastric junction cannot totally exclude the presence of reflux esophagitis, patients without hiatal hernia are unlikely to have the severer forms of endoscopic esophagitis.[17] Hiatal hernia is therefore a common but nonspecific radiographic finding since it poorly predicts the presence of GERD. Conversely, patients with GERD are likely to have an associated hiatal hernia, while absence of hiatal hernia tends to exclude the severer forms of this disease.

In summary, current evidence suggests that hiatal hernia is not the primary cause of abnormal gastroesophageal reflux. However, other causative factors promoting excessive gastroesophageal reflux may be affected by the presence of hiatal hernia. Perhaps, hiatal hernia enhances the likelihood of LES dysfunction in some individuals, thus playing a permissive role in the development of GERD. Clarification of this potential relationship between hiatal hernia and abnormal LES function appears to warrant further investigation.

Physiology of Esophagogastric Region

Physiologically, there are two components that constitute barriers to gastroesophageal reflux. Anatomatic factors appear to act entirely as a mechanical barrier against reflux. These proposed factors include: a mucosal flap, flutter valve, acute esophagogastric angle, compression by the gastric sling fibers, diaphragmatic pinchcock mechanism, hiatal tunnel, and sling action of the right diaphragmatic crus. We agree with Dodds et al.[41] that further studies need to be done before any conclusions can be made concerning the importance of these factors in the pathogenesis of GERD. On the other hand, the role of the LES as an anti-reflux barrier is far better defined.

Lower Esophageal Sphincter

Although the pathogenesis of GERD is multifactorial, there is no doubt that the LES plays a significant role as an anti-reflux barrier.

Esophageal manometry has served as a major research tool in investigation of the pathogenesis and pharmacology of the sphincter and its role in reflux disease. A brief review of the characteristics of the LES and evidence for its potential role in reflux is useful in understanding the pathogenesis of GERD.

Though an anatomically distinct sphincter has been difficult to demonstrate in man, there is little question that a physiological sphincter exists. Manometric studies have characterized the sphincter as a high pressure zone, approximately 3 cm in length, located in the area of the diaphragmatic hiatus. It relaxes during esophageal peristalsis, vagal stimulatory maneuvers, and esophageal distension. It has quantitative and qualitative responses to drugs, gastrointestinal hormones, and stretch, allowing it to be distinguished from adjacent smooth muscle.

The sphincter was first identified manometrically in 1956 by Fyke et al.,[42] but accurate measurements were not possible until the development of infused catheters in the mid-1960s. Using radially oriented catheters, investigators have found asymmetry of the sphincter, with pressures higher on the left and posteriorly than in other directions. This fact should be kept in mind when measuring sphincter pressures.

The asymmetry of the LES and controversy about the methods of measurement have called into question the value of basal or resting sphincter pressures in assessing reflux disease. Early studies with perfused catheters found a clear separation in LES pressures between normals and patients with severe reflux.[43] Further studies, using larger numbers of patients, failed to confirm the clear-cut distinction found by early investigators. In 1970 Haddad showed separation of mean resting LES pressure between heartburn patients and normals, but found considerable overlap in the range of 5–11 mmHg.[44] Miller (1974) found overlap as well, but suggested that isolated LES pressures below 6 mmHg could identify patients with moderate-to-severe esophagitis.[45] A recent study, comparing patients with Barrett's esophagus (a lesion associated with chronic reflux disease), patients with reflux disease and normals, found lower resting LES pressures in reflux patients and those with Barrett's esophagus as compared with normals (Figure 7).[46] Other investigators have demonstrated that patients with low resting sphincter pressures have reflux at low volumes of gastric acid (120 cc), while those with high sphincter pressures do not reflux, even with large volumes of gastric acid (500 cc).[47] In addition, another report found good correlation between patients with low resting sphincter pressures and histologic evidence of esophagitis.[48] A recent review of GERD showed considerable overlap of LES pressures in normals and reflux patients, suggest-

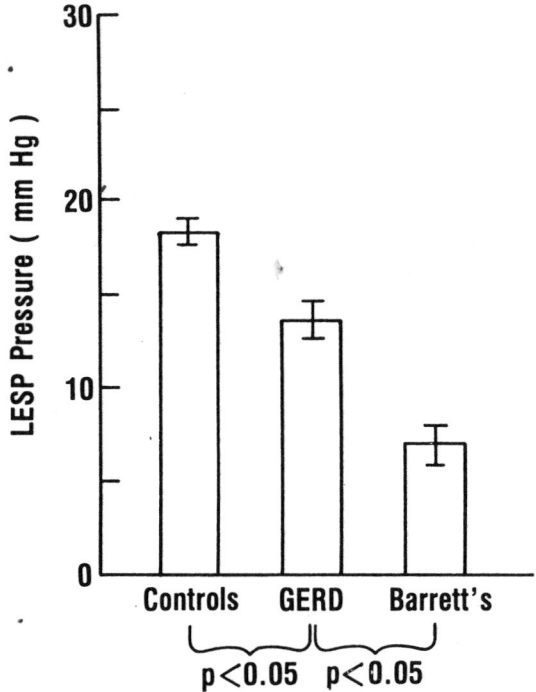

Figure 7: *Comparison of LES pressures in normals (controls), reflux patients (GERD), and patients with Barrett's esophagus.*

ing that an isolated average LES pressure has little predictive value in diagnosing GERD, except at extremes of LES pressure.[49] Overall, an isolated LES pressure of 10 or less has low sensitivity (58%) but reasonably high specificity (84%) in the diagnosis of reflux.

Continuous measurement of LES pressure, using a sleeve device over a 12-hour period in healthy volunteers and patients with reflux disease provides further support of the importance of the LES in the pathogenesis of reflux disease.[50] Patients with reflux had lower mean resting sphincter pressures (13 ± 8 mmHg) than did controls (29 ± 9 mmHg), though some overlap did exist. Reflux occurred by three different mechanisms: (a) transient complete relaxation of the LES; (b) transient increase in intra-abdominal pressure; and (c) spontaneous reflux associated with low resting LES pressure. Almost all episodes of reflux in normals were related to complete relaxation of the LES. All normals had resting pressures above 11 mmHg prior to relaxation and reflux did not occur with incomplete relaxation of the sphincter. Transient increase in intra-abdominal pressure caused acid reflux in a few instances, with resting pressures ranging from 5–13 mmHg prior to reflux (Table 1). Patients with esophagitis exhibited more reflux episodes, as well as lower resting pressures. Transient relaxation of the sphincter was also found in greater frequency than in controls. In addition, there was a greater incidence of spontaneous free reflux, and reflux occurring after increase in intra-abdominal pressure, as compared with controls. Like controls, however, most episodes of reflux occurred with transient complete relaxation of the sphincter (Table 2). The common denominator in almost all episodes of reflux was low or absent sphincter pressure, whether transient or persistent. In esophagitis patients, reflux occurs by the three previously mentioned mechanisms.

Table 1. Comparison of GE Reflux and LES Pressure in Patients with Esophagitis and Controls		
	Patients	**Controls**
1. Mean LES pressure during 12 hrs. (mean ± S.D.)	13 ± 8 mmHg*	29 ± 9 mmHg
2. Resting LES pressure 1 min prior to reflux (mean ± S.D.)		
a. complete relaxation	9 ± 7 mmHg*	23 ± 12 mmHg
b. stress-induced reflux	7 ± 8	9 ± 4
c. free reflux	1 ± 2	1 ± 0

*indicates significant change from controls
(Modified from Dodds et al: *N Engl J Med* 1982; 307:1547)

Table 2. Mechanisms of GE Reflux in Esophagitis Patients and Normals		
	Patients no. of episodes (%)	**Controls** no. of episodes (%)
1. Transient LES relaxation	228 (65)*	84 (94)
2. Transient intra-abdominal pressure increase	59 (17)*	4 (5)
3. Spontaneous free reflux	65 (18)*	1 (1)
4. Total episodes of reflux	352*	89

*Significant at P < 0.01
(Modified from Dodds et al: *N Engl J Med* 1982; 307:1550)

It is apparent that the average resting LES pressure is of little value in diagnosing most patients with suspected GERD. Those with extremely low sphincter pressures (≤ 6 mmHg) have a greater potential for development of reflux disease, while patients with sphincter pressures above $20-25$ mmHg should be adequately protected from GERD in most situations.

Agents

A study of the effects of gastrointestinal hormones, drugs, and other agents on the LES has provided a greater understanding of both the mechanisms and agents involved in the production of reflux, as well as evaluation of potential therapeutic modalities in reflux disease.

Many gastrointestinal and other hormones, when given intravenously, have been shown to affect LES pressure (Table 3), though their clinical importance is subject to debate. The most directly important effect is probably that of progesterone. LES pressures are greatly decreased in pregnancy[51] and in women on birth-control pills containing progesterone,[49] conditions associated with increased heartburn.

Various drugs, including theophylline, anticholinergic agents, diazepam, meperidine, morphine, and the calcium channel blockers all decrease sphincter pressure.[25] Foods such as chocolate, alcohol, and carminatives (peppermint) also lower LES pressure and may cause increased reflux.[49] A sustained decrease in LES pressure occurs after a fatty meal, suggesting an explanation for fatty-food intolerance in some patients. Cigarettes, probably through the anticholinergic effect of nicotine, also cause a decrease in sphincter pressure (Table 4).

Perhaps of greater importance, particularly in the therapy of heartburn, are the agents which have been shown to augment LES pressure, many of which are useful in anti-reflux therapy. Pharmacologic doses of gastrin and pentagastrin have been shown to increase LES pressures. A protein meal given to normals is found to exert a definite augmentation of sphincter pressure. This effect has been documented in esophagitis patients, though the effect is not as pronounced as in normals. Bethanechol, a cholinergic agent, has been found to increase LES pressure, and has proved to be a useful addition to anti-reflux therapy. Antacids, the mainstay of treatment for reflux disease, have been shown to have an augmenting effect on LES pressure, probably secondary to gastric alkalinization. Metoclopramide has been shown to increase LES pressure as well (Table 4).

Table 3. Hormones Affecting LES Pressure	
Increased	**Decreased**
Gastrin/Pentagastrin	Secretin
Motilin	Cholecystokinin
Pancreatic polypeptide	Glucagon
Bombesin	Vasoactive intestine
	peptide (VIP)
Pitressin	Progesterone
Angiotensin II	

Table 4. Other Agents Affecting LES Pressure	
Increased	**Decreased**
*Cholinergic stimulation	Theophylline
(Bethanechol)	Caffeine
*Gastric alkalinization	gastric acidification
*Metoclopramide	*Fatty meal
Anticholinesterases	*Chocolate
Protein meal	*Smoking
	*Ethanol
	β adrenergic agonists
	α adrenergic antagonists
	Anticholinergics (atropine)
	Calcium channel blocking
	agents
	Nitrates?

*therapeutic importance

Summary

Although the anatomy and physiology of the EGR has been clarified in recent decades, the exact nature of the anti-reflux barrier in this region remains elusive. Furthermore, elucidation of the relationship between the anti-reflux barrier and GERD is complicated by the multifactorial pathogenesis of the disease. Abnormalities in esophageal body function, esophageal tissue resistance, and gastric factors, along with sphincteric dysfunction, may all contribute to the development of GERD. Thus, the contribution of the anti-reflux barrier in GERD probably varies from one patient to the next.

The presence of a physiologic sphincter at the lower end of the esophagus, called the LES, is currently accepted as the major candidate for the anti-reflux barrier. Though the functional characteristics of the LES have become better understood, an anatomic counterpart corresponding to the sphincter has not been convincingly demonstrated. The uncertain relationship between esophagogastric morphology and sphincteric function continues to confound correlation of LES dysfunction to abnormal anatomy of the EGR. Further study of the EGR and LES using a combination of disciplines is needed to better define the true nature of the anti-reflux barrier.

References

1. Friedland GW: Historical review of the changing concepts of lower esophageal anatomy: 430 B.C. – 1977. *AJR* 1978; 131:373–388.
2. Ott DJ, Gelfand DW, Wu WC, Castell DO: Esophagogastric region and its rings. *AJR* 1984; 142:281–287.
3. Gould DM, Barnhard HJ: Changing concepts in the structure, function and disease of the lower esophagus. *Am J Med Sci* 1957; 233:581–595.
4. Wolf BS: Roentgen features of the normal and herniated esophagogastric region. *Am J Dig Dis* 1960; 5:751–769.
5. Berridge FR, Friedland GW, Tagart REB: Radiological landmarks at the oesophago-gastric junction. *Thorax* 1966; 21:499–510.
6. Friedland GW, Melcher DH, Berridge FR, Gresham GA: Debatable points in the anatomy of the lower oesophagus. *Thorax* 1966; 21:487–498.
7. Zboralske FF, Friedland GW: Diseases of the esophagus: Present concepts. *West J Med* 1970; 112:33–51.
8. Wolf BS: The inferior esophageal sphincter-anatomic, roentgenologic and manometric correlation, contradictions, and terminology. *AJR* 1970; 110:260–277.
9. Dodds WJ: Current concepts of esophageal motor function: Clinical implications for radiology. *AJR* 1977; 128:549–561.
10. Palmer ED: An attempt to localize the normal esophagogastric junction. *Radiology* 1953; 60:825–831.
11. Botha GSM: Radiological localisation of the diaphragmatic hiatus. *Lancet* 1957; 1:662–664.
12. Berridge FR, Friedland GW: The anatomical basis for the radiological diagnosis of minimal hiatal herniation. *Ir J Med Sci* 1967; 6:51–62.
13. Wolf BS: Sliding hiatal hernia: The need for redefinition. *AJR* 1973; 117:231–247.
14. Lewicki AM, Brooks JR, Meguid M, Membreno A, Kia D: pH-tested reflux without hiatus hernia. *AJR* 1978; 130:43–45.
15. Lindell D, Sandmark S: Hiatal incompetence and gastro-oesophageal reflux. *Acta Radiol Diagn* 1979; 20:626–636.
16. Wright RA, Hurwitz AL: Relationship of hiatal hernia to endoscopically proved reflux esophagitis. *Dig Dis Sci* 1979; 24:311–313.

17. Ott DJ, Wu WC, Gelfand DW: Reflux esophagitis revisited: Prospective analysis of radiologic accuracy. *Gastrointest Radiol* 1981; 6:1–7.
18. Ott DJ, Dodds WJ, Wu WC, Gelfand DW, Hogan WJ, Stewart ET: Current status of radiology in evaluating for gastroesophageal reflux disease. *J Clin Gastroenterol* 1982; 4:365–375.
19. Pettersson GB, Bombeck CT, Nyhus LM: Influence of hiatal hernia on lower esophageal sphincter function. *Ann Surg* 1981; 193:214–220.
20. Joelsson BE, DeMeester TR, Skinner DB, LaFontaine E, Waters PF, O'Sullivan GC: The role of the esophageal body in the antireflux mechanism. *Surgery* 1982; 92:417–424.
21. Lerche W: *The Esophagus and Pharynx in Action.* Springfield, IL: Charles C. Thomas, 1950.
22. Poppel MH, Zaino C, Lentino W: Roentgenologic study of the lower esophagus and esophagogastric junction. *Radiology* 1955; 64:690–700.
23. Johnstone AS: Observations on the radiologic anatomy of the esophagogastric junction. *Radiology* 1959; 73:501–509.
24. Heitmann NP, Wolf BS, Sokol EM, Cohen BR: Simultaneous cineradiographic-manometric study of the distal esophagus: Small hiatal hernias and rings. *Gastroenterology* 1966; 50:737–753.
25. Castell DO: The lower esophageal sphincter: Physiologic and clinical aspects. *Ann Intern Med* 1975; 93:390–401.
26. Goyal RK, Cobb BW: Motility of the pharynx, esophagus, and esophageal sphincters. In: Johnson LR, ed. *Physiology of the Gastrointestinal Tract,* Vol. 1. New York: Raven, 1981: 359–391.
27. Liebermann-Meffert D, Allgöwer M, Schmid P, Blum AL: Muscular equivalent of the lower esophageal sphincter. *Gastroenterology* 1979; 76:31–38.
28. Gelfand DW, Ott DJ: Anatomy and technique in evaluating the esophagus. *Semin Roentgenol* 1981; 16:168–182.
29. Ott DJ: Radiologic evaluation of the esophagus. In: Castell DO, Johnson LF, eds. *Esophageal Function in Health and Disease.* New York: Elsevier Biomedical, 1983: 211–235.
30. Goyal RK, Glancy JJ, Spiro HM: Lower esophageal ring. *N Engl J Med* 1970; 282:1298–1305, 1355–1362.
31. Hendrix TR: Schatzki ring, epithelial junction, and hiatal hernia—An unresolved controversy. *Gastroenterology* 1980; 79:584–585.
32. Gelfand, DW, Ott DJ: Areae gastricae traversing the esophageal hiatus: A sign of hiatus hernia. *Gastrointest Radiol* 1979; 4:127–129.
33. Wolf BS, Brahams SA, Khilnani MT: The incidence of hiatus hernia in routine barium meal examination. *Mt Sinai J Med NY* 1959; 26:598–600.
34. Ott DJ, Gelfand DW, Wu WC: Reflux esophagitis: Radiographic and endoscopic correlation. *Radiology* 1979; 130:583–588.
35. Koehler RE, Weyman PJ, Oakley HF: Single- and double-contrast techniques in esophagitis. *AJR* 1980; 135:15–19.
36. Creteur V, Thoeni RF, Federle MP, et al: The role of single and double-contrast radiography in the diagnosis of reflux esophagitis. *Radiology* 1983; 147:71–75.
37. Maglinte DDT, Schultheir TE, Krol KL, Caudill LD, Chernish SM, McCune WM: Survey of the esophagus during the upper gastrointestinal examination in 500 patients. *Radiology* 1983; 147:65–70.
38. Kaufmann HJ: Esophageal roentgenographic "abnormalities" in patients without symptoms. *J Clin Gastroenterol* 1979; 1:313–316.

39. Behar J, Biancani P, Sheahan DG: Evaluation of esophageal tests in the diagnosis of reflux esophagitis. *Gastroenterology* 1976; 71:9–15.
40. Johnson LF, DeMeester TR, Haggitt RC: Endoscopic signs for gastroesophageal reflux objectively evaluated. *Gastrointest Endosc* 1976; 22:151–155.
41. Dodds WJ, Hogan WJ, Helm JF, Dent J: Pathogenesis of reflux esophagitis. *Gastroenterology* 1981; 81:376–384.
42. Fyke FE Jr, Code CF, Schlegel JF: The gastroesophageal sphincter in healthy human beings. *Gastroenterology* (Basel) 1956; 86:135–150.
43. Pope CE: A dynamic test of sphincter strength: Its application to lower esophageal sphincter pressure. *Gastroenterology* 1967; 52:779–786.
44. Haddad JK: Relation of gastroesophageal reflux to yield sphincter pressures. *Gastroenterology* 1970; 58:175–184.
45. Miller WN, Hogan WJ, Dodds WJ, Arndorfer RC, Stef JJ: A comprehensive investigation of patients with symptoms of gastroesophageal reflux (GER). *Gastroenterology* 1974; 66:747 (abstract).
46. Knuff TE, Benjamin SB, Worsham GF, Hancock JE, Castell DO: Histologic evaluation of chronic gastroesophageal reflux. *Dig Dis Sci* 1984; 29:194–201.
47. Ahtaridis G, Snape WJ, Cohen S: Lower esophageal sphincter pressure as an index of gastroesophageal acid reflux. *Dig Dis Sci* 1981; 26:993–998.
48. Welch RW, Lackmann K, Racks P, et al: Lower esophageal sphincter pressure in histologic esophagitis. *Dig Dis Sci* 1980; 25:420–426.
49. Richter JE, Castell DO: Gastroesophageal reflux. *Ann Intern Med* 1982; 97:93–103.
50. Dodds WJ, Dent J, Hogan WJ, et al: Mechanism of gastroesophageal reflux in patients with reflux esophagitis. *N Engl J Med* 1982; 307:1547–1552.
51. Dodds WJ, Dent J, Hogan WJ: Pregnancy and the lower esophageal sphincter (Editorial). *Gastroenterology* 1978; 74:1334–1335.

4

Esophageal Epithelial Resistance

Roy C. Orlando, M.D.

Chapter Contents

Recent studies with 24-hour pH monitoring leave little doubt that gastroesophageal (acid) reflux is an almost universal and daily occurrence even in asymptomatic healthy subjects.[1,2] Nevertheless, only a small percentage of the population at risk develop reflux esophagitis and an even smaller number demonstrate evidence of severe (macroscopic) disease. These observations serve to emphasize the importance of mechanisms other than the anti-reflux barriers (e.g., the lower esophageal sphincter, diaphragmatic pinchcock, acute angle

From Castell DO, Wu WC, Ott DJ (eds): *Gastroesophageal Reflux Disease: Pathogenesis, Diagnosis, Therapy.* Mount Kisco, NY, Futura Publishing Co., Inc., 1985.

of His, among others) as determinants of reflux disease. In effect, the anti-reflux barriers are the first line of defense designed only to limit the *frequency and volume* of contact between gastric contents and the esophageal epithelium. When this fails, a second line of defense known as esophageal clearance comes into play. This defense, composed of esophageal peristalsis for volume removal and swallowed salivary secretions for acid neutralization, is designed to limit the *duration* of contact between gastric contents and the esophageal epithelium.[3,4] However, esophageal clearance is not instantaneous, and perhaps more important, is inoperable when subjects are asleep.[5-7] Thus, the total daily dwell time for acid contact with the esophagus may be considerable, necessitating an additional defense to avoid significant injury to the epithelium. This third line of defense is commonly referred to as "tissue resistance."[8-10] That "tissue resistance" is effective in epithelial protection against acid is best illustrated by experimental studies in which anti-reflux barriers and esophageal clearance mechanisms are bypassed. In such studies the esophageal epithelium may be exposed to acid for substantial periods of time, but despite this, exhibits little if any morphologic evidence of injury.[11-16] In this chapter the term "tissue resistance" is used to encompass a number of pre-epithelial, epithelial, and post-epithelial factors that may contribute to epithelial protection (Table 1). The approach taken is based on three premises: (a) that gastroesophageal reflux leads to an attack by acid upon the esophageal epithelium from the luminal surface; (b) that the hydrogen ion (H^+) is the major ion responsible for epithelial necrosis; and (c) that for significant epithelial injury to result from this attack, H^+ must reach the mid to lower layers of the tissue. It is the goal of this discussion to provide a greater appreciation for "tissue resistance" as a dynamic and complex group of epithelial processes with an important and perhaps crucial role in the prevention of reflux esophagitis.

Pre-epithelial Defenses

Mucus, Unstirred Water Layer, and Surface Bicarbonate

When gastroesophageal reflux occurs, gastric juice is introduced into the esophageal lumen. However, this alone doesn't ensure epithelial contact with noxious gastric contents because of the existence of pre-epithelial defenses such as mucus, the unstirred water layer, and surface bicarbonate ions (HCO_3^-) (Figure 1). The esophagus, like the remainder of the gastrointestinal tract, has a surface layer of

---

Table 1.
Esophageal Defenses Against Acid Injury

Pre-epithelial

1. Mucous layer
2. Unstirred water layer
3. Surface bicarbonate ion concentration

Epithelial

4. Structures (uppermost living cell layer)
   a. cell membranes
   b. intercellular junctional complexes

5. Functions
   a. epithelial transport
   b. intracellular buffering
   c. cellular uncoupling
   d. cell replication

Post-epithelial

6. Blood flow
7. Tissue acid-base status

PRE-EPITHELIAL DEFENSES

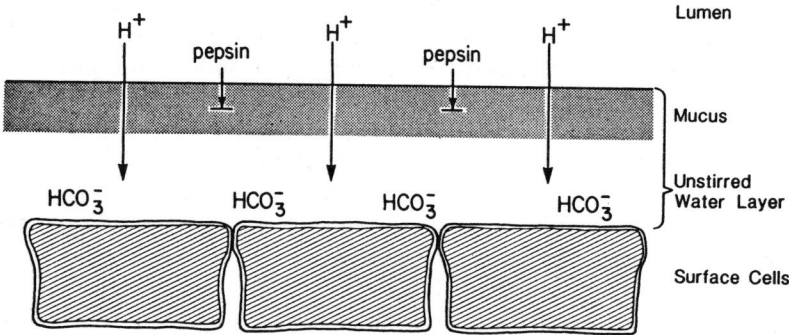

Figure 1: H^+ *must pass through the pre-epithelial defenses (mucus, unstirred water layer, and surface bicarbonate ions) before contact can be made with epithelial cells. Diffusion of pepsin toward the tissue can be blocked by mucus.* H^+, *which penetrates the mucous layer, can be neutralized by bicarbonate ions in the unstirred water layer.*

mucus that serves as both lubricant and protective barrier against mechanical and to some extent chemical injury.[17-21] Mucus, due to its composition of high molecular weight glycoproteins, has both viscoelastic and gel properties. These properties enable it to effectively prevent large protein molecules like pepsin from gaining access to the underlying epithelium.[17] However, mucus itself is not an effective barrier to H^+,[22,23] though one report suggests that it slows the rate of H^+ diffusion toward the tissue.[24] Yet mucus participates indirectly in epithelial protection against H^+ by contributing to an area of low turbulence adjacent to the tissue[25]—the unstirred water layer.[26,27] The unstirred water layer is significant because of its capacity to act as a sink for bicarbonate ions (HCO_3^-), which establishes an alkaline microenvironment close to the epithelial surface.[23,28] Although not defined for esophagus, the potential sources of HCO_3^- in this layer include: (a) HCO_3^- from secretions of the salivary and/or submucosal glands, (b) HCO_3^- diffusing from blood, or (c) HCO_3^- actively secreted by the stratified squamous epithelium. Regardless of source, the presence of HCO_3^- in the unstirred water layer can serve as an effective barrier to acid by neutralizing H^+ as it penetrates the mucous layer en route to the epithelium. The capacity to sustain a significant pH gradient across these layers has been demonstrated previously for stomach[29] and duodenum.[30] In these studies the passage of pH-sensitive microelectrodes from lumen to epithelium show that the mucus and unstirred water layers are capable of supporting a pH of 7 at the epithelial surface in the presence of a luminal pH of 2.

The mucous layer in the esophagus of humans is probably derived from secretions of the submucosal and salivary glands. However, the submucosal glands whose secretory ducts open directly onto the surface of the epithelium are found only in the proximal esophagus near the upper esophageal sphincter and in the distal esophagus near the esophagogastric junction.[18,20] Thus the secretions of the proximal glands could coat the upper and, by virtue of peristaltic activity sweeping mucus distally, the middle and lower esophagus. The distal glands, on the other hand, appear strategically located to ensure an adequate mucous coat in that region most susceptible to reflux injury. While in humans swallowed salivary mucus probably contributes to the esophageal mucous layer, this may be especially important for the rabbit whose esophagus is devoid of submucosal glands.[31] In contrast, the mucous layer for the opossum esophagus appears to be provided for by an abundance of submucosal glands widely distributed along the length of the organ.[31] It is of interest that secretions from the salivary and esophageal submucosal glands are increased by stimulation of the vagus nerve or administration of cholinergic agonists.[31-33] This observation could account for some of the beneficial effects reported for the cholinergic agonist, bethanechol, in reflux esophagitis.[34,35] Similarly, the success reported for carbenoxolone[36] and methyl prostaglandin E_2[37] in the treatment or prevention of reflux esophagitis may result at least in part from their ability to enhance salivary and esophageal submucosal gland mucus and/or HCO_3^- secretion. This contrasts with agents like aspirin, whose ability to inhibit mucus secretion may contribute to its toxicity for upper gastrointestinal epithelia.[38,39]

Epithelial Defenses

Esophageal Epithelial Structure

The lining of the esophagus is a partially or non-keratinized stratified squamous epithelium[20,40] that more closely resembles in structure and function the epithelia of skin, rumen, oral cavity, and cervix than it does the (columnar) epithelium lining the remainder of the gastrointestinal tract. In most species esophageal stratified squamous epithelium is subdivided into three layers: stratum corneum, stratum spinosum, and stratum germinativum or basalis (Figure 2). Less frequently a fourth layer, the stratum granulosum, is present and is identified by the presence of keratohyalin granules in the cytoplasm of its cells. The stratum corneum, depending on species, consists of one or more cell layers lining the luminal surface. Since these cells, which are the oldest within the epithelium, are in varying stages of degeneration,[40] they provide no effective barrier to H^+ penetration of the tissue. Below the stratum corneum is the stratum spinosum. This stratum is composed of multiple layers of flattened cells with numerous desmosomal connections producing a characteristic spiculated appearance on microscopy. Within this stratum, lies the *uppermost living cell layer*, a layer whose importance resides in its role as the major structural barrier to the permeation of ions and molecules into the epithelium.[41-43] This cell layer thus provides the next line of defense against the advance of H^+ into the tissue— these H^+ having successfully eluded the more luminal defenses consisting of mucus, the unstirred water layer, and surface HCO_3^-.

Morphologically, the two structural components of the uppermost living cell layer which constitute the permeability barrier are the cell membranes and the intercellular junctional complexes (Figure 3). These structures combine to produce an electrical resistance

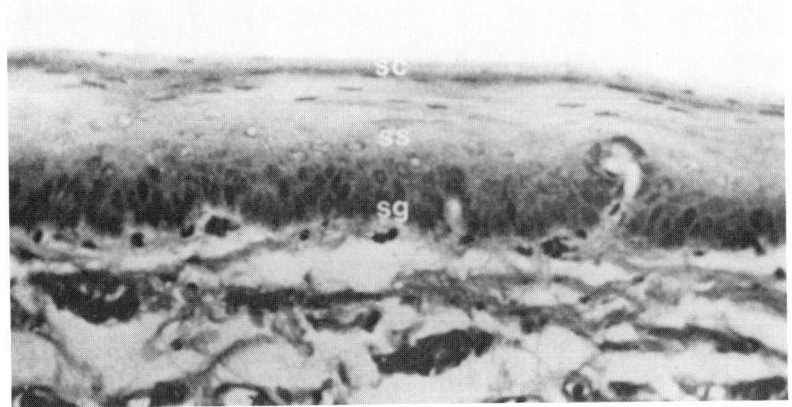

Figure 2: *Stratified squamous epithelium, rabbit esophagus. One-cell thick basal layer is the stratum germinativum (sg). Other two-cell layers are a continuum progressing from the stratum spinosum (ss) to stratum corneum (sc); distinction between the two is not well defined. Hematoxylin and eosin;* × *160. (Reproduced from* Laboratory Investigation, *1981; 45: 198−208, by copyright permission of US-Canadian Division of the Internal Academy of Pathology).*

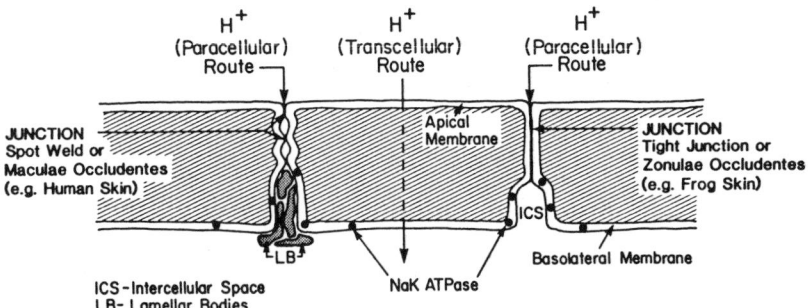

Figure 3: *The structural barriers to the permeation of H⁺ across stratified squamous epithelia are the cell membranes (transcellular route) and intercellular junctions (paracellular route). Two types of intercellular junctions are illustrated since it is not clear which predominates in esophageal epithelium.*

for human and rabbit esophageal epithelium in the range of 1,000–2,500 ohm · cm^2.[31,41,44,45] Electrical resistances in this range characterize the esophagus as having a "tight" epithelium. In contrast, "leaky" epithelia like gallbladder and small intestine have electrical resistances of < 500 ohm · cm^2.[46,47] Since the resistances of the cell membranes in "tight" and "leaky" epithelia are similar, the intercellular junctional complex is the major factor determining permeability (and overall electrical resistance). Presently, the nature of the intercellular junction in esophageal stratified squamous epithelium is unknown although the candidates are tight junctions and/or lamellar bodies.[45,46] In frog skin, the permeability of the intercellular junction is determined by tight junctions (also known as zonulae occludentes).[42,46,48] These structures, formed by the interaction of integral membrane proteins from adjacent cell membranes, encircle the cells of the layer to seal off the lumen from the intercellular space much as the plastic wrapping around a six-pack of canned beverage seals off the space above and below the plane of the cans' surface.[47] Thus, tight junctions act as a barrier to molecules passing between the cells from lumen to blood and vice versa (Figure 4). Tight junctions, however, are not impermeable nor are they equally permeable to all ions, a characteristic known as its permselectivity.[46,47] Since most tissues have negatively charged ions (e.g., carboxyl, phosphate, and sulfate groups) lining the junctions and intercellular space, they are usually more permeable to cations that to anions. However, H^+ can titrate the negatively charged ions as they enter the path and this changes the permselectivity from cation to anion selective.[46,47,49] Thus, the penetration of H^+ into the tissue via this pathway may be to some degree self-limited. In contrast to frog skin, human skin has only rudimentary tight junctions called maculae occludentes or spot welds.[50,51] Since spot welds represent only small areas of apposition between adjacent cell membranes, they are ineffective barriers to the diffusion of ions through the intercellular junction. Instead of tight junctions as in frog skin, the permeability of this pathway in human skin is governed by intercellular lipid-rich lamellar bodies.[50–52] These bodies appear to be formed in the cells of the stratum spinosum where they are packaged in round membrane-bound structures known as membrane coating granules. Contents of the membrane coating granules are subsequently secreted into the intercellular space where they act as an intercellular plug or cement (Figure 5).[50,51] Evidence that lamellar bodies are the permeability barrier in human skin also comes from experimental studies in fatty-acid deficient animals. These animals fail to produce lameller bodies and consequently can be shown to have markedly increased permeability through their

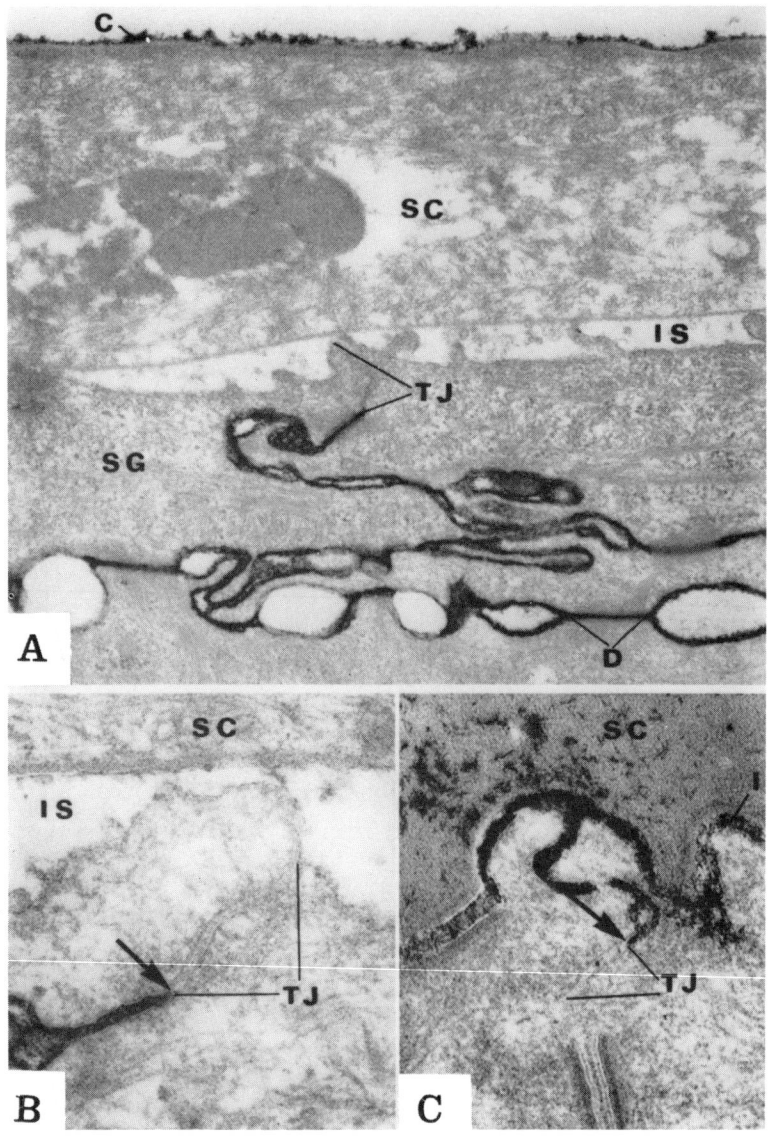

Figure 4A: *Outer region of an isolated frog epidermis treated with ruthenium red. Notice the presence of ruthenium red-positive material at the surface coat (C) of a cornified cell (SC). Ruthenium red penetrates from the interior of the epidermis and forms dense deposits at the outer surface of cell membranes in the stratum granulosum (G) but it does not permeate a tight junction (TJ) located beneath the intercellular space (IS) separating the stratum corneum (SC) from the stratum granulosum (SG). D, desmosome. ×23,000.* **B.** *Tight junctions (TJ) between two cells of the stratum granulosum.*

Continued

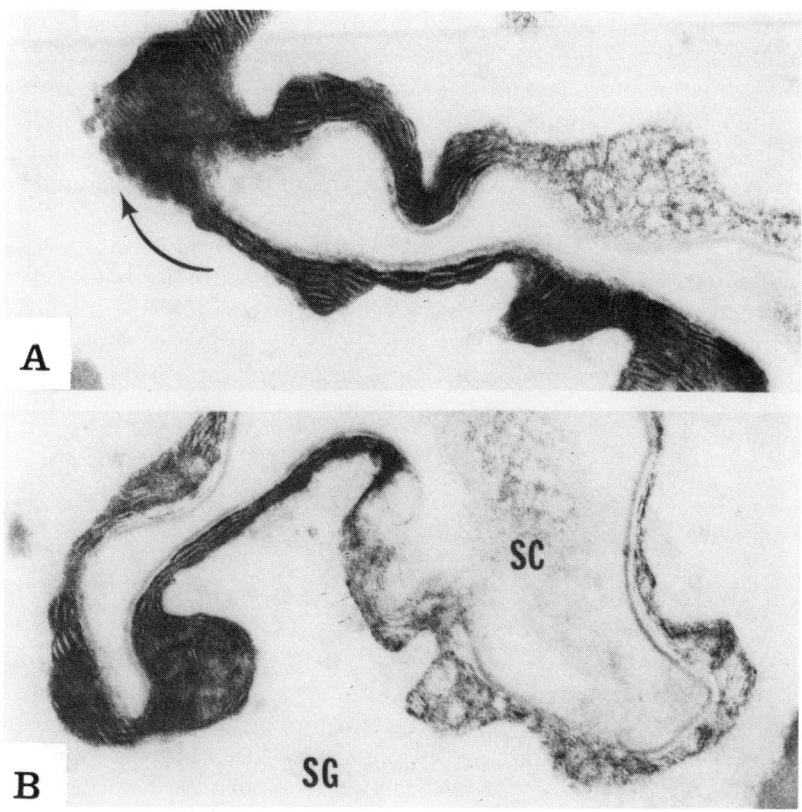

Figure 5: *Thin sections of adult mouse esophagus. Lanthanum percolates upward to the mid-stratum granulosum and permeates discs (lamellar bodies) lying within the intercellular spaces for variable distances until egress ceases. Lanthanum rarely appears to reach the interface of the stratum granulosum (SG) and stratum corneum (SC). Figure 5A × 60,000; 5B × 90,000 (Reproduced from* **Anat Rec** *1977; 189:577–594 by copyright permission of Alan R. Liss, Inc.)*

The junction is not permeated by ruthenium red (arrow), which had penetrated the intercellular space from the basal region of the epidermis. The intercellular space (IS) between the stratum granulosum and the stratum corneum (SC) is devoid of ruthenium red precipitate. × 90,000. C. Tight junction (TJ) in a location similar to that shown in Figure 4B. Colloidal lanthanum has penetrated into the cytoplasm of a cornified cell (SC) and into the intercellular space (IS) separating cornified cells from the stratum granulosum. However, the tracer is prevented from entering into the lateral intercellular spaces between two cells of the s. granulosum by the tight junction (TJ). (Reproduced from The Journal of Cell Biology, *1981; 50: 277–287, by copyright permission of The Rockefeller University Press.)*

intercellular junctions.[53] The failure to form lamellar bodies in this condition may be due to a lack of linoleic acid, a compound needed to form the molecules (acylglycosylceramides) necessary for assembly of the lamellar granules.[54] Since a method for isolation of lamellar bodies from tissue has recently been reported,[55] a more complete understanding of the nature and properties of this material should be forthcoming.

Whether the structural barriers to the diffusion of ions into a tissue are cell membranes, tight junctions, or lamellar bodies, the penetration of H^+ across them creates a major threat to the integrity of the tissue. This occurs because H^+ gains access to the transporting cells of the stratum spinosum. Before describing the effects of H^+ on this layer, a brief review of transport in stratified squamous epithelium is presented.

Esophageal Epithelial Transport

The stratified squamous epithelium of the esophagus exhibits *in vivo* a lumen negative potential difference (PD) of approximately –30 mV in rabbit and –15 mV in humans.[56] *In vitro* studies in the Ussing chamber have established that this PD for both man[45] and rabbit[44] primarily results from the active transport of Na^+ from lumen to blood. Since net Na^+ transport is reduced by either mucosal application of amiloride or serosal application of ouabain,[44] the transport characteristics of the esophageal epithelium closely resemble that of the more extensively studied stratified squamous epithelium of frog skin. Based on the frog skin model[57] (Figure 6), transport in esophageal epithelium can be summarized as followed: initially luminal Na^+ passively enters the cells of the uppermost living cell layer by passing through Na^+ channels in the apical cell membrane along a concentration gradient. After entering these cells, Na^+ diffuses to adjacent cells through cell to cell connections called gap junctions. NaK ATPase, an enzyme located on the basolateral cell membranes, then pumps Na^+ into the intercellular space below the level of the permeability barrier (tight junctions and/or lamellar bodies). Because the permeability barrier effectively limits Na^+ movement toward the lumen, its net movement is toward the serosal surface of the tissue and into blood. While the net movement of Na^+ from mucosal to serosal surface is accomplished relatively rapidly by the expenditure of cellular energy, the accompanying anion (usually Cl^-) moves passively and more slowly in the same direction along its electrical gradient. Thus the active movement of Na^+ from mucosal to serosal

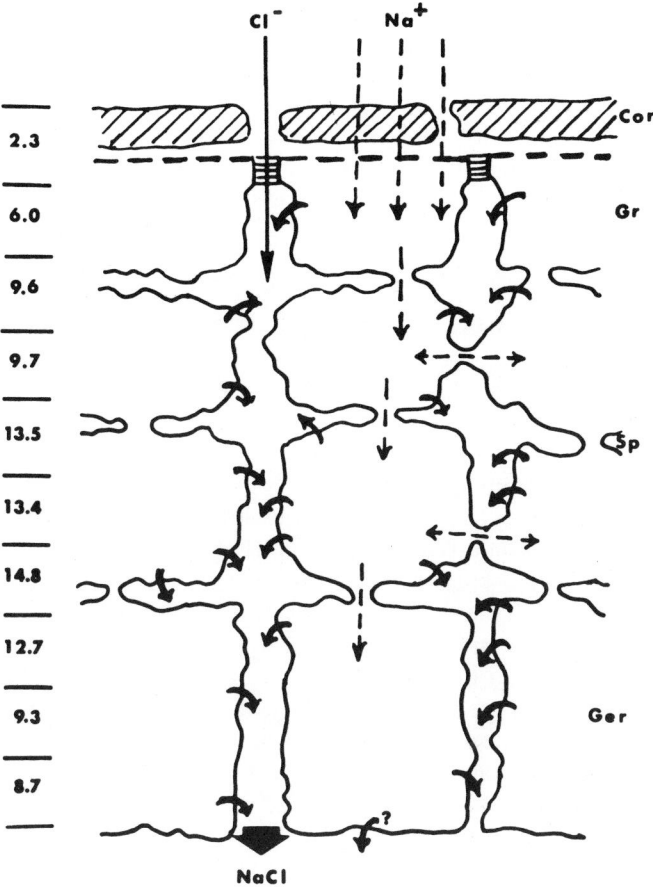

Figure 6: *A model for active Na⁺ transport by the frog skin. Na⁺ diffuses across or between the dead cells of the stratum corneum (Cor) and into the first living cell layer (stratum granulosum (Gr), whose apical cell membranes are selectively permeable to Na⁺. Tight junctions surround the cells of this layer and serve as a barrier to passive diffusion. The intracellular Na⁺ is then either actively pumped out of the cells by the Na pump (Na-K ATPase) located on the basolateral cell membranes, or else Na⁺ flows laterally or horizontally to adjacent cells of the stratum spinosum (Sp), probably via gap junctions. Na⁺ pumped into the intercellular spaces causes a flow of water, and both electrolytes and water then make their way across the basement membrane (not shown) to the interstitium. Ger, stratum germinativum. (Reproduced from* The Journal of Cell Biology, *1977; 73: 88–110, by copyright permission of The Rockefeller University Press.)*

surface, the slower passive movement of Cl^- in the same direction, and the limited back diffusion of ions due to structural barriers combine to separate charges in space, a process creating a measurable PD. Understanding these factors that determine PD are of more than theoretical interest since the transmural PD has been used to study the pathogenesis of acid injury to the esophageal epithelium[40,58,59] and to identify patients with esophagitis and Barrett's esophagus.[60,61]

Effects of H^+ on Esophageal Structure and Function

Since *in vivo* measurement of esophageal PD in healthy animals reflects the structural and functional integrity of the tissue, it is not surprising that acid-injured epithelia have an altered PD.[60,62–64] However, changes in PD may not only reflect epithelial injury but physiologic changes in epithelial permeability and transport. In addition, the PD may be altered by non-epithelial factors such as liquid junction (diffusion) potentials that develop when the luminal solution and recording electrode differ in ionic composition.[59,60,65] Thus *in vivo* PD changes need to be interpreted cautiously and should be validated with *in vitro* techniques where variables can be better controlled. In a recent series of studies, the effects of acid on esophageal epithelial structure and function have been reported.[40,58,59] In these studies, esophageal PD was monitored *in vivo* before and after acid exposure and changes in PD were documented. Subsequently, studies of epithelial morphology and transport were performed *in vitro* to determine the cause for the *in vivo* PD alterations induced by acid exposure. Thus, exposing the esophageal epithelium of a healthy rabbit to acid (80 mM HCl-80 mM NaCl) results in a biphasic response of the *in vivo* esophageal PD (Figure 7). Initially there is a transient increase in PD followed by a gradual but progressive fall in PD toward zero.[58] A similar pattern can be discerned in human subjects who have had esophageal PD monitored during acid-perfusion (Bernstein) tests[45] and PDs measured in the presence of gross esophagitis (evidence of prolonged acid exposure).[60] From studies of rabbit esophagi exposed to acid in the Ussing chamber, it is evident that the initial increase in esophageal PD in the presence of luminal acid results from a H^+ diffusion potential from lumen to blood.[59] Since H^+ diffusion across the tissue also results in its disappearance from the lumen, some investigators have utilized H^+ disappearance as a marker of altered epithelial permeability or epithelial injury.[11,66–68]

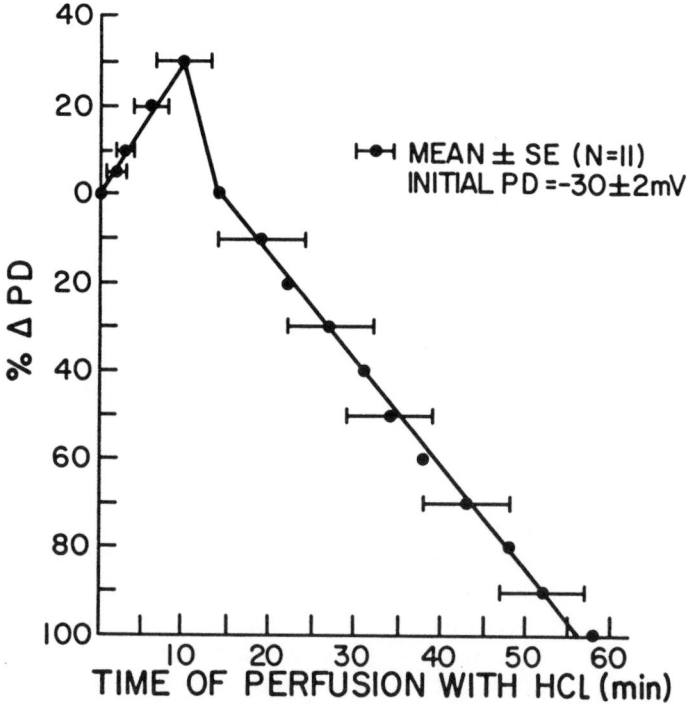

Figure 7: *The percent change in esophageal transmural potential differ-ence (Δ PD) is shown plotted against the time of exposure to 80 mM HCl-80 mM NaCl. A transient increase in PD occurs during the first 10 min. This is followed by a progressive linear decline in PD until it reaches zero at 1 h. •, Mean ± SE (n = 11); initial PD = –30 ± 2 mV. (Reproduced from* The Journal of Clinical Investigation, *1981; 68:286–293, by copyright permission of The American Society for Clinical Investigation.)*

The path that H^+ takes across the tissue is unclear, but it may be via the cell membranes (transcellular route), intercellular junctions (paracellular route), or both.[59,69] There is evidence that it materially alters structures in both paths. After brief exposure of the esophageal epithelium to acid, short-circuit current increases.[59] Since this increase in current has been shown to be due to increased net Na^+ absorption through an amiloride-sensitive pathway, it indicates that H^+ had altered the entry site for Na^+ (presumably the Na^+ channels) in the apical cell membrane. That H^+ may travel through the Na^+ channel (and thereby possibly alter its function) has been previously reported in toad bladders.[70] Additional transcellular routes for H^+ to take across the apical cell membrane might include: (a) Na:H exchange, an electroneutral amiloride-sensitive pathway, (b) movement along the peptide backbone of integral membrane proteins, and/or (c) movement assisted by adsorbed membrane surfactants acting as protonophores.[69] After the esophageal PD has fallen to 50% of its initial value in acid-exposed rabbit esophagi, there is evidence that H^+ alters the intercellular junctions. At this stage the decline in PD results from a reduction in electrical resistance, a finding paralleled by increased mannitol flux from lumen to blood.[58] These results are consistent with an increase in epithelial permeability through the paracellular pathway. Morphologic studies also corroborate this interpretation by showing dilated intercellular spaces in acid-exposed rabbit esophagi and separation of epithelial tight junctions in acid-exposed frog skin.[71] In contrast to the postulated mechanisms by which H^+ may cross the apical cell membrane, H^+ probably traverses the paracellular pathway by hopping from water molecule to water molecule through rearrangement of hydrogen bonds.[72]

At this point it should be noted that the effects of H^+ on the apical cell membrane and the permeability of the intercellular junctions described above are reversible and unassociated with either impaired epithelial transport or morphologic evidence of cell necrosis.[58] Therefore, even after H^+ penetration across the permeability barriers of the uppermost living cell layer, mechanisms exist to protect the epithelium from injury. Based on studies in other epithelia requiring protection from H^+, one important mechanism may be the removal of H^+ through neutralization with intracellular HCO_3^-. The generation of intracellular HCO_3^- appears to result from an exchange for intracellular Cl^- across the nutrient membrane (Figure 8).[73-76] H_2CO_3, the product of H^+ neutralization, is then dehydrated to H_2O and the readily diffusible CO_2, a reaction catalyzed by the enzyme, carbonic anhydrase. Although carbonic anhydrase has not been sought in esophagus, there is evidence for its presence in frog skin[77] and ox rumen.[78] In addition, studies by Schiessel and colleagues indicate that prostaglandins stimulate the exchange of cellular Cl^- for nutrient HCO_3^-,[79] a process that could contribute to their recognized cytoprotective effect against H^+ injury in gastric epithelium. Although prostaglandins are protective in stomach, their protective role in esophagus remains controversial. In one study the administration of 16, 16, dimethyl PGE_2 to opossums increased the severity of radiation-induced esophagitis while indomethacin, a potent blocker of prostaglandin synthesis, reduced it.[80] Similarly, the potential for prostaglandins to be harmful rather than beneficial for esophagus was suggested by the observation that treatment with indomethacin increased the rate of healing in acid-injured epithelia

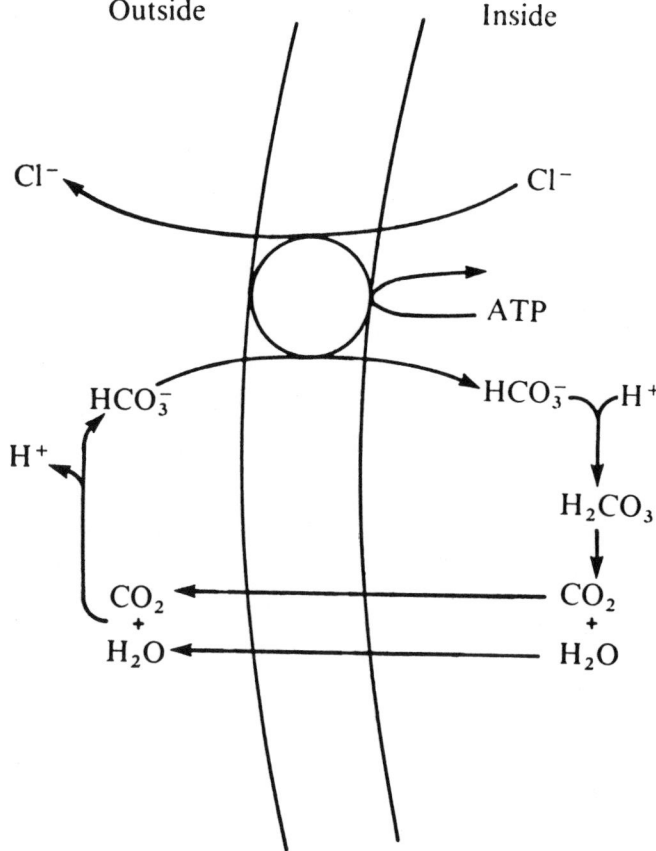

Figure 8: *Proposed scheme for acid extrusion. An ATP-dependent mechanism would inject external HCO_3^- in exchange for internal Cl^-. Once inside, the HCO_3^- would combine with H^+ to produce $CO_2 \cdot H_2O$, which would then leave the cell and yield $H^+ + HCO_3^-$ once again. The net effect is to eject HCl from the cell. (Reprinted by permission from* Nature, 264: *73–74, Copyright © 1976, Macmillan Journals Limited.)*

of cats.[81] In contrast, the administration of methyl PGE_2 to baboons was reported to enhance the rate of healing in acid-injured esophageal epithelia.[37] A second mechanism that may assist in epithelial protection after H^+ entry is the process of cellular uncoupling.[82,83] This occurs because the permeability of gap junctions, the channels for cell to cell communication, are controlled by the concentration of intracellular Ca^{++}. When intracellular pH falls as a result of H^+ entry, Ca^{++} ions are displaced from their membrane binding sites. Since the resultant increase in intracellular Ca^{++} reduces the permeability of gap junctions, adjacent cells are protected from exposure to low pH. However, when acid exposure is prolonged, these mechanisms can be overwhelmed, leading to a further decline in intracellular pH and cell injury. This process is illustrated by exposing the esophageal epithelium to acid until the *in vivo* PD declines to 80–100% of its initial value (i.e., PD approaches zero). When this occurs, *in vitro* studies have shown severe and irreversible damage to epithelial structure and function.[40,58] Functionally net Na^+ transport and NaK ATPase activity are inhibited[58,59] while structurally cellular edema and necrosis are identified most prominently in the stratum spinosum (Figure 9). The stratum spinosum has a high concentration of NaK ATPase.[57] Since this enzyme is inhibited in acid-exposed esophagi with low PD,[59] this may account for the severity of cell necrosis in this layer. However H^+-inhibition of NaK ATPase alone cannot account for edema and necrosis since similar changes do not occur in epithelia exposed to ouabain.[84] The lack of cell edema and necrosis with ouabain may be due to feedback mechanisms involving apical cell membrane permeability to Na^+.[85,86] Thus when intracellular Na^+ increases as a result of NaK ATPase inhibition by ouabain, intracellular Ca^{++} increases through $Na^+:Ca^{++}$ exchange across the basolateral cell membrane.[86] The resulting increase in cellular Ca^{++} acts to reduce Na^+ entry across the apical cell membrane and by so doing maintains a constant intracellular volume. However, in contrast to ouabain, H^+ inhibition of NaK ATPase not only reduces Na^+ exit but enhances apical cell membrane entry for Na^+[59]. Thus H^+ interference with the negative feedback for Na

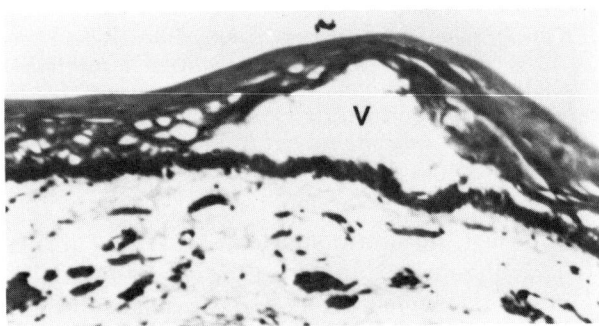

Figure 9: *Light-micrograph of acid-perfused esophageal mucosa (PD ↓ 80–100%) showing cellular necrosis, edema, and vesicle formation (V) in the mid-zone of the epithelium (stratum spinosum). The stratum corneum and stratum germinativum remain intact. Hematoxylin and eosin stain × 360. (Reproduced from* The Journal of Clinical Investigation *1981; 68:286–293, by copyright permission of the American Society for Clinical Investigation.)*

entry results in the loss of cell volume regulation, cell edema, and necrosis. That altered Na^+ transport may be responsible for cell swelling and death is readily understandable in view of its acknowledged importance in volume regulation.[84,87]

In summary, these studies indicate that H^+ injury to the stratified squamous epithelium may be considered a three-stage process: the first reflected by increased PD is due to H^+ diffusion into the tissue and enhanced apical cell membrane permeability to Na^+. The second, identified by the initial decline in PD, results from H^+ effects on the intercellular junctions leading to increased epithelial permeability through the paracellular pathway and access of H^+ to NaK ATPase on the basolateral cell membranes. The third, characterized by the fall in PD to zero, reflects H^+ inhibition of NaK ATPase activity with subsequent inhibition of Na^+ exit from cells. This effect, when associated with enhanced Na^+ entry (stage I), leads to loss of cell volume regulation, edema, and necrosis.

Post-epithelial Defenses

As in all tissues, an adequate flow of blood to the esophagus and normal tissue acid-base status are essential for maintenance of a viable and healthy epithelium. Through the blood, nutrients and oxygen are provided for cell functions including cell replication, and in the event of cell injury, cell repair. In addition, blood flow is important for preservation of a normal acid-base status in the tissue. For this capacity it brings HCO_3^- and other molecules to serve as buffers for the byproducts of cellular metabolism. In the event of epithelial injury as in reflux esophagitis, an increase in epithelial blood flow would be desirable to provide additional nutrients for epithelial repair and replication and HCO_3^- for H^+ neutralization. Although no direct measurements of esophageal blood flow have been reported, Geboes and colleagues have provided evidence that this occurs by demonstrating on esophageal biopsy an ingrowth of capillaries into the epithelium of patients with reflux esophagitis.[88] The ability of an increase in blood flow to protect epithelia from H^+ injury has previously been shown for gastric mucosa.[89,90] Studies in gastric mucosa have also shown the importance of tissue acid-base status in epithelial protection from H^+ injury.[73-75] For example, Kivilaakso[73] has demonstrated that the systemic administration of $NaHCO_3$ protected the rat gastric epithelium from ulceration. Since hyperventilating the experimental animal elevated the systemic pH to the same degree as $NaHCO_3$ administration but failed to prevent ulceration, it was concluded that HCO_3^- concentration in the tissue and not the elevated pH per se was the important factor in epithelial protection against H^+ back-diffusion. The mechanism by which high HCO_3^- concentration in the tissue protects the epithelium has not been established but it may be through the generation of intracellular HCO_3^- (discussed above). This possibility is supported by studies in frog gastric mucosa showing that SITS, an inhibitor of anion transport across cell membranes, abolished the protection afforded by high concentration of HCO_3^- in the nutrient solution.[75]

Epithelial Regeneration

Despite the intrinsic capability of the esophagus to resist acid injury, as described above, prolonged exposure produces epithelial cell necrosis. Since cell necrosis further increases epithelial permeability to H^+, a vicious cycle is set in motion which could lead to complete destruction of the epithelium, including the stratum germinativum. The stratum germinativum, a single cell layer located along the basement membrane, is important because it contains the only population of cells within the stratified squamous epithelium capable of mitosis and replication.[91–94] It is therefore critical that this layer survive if epithelial regeneration is to take place normally following injury. Although not experimentally proven, the destruction of the stratum germinativum and/or its basement membrane appears to be a necessary prelude to the development of such serious complications of reflux esophagitis as esophageal strictures, ulcers, and Barrett's esophagus. Thus, the location of this layer furthest from the lumen appears designed to provide maximal protection from attack by refluxed H^+ or other noxious agents in gastric juice.

Although the mechanisms that control the rate of cell replication in the esophagus are unknown, there is evidence that it can be increased after H^+ injury. Thus Livstone and colleagues showed that thymidine uptake, a marker of epithelial turnover, was increased in human mucosal biopsies from patients with severe esophagitis.[95] Also, since basal cell hyperplasia has been considered one of the biopsy hallmarks of reflux esophagitis,[96] this adds morphologic support for increased cell replication in H^+ injured tissue. Based on studies in mouse and man, a normal turnover rate for the esophageal epithelium appears to be 5–8 days.[94,97] With the increased rate of replication identified with H^+ injury, it would seem possible for the epithelium to regenerate in as few as 2–4 days. From a therapeutic standpoint, this would mean that epithelial protection from H^+ for even short periods of time might be sufficient for recovery.

Effects of Bile Salts and Other Noxious Agents on the Esophageal Epithelium

Although the primary focus of this discussion has been on H^+ injury to the esophageal epithelium, there is no doubt that other agents contribute to the injury in reflux esophagitis. Indeed, most investigations indicate that the addition of conjugated bile salts, alcohol, or pepsin to an acid solution produces greater injury in a shorter time than that of the acid solution alone.[11,12,15,16,67,98-100] However, it is also important to recognize that these agents are relatively innocuous in the esophagus when acid is absent. Therefore, their propensity to produce damage appears to rest on their ability to act as "barrier breakers"—thereby enhancing epithelial permeability to H^+. How they break the barrier may differ from agent to agent. For example, a detailed study in dogs indicates that bile salts disrupt the gastric mucosal barrier by micellar dissolution of the lipids in cell membranes.[101] The same process may be operative in esophagus since Salo and colleagues provide morphologic evidence that bile salts attack primarily the cell membranes and intracellular organelles of this tissue.[12] In contrast to the effects of bile salts, these investigators observed that the proteolytic enzyme, pepsin, acted on the intercellular substance causing the epithelial cells to shed intact.[12] Alcohol is another agent noxious to the esophageal epithelium. This may be due to its ability to solubilize lipids or to its presence as a hyperosmolar solution. Since hyperosmolar solutions open tight junctions in stratified squamous epithelia[102,103] and induce heartburn in patients with an acid-sensitive esophagus,[104] alcohol may increase the permeability to H^+ through the paracellular path as well as the transcellular path.[99,105] Regardless of mechanism(s), however, ultimately the entry of H^+ into the tissue is responsible for cell death. Yet the ability of "barrier breakers" to increase permeability may be crucial in determining the success or failure of the epithelium to defend against H^+ injury.

Acknowledgment: The author wishes to thank Mrs. Sandra F. Woody for her expert technical assistance in the preparation of this manuscript.

References

1. Johnson LF, DeMeester TR: Twenty-four hour pH monitoring of the distal esophagus. *Am J Gastroenterology* 1974; 62:325-332.

2. DeMeester TR, Johnson LF, Joseph GJ, et al: Patterns of gastroesophageal reflux in health and disease. *Ann Surg* 1976; 184:459–469.
3. Helm JF, Dodds WJ, Riedel DR, et al: Determinants of esophageal acid clearance in normal subjects. *Gastroenterology* 1983; 85:607–612.
4. Helm JF, Dodds WJ, Pelc LR, et al: Effect of esophageal emptying and saliva on clearance of acid from the esophagus. *N Engl J Med* 1984; 310:284–287.
5. Dent J, Dodds WJ, Friedman RH, et al: Mechanism of gastroesophageal reflux in recumbent asymptomatic subjects. *J Clin Invest* 1980; 65: 256–267.
6. Lichter I, Muir RC: The pattern of swallowing during sleep. *Electroencephalogr Clin Neurophysiol* 1975; 38:427–432.
7. Schneyer LH, Pigman W, Hanahan L, Gilmore RW: Rate of flow of human parotid, sublingual and submaxillary secretions during sleep. *J Dental Res* 1956; 35:109–114.
8. Richter JE, Castell DO: Gastroesophageal reflux: Pathogenesis, diagnosis and therapy. *Ann Intern Med* 1982; 97:93–103.
9. Dodds WJ, Hogan WJ, Helm JF, Dent J: Pathogenesis of reflux esophagitis. *Gastroenterology* 1981; 81:376–394.
10. Pope CE II: Pathophysiology and diagnosis of reflux esophagitis. *Gastroenterology* 1976; 70:445–454.
11. Salo J, Kivilaakso E: Role of luminal H^+ in the pathogenesis of experimental esophagitis. *Surgery* 1982; 92:61–68.
12. Salo JA, Lehto VP, Kivilaakso E: Morphologic alterations in experimental esophagitis: Light microscopic and scanning and transmission electron microscopic study. *Dig Dis Sci* 1983; 28:440–448.
13. Safaie-Schirazi S: Effect of pepsin on ionic permeability of canine esophageal mucosa. *J Surg Res* 1977; 22:5–8.
14. Bateson MC, Hopwood D, Milne G, Bouchier AD: Oesophageal epithelial ultrastructure after incubation with gastrointestinal fluids and their components. *J Pathol* 1981; 133:33–51.
15. Lillemoe KD, Johnson LF, Harmon JW: Role of the components of the gastroduodenal contents in experimental acid esophagitis. *Surgery* 1982; 92:276–284.
16. Redo SF, Barnes WA, de la Sierra OA: Perfusion of the canine esophagus with secretions of upper gastrointestinal tract. *Ann Surg* 1959; 149: 556–564.
17. Allen A, Phil D: The structure and function of gastrointestinal mucus. In: Harmon JW, ed. *Basic Mechanisms of Gastrointestinal Mucosal Cell Injury and Protection.* Baltimore: Williams and Wilkins, 1981: 351–367.
18. Hafez ESE: Functional anatomy of mucus-secreting cells. In: Elstein M, Parke DV, eds. *Mucus in Health and Disease.* New York: Plenum Press, 1977: 19–38.
19. Logan K, Hopwood D, Milne G: Ultrastructural demonstration of cell coat on the surface of normal oesophageal epithelium. *Histochem J* 1977; 9:495–504.
20. Al Yassin T, Toner PG: Fine structure of squamous epithelium and submucosal glands of human esophagus. *J Anat* 1977; 123:705–721.
21. Kiriluk LB, Merendino KA: The comparative sensitivity of the mucosa of the various segments of the alimentary tract in the dog to acid-peptic action. *Surgery* 1954; 35:547–556.

22. Heatley NG: Mucosubstance as a barrier to diffusion. *Gastroenterology* 1959; 37:313–317.
23. Williams SE, Turnberg LA: Studies of the "protective" properties of gastric mucus: Evidence for mucus bicarbonate barrier. *Gut* 1979; 20:A922–923.
24. Pfeiffer CJ: Experimental analysis of hydrogen ion diffusion in gastrointestinal mucus glycoprotein. *Am J Physiol* 1981; 240:G176–182.
25. Mantle M, Mantle D, Allen A: Polymeric structure of pig small-intestinal mucus glycoprotein. *Biochem J* 1981; 195:277–285.
26. Thomson ABR: Unstirred water layers: A basic mechanism of gastrointestinal mucosal cell cytoprotection. In: Harmon JW, ed. *Basic Mechanisms of Gastrointestinal Mucosal Cell Injury and Protection.* Baltimore: Williams and Wilkins, 1981: 327–350.
27. Thomson ABR: Unstirred water layers: Possible adaptive and cytoprotective function. In: Allen A, Flemstrom G, Garner A, Silen W, Turnberg LA, eds. *Mechanisms of Mucosal Protection in the Upper Gastrointestinal Tract.* New York: Raven Press, 1984: 233–239.
28. Allen A, Garner A: Mucus and bicarbonate secretion in the stomach and their possible role in mucosal protection. *Gut* 1980; 21:249–262.
29. Williams SE, Turnberg LA: The demonstration of a pH gradient across mucus adherent to rabbit gastric mucosa: Evidence for a mucus-bicarbonate barrier. *Gut* 22:94–96.
30. Kivilaakso E, Flemstrom G: HCO_3^- secretion and pH gradient across the surface mucus gel in rat duodenum (abstract). *Gastroenterology* 1982; 82:1101.
31. Boyd DD, Carney CN, Powell DW: Neurohumoral control of esophageal epithelial electrolyte transport. *Am J Physiol* 1980: 239:G5–11.
32. Helm JF, Dodds WJ, Hogan WJ, et al: Acid neutralizing capacity of human saliva. *Gastroenterology* 1982; 83:69–74.
33. Emmelin N: Nervous control of salivary glands. In: Code CF, ed. *Handbook of Physiology.* Section 6: Alimentary canal, Vol. II. Washington, D.C.: American Physiological Society 1967: 595–632.
34. Farrell RL, Roling GT, Castell DO: Cholinergic therapy of chronic heartburn. *Ann Intern Med* 1974; 80:573–576.
35. Thanik KD, Chey WY, Shah AN, Gutierrez JG: Reflux esophagitis: Effect of oral bethanechol on symptoms and endoscopic findings. *Ann Intern Med* 1980; 93:805–808.
36. Reed PI, Davies WA: Controlled trial of a new dosage form of carbenoxolone (pyrogastrone) in the treatment of reflux esophagitis. *Dig Dis* 1978; 23:161–165.
37. Sinar DR, Fletcher JR, Castell DO: The beneficial effect of methyl PGE_2 to diminish caustic esophageal injury. *Clin Res* 1982; 30:498A.
38. Menguy R, Masters YF: The effects of aspirin on gastric mucus production. *Surg Gynecol Obstet* 1965; 92:1–7.
39. Kent PW, Allen A: The biosynthesis of intestinal mucins: Effect of salicylate on glycoprotein biosynthesis by sheep colonic and human gastric mucosal tissues *in vitro. Biochem J* 1967; 106:645–658.
40. Carney CN, Orlando RC, Powell DW, Dotson MM: Morphologic alterations in early acid-induced epithelial injury of the rabbit esophagus. *Lab Invest* 1981; 45:198–208.
41. Powell DW, Orlando RC, Carney CN: Acid injury of the esophageal epithelium. In: Harmon JW, ed. *Basic Mechanisms of Gastrointestinal*

Mucosal Cell Injury and Protection. Baltimore: Williams and Wilkins, 1981: 155–177.

42. Martinez-Palomo A, Erlij D, Bracho H: Localization of permeability barriers in the frog skin epithelium. *J Cell Biol* 1971; 50:277–287.

43. Rick R, Dorge A, VonArnim E, Thurau K: Electron microprobe analysis of frog skin epithelium: Evidence for a synctial sodium transport compartment. *J Membr Biol* 1978; 39:313–331.

44. Powell DW, Morris SM, Boyd DD: Water and electrolyte transport by rabbit esophagus. *Am J Physiol* 1975; 229:438–443.

45. Orlando RC, Powell DW: Studies of esophageal epithelial electrolyte transport and potential difference in man. In: Allen A, Flemstrom G, Garner A, Silen W, Turnberg LA, eds. *Mechanisms of Mucosal Protection in the Upper Gastrointestinal Tract.* New York: Raven Press, 1984: 75–79.

46. Powell DW: Barrier function of epithelia. *Am J Physiol* 1981; 241: G275–G288.

47. Diamond JM: Channels in epithelial cell membranes and junctions. *Fed Proc* 1978; 37:2639–2644.

48. Farquhar MG, Palade GE: Functional organization of amphibian skin. *Proc Natl Acad Sci* 1964; 51:569–577.

49. Moreno JH, Diamond JM: Discrimination of monovalent inorganic cations by "tight" junctions of gallbladder epithelium. *J Membr Biol* 1974; 15:277–318.

50. Elias PM, Friend DS: The permeability barrier in mammalian epidermis. *J Cell Biol* 1975; 65:180–201.

51. Elias PM, McNutt NS, Friend DS: Membrane alterations during cornification of mammalian squamous epithelia: A freeze-fracture, tracer and thin-section study. *Anat Rec* 1977; 189:577–594.

52. Elias PM, Goerke J, Friend DS: Mammalian epidermal barrier layer lipids: Composition and influence on structure. *J Invest Derm* 1977; 69:535–546.

53. Elias PM, Brown BE: The mammalian cutaneous permeability barrier: Defective barrier function in essential fatty acid deficiency correlates with abnormal intercellular lipid deposition. *Lab Invest* 1978; 39: 574–583.

54. Wertz PW, Downing DT: Glycolipids in mammalian epidermis: Structure and function in the water barrier. *Science* 1982; 217:1261–1262.

55. Grayson S, Johnson-Winegar AD, Elias PM: Isolation of lamellar bodies from neonatal mouse epidermis by selective sequential filtration. *Science* 1983; 221:962–964.

56. Turner KS, Powell DW, Carney CN, et al: Transmural electrical potential difference in the mammalian esophagus in vivo. *Gastroenterology* 1978; 75:286–291.

57. Mills JW, Ernst SA, DiBona DR: Localization of Na^+-pump sites in frog skin. *J Cell Biol* 1977; 73:88–110.

58. Orlando RC, Powell DW, Carney CN: Pathophysiology of acute acid injury in rabbit esophageal epithelium. *J Clin Invest* 1981; 68:286–293.

59. Orlando RC, Bryson JC, Powell DW: Mechanisms of H^+ injury in rabbit esophageal epithelium. *Am J Physiol* 1984; 246:G718–G724.

60. Orlando RC, Powell DW, Bryson JC, et al: Esophageal potential difference measurements in esophageal disease. *Gastroenterology* 1982; 83:1026–1032.

61. Herlihy KJ, Orlando RC, Bryson JC, et al: Barrett's esophagus: Clinical, endoscopic, histologic, manometric and electrical potential difference characteristics. *Gastroenterology* 1984; 86:436–444.
62. Vidins EI, Fox JEF, Beck IT: Transmural potential difference (PD) in the body of the esophagus in patients with esophagitis, Barrett's epithelium and carcinoma of the esophagus. *Am J Dig Dis* 1971; 16:991–999.
63. Khamis B, Kennedy C, Finucane J, et al: Transmural potential difference: Diagnostic value in gastro-oesophageal reflux. *Gut* 1978; 19:396–398.
64. Eckardt VF, Adami B: Esophageal transmural potential difference in patients with symptomatic gastroesophageal reflux. *Klin Wochenschr* 1980; 58:293–297.
65. Read NW, Fordtran JS: The role of intraluminal junction potentials in the generation of the gastric potential difference in man. *Gastroenterology* 1979; 76:932–938.
66. Kivilaakso E, Fromm D, Silen W: Effect of bile salts and related compounds on isolated esophageal mucosa. *Surgery* 1980; 87:280–285.
67. Harmon JW, Johnson LF, Maydonovitch CL: Effects of acid and bile salts on the rabbit esophageal mucosa. *Dig Dis Sci* 1981; 87:280–285.
68. Chung RSK, Magri J, DenBesten L: Hydrogen ion transport in the rabbit esophagus. *Am J Physiol* 1975; 229:496–499.
69. Powell DW: Physiological concept of epithelial barriers. In: Allen A, Flemstrom G, Garner A, Silen W, Turnberg LA, eds. *Mechanisms of Mucosal Protection in the Upper Gastrointestinal Tract.* New York: Raven Press, 1984: 1–6.
70. Palmer LG: Ion selectivity of the apical membrane Na channel in the toad urinary bladder. *J Membr Biol* 1982; 67:91–98.
71. Ferreira KG, Hill BS: The effect of low external pH on properties of the paracellular pathway and junctional structure in frog skin. *J Physiol* 1982; 332:59–67.
72. Sachs G: H^+ pathways and pH changes in gastric tissue. *Gastroenterology* 1978; 75:750–752.
73. Kivilaakso E: High plasma HCO_3^- protects gastric mucosa against acute ulceration in the rat. *Gastroenterology* 1981; 81:921–927.
74. Schiessel R, Merhav A, Matthews J, et al: Role of nutrient HCO_3^- in the protection of amphibian gastric mucosa. *Am J Physiol* 1980; 239:G536–542.
75. Kivilaakso E, Barzilai A, Schiessel R, et al: Ulceration of isolated amphibian gastric mucosa. *Gastroenterology* 1979; 77:31–37.
76. Russell JM, Boron WF: Role of chloride transport in regulation of intracellular pH. *Nature* 1976; 264:73–74.
77. Emilio MG, Machado MM, Menano HP: The production of a hydrogen ion gradient across the isolated frog skin. *Biochemica et Biophysica Acta* 1970; 203:394–409.
78. Carter MJ: Carbonic anhydrase: Isoenzymes, properties, distribution, and functional significance. *Biol Rev* 1972; 47:465–513.
79. Schiessel R, Matthew J, Barzilai A, Merhav A, Silen W: PGE_2 stimulates gastric chloride transport: Possible key to cytoprotection. *Nature* 1980; 283:671–673.
80. Northway MG, Libshitz HI, Osborne BM, et al: Radiation esophagitis in the opossum: Radioprotection with indomethacin. *Gastroenterology* 1980; 78:883–892.

81. Eastwood GL, Beck BD, Castell DO, et al: Beneficial effect of indomethacin on acid-induced esophagitis in cats. *Dig Dis Sci* 1981; 26:601–608.
82. Rose B, Rick R: Intracellular pH, intracellular Ca and junctional cell to cell coupling. *J Membr Biol* 1978; 44:377–415.
83. Turin L, Warner A: Carbon dioxide reversibly abolishes ionic communication between cells of early amphibian embyro. *Nature* 1977; 270: 56–57.
84. MacKnight ADC, Leaf A: Regulation of cellular volume. *Physiol Rev* 1977; 57:510–573.
85. Cuthbert AW, Shum WK: Does intracellular sodium modify membrane permeability to sodium ions? *Nature* 1977; 266:468–469.
86. Taylor A, Windhager EE: Possible role of cytosolic calcium and Na–Ca exchange in regulation of transepithelial sodium transport. *Am J Physiol* 1979; 236:F505–512.
87. Spring KR, Ericson AC: Epithelial cell volume modulation and regulation. *J Membr Biol* 1982; 69:167–176.
88. Geboes K, Desmet V, Vantrappan G, Mebis J: Vascular changes in the esophageal mucosa: An early histologic sign of esophagitis. *Gastrointest Endosc* 1980; 26:29–32.
89. Guth PH: Local metabolism and circulation in mucosal defense. In: Harmon JW, ed. *Basic Mechanisms of Gastrointestinal Mucosal Cell Injury and Protection.* Baltimore: Williams and Wilkins, 1981: 253–258.
90. Bowen JC, Fairchild RB: Oxygen in gastric mucosal protection. In: Harmon JW, ed. *Basic Mechanisms of Gastrointestinal Mucosal Cell Injury and Protection.* Baltimore: Williams and Wilkins, 1981: 259–266.
91. Eastwood GL: Gastrointestinal epithelial renewal. *Gastroenterology* 1977; 72:962–975.
92. Marques-Pereira JP, Leblond CP: Mitosis and differentiation in the stratified-squamous epithelium of the rat esophagus. *Am J Anat* 1965; 117:73–90.
93. Messier B, Leblond CP: Cell proliferation and migration as revealed by radioautography after injection of thymidine-H[3] into rats and mice. *Am J Anat* 1960; 106:247–285.
94. Leblond CP, Greulich RC, Pereira JPM: Relationship of cell formation and cell migration in the renewal of stratified squamous epithelia. In: Montagna W, Billingham RE, eds. *Advance in Biology of Skin, Vol. 5, Wound Healing.* New York: Pergamon Press, 1974: 39–67.
95. Livstone EM, Sheahan DG, Behar J: Studies of esophageal epithelial cell proliferation in patients with reflux esophagitis. *Gastroenterology* 1977; 73:1315–1319.
96. Ismail-Beigi F, Horton PF, Pope CE II: Histological consequences of gastroesophageal reflux in man. *Gastroenterology* 1970; 58:163–174.
97. Bell B, Almy TP, Lipkin M: Cell proliferation kinetics in the gastrointestinal tract of man. III. Cell renewal in esophagus, stomach and jejunum of a patient with treated pernicious anemia. *J Natl Cancer Inst* 1967; 38:615–623.
98. Chung RSK, Johnson GM, DenBesten L: Effect of Na taurocholate and ethanol on hydrogen ion absorption in rabbit esophagus. *Am J Dig Dis* 1975; 20:582–588.

99. Safaie-Shirazi S, DenBesten L, Zike WL: Effect of bile salts on the ionic permeability of the esophageal mucosa and their role in the production of esophagitis. *Gastroenterology* 1975; 68:728–733.

100. Lillemoe KD, Johnson LF, Harmon JW: Alkaline esophagitis: A comparison of the ability of components of gastroduodenal contents to injure the rabbit esophagus. *Gastroenterology* 1983; 85:621–628.

101. Duane WC, Weigand DM: Mechanism by which bile salt disrupts the gastric mucosal barrier in the dog. *J Clin Invest* 1980; 66:1044–1049.

102. Erlij D, Martinez-Palomo A: Opening of tight junctions in frog skin by hypertonic urea solutions. *J Membr Biol* 1972; 9:229–240.

103. Fischbarg J, Whittembury G: The effect of external pH on osmotic permeability, ion and fluid transport across isolated frog skin. *J Physiol* 1978; 275:403–417.

104. Lloyd DA, Borda IT: Food-induced heartburn: Effect of osmolality. *Gastroenterology* 1981; 80:740–741.

105. Shirazi SS, Platz CD: Effect of alcohol on canine esophageal mucosa. *J Surg Res* 1978; 25:373–379.

5

Role of Gastric Factors in the Pathogenesis of Gastroesophageal Reflux: Emptying, Acid and Pepsin, Bile Reflux

Andre Dubois, M.D., Ph.D.

Chapter Contents

From Castell DO, Wu WC, Ott DJ (eds): *Gastroesophageal Reflux Disease: Pathogenesis, Diagnosis, Therapy.* Mount Kisco, NY, Futura Publishing Co., Inc., 1985.

Acknowledgments: I wish to thank Drs. D.O. Castell and L.F. Johnson for their valuable advice during the preparation of this review.
This work was supported in part by the Uniformed Services University of the Health Sciences Protocol No. R08342.

81

The esophagus is exposed to the deleterious effect of the many materials that can reach it, although it is normally protected by two natural defenses. The first one is the oropharyngeal region, which reflexively rejects any damaging agent. The other is the lower esophageal sphincter which, along with the peristaltic activity of the lower esophagus, prevents gastroesophageal reflux. This latter defense is relative, however, and its efficacy depends in part on the gastric milieu. Gastroesophageal reflux can only occur if there is a positive pressure gradient between stomach and esophagus and if the stomach contains fluids or solids, available for reflux. In addition, this reflux will be damaging only if the material flowing back has a composition that is harmful to the esophageal mucosa. This chapter will deal with the six gastric factors that may play a role in the pathogenesis of gastroesophageal reflux: (1) gastroesophageal pressure gradient; (2) intragastric volume and its determinants; (3) gastric emptying; (4) gastric secretion; (5) duodenogastric reflux; and finally (6) composition of gastric fluids.

Gastroesophageal Pressure Gradient

Intragastric pressure is usually higher than resting intraesophageal pressure, this gradient being maintained because of the tonic contraction of the lower esophageal sphincter (LES). Reflux occurs if the pressure gradient increases or if the resistance of the LES decreases. As the role of the esophagus and LES are discussed elsewhere in this book (Chapters 2–4), we will examine only the factors affecting intragastric pressure. It is well known that reflux may be initiated by bending forward and that raising the head of the bed relieves this symptom by facilitating esophageal emptying. These observations clearly illustrate the importance of the intragastric pressure and hydrostatic gradient between esophagus and stomach. In contrast, the role of physiological changes of intragastric pressure in the pathophysiology of reflux remains largely unknown.

Under normal conditions, phasic rises of intragastric pressure are recorded only in the distal stomach where they are thought to play a role in gastric emptying (see below). In contrast, intraluminal pres-

The opinions and assertions contained herein are the private ones of the author and are not to be construed as official or reflecting the views of the Department of Defense or the Uniformed Services University of the Health Sciences.

sures recorded in the proximal stomach normally remain stable and almost at basal levels at all times, even after food intake, because chewing and swallowing are normally followed by vagally mediated receptive relaxation of the stomach. The neurotransmitter involved is neither adrenergic nor cholinergic, but its exact nature is unknown, the most probable candidate currently being VIP. Following vagotomy, gastric relaxation is absent or insufficient, resulting in an increase of intragastric pressure which, in turn, may produce the potential for reflux occurrence in some operated patients. It is important to know that this potential problem will occur both after truncal and highly selective vagotomy. However, no data are currently available concerning the exact role of this factor.

Intragastric Volume

Intragastric volume appears to be an important determinant of gastroesophageal reflux. In a recent study, acid refluxed in the esophagus only after intragastric injection of 140 ml 0.1 N HCl if LES pressure was 7.5 mmHg (symptomatic refluxers) but 308 ml were necessary to produce reflux in healthy controls with a LES pressure of 13.8 mmHg.[1]

The volume of the intragastric contents reflects the balance between inputs and outputs. The inputs result from swallowing of foods and saliva, gastric secretion, and duodenogastric reflux while the outputs correspond to gastroesophageal reflux and gastric emptying (Figure 1). Under basal fasting conditions, normal subjects have a steady state resting volume of approximately 10 ml, which results from secretory and emptying rates of 1 ml/min; by dividing the emptying rate by the intragastric volume, one can calculate the fractional rate of gastric emptying which, in this case, is 10%/min.[2] After a meal, intragastric volume increases by the amount of food and liquids swallowed, which can be 1,000 ml or more. During the early postprandial period, the contribution of gastric output is negligible, even if it is maximally stimulated to 4 ml/min. While emptying of the meal progresses, however, the participation of fluid output becomes more and more important and eventually represents the total intragastric volume, i.e., 10 ml, when the fasting steady state level is reached, usually in 3 to 6 hours.

Thus, the intragastric volume available for gastroesophageal reflux depends on gastric emptying, on duodenogastric reflux, and on gastric secretion, in addition to the volume of food consumed. It may

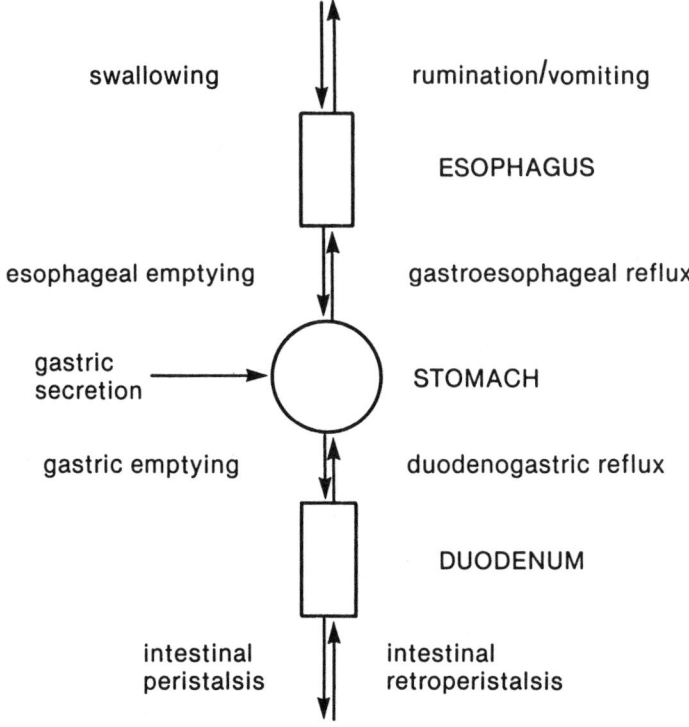

Figure 1: *Schematic representation of the esophago-gastroduodenal kinetics.*

be important, therefore, to examine whether patients with reflux have alterations of these three parameters.

Gastric Emptying (See also summary of results in Table 1)

The possible role played by abnormalities of gastric emptying in the pathogenesis of gastroesophageal reflux is at present unclear. It is tempting to postulate that gastric retention should facilitate reflux, but the published evidence demonstrates that only a fraction of patients with reflux have significant gastric retention. Furthermore, most patients with gastric retention caused by functional or mechanical outlet obstruction do not have reflux esophagitis.

Results published in the literature led to variable and confusing conclusions, possibly because of methodological problems. In an attempt to clarify this question, I have divided this section into three

Table 1.
Gastric Emptying Rate of Various Meals (GE) in all or in a
Majority of Patients Compared with Controls

Type of Meal	Marker for		Gastric Emptying (GE) of		Reference
	Liquids	Solids	Controls	Refluxers	
Ensure	^{99m}Tc-DTPA	—	GE = GE $\wedge$	$\vee$	(3)
Egg salad sandwich	^{99m}Tc-DTPA	—	GE > GE		(3)
Cornflakes/ milk	^{99m}Tc-DTPA	—	GE = GE		(4)
Egg salad sandwich	^{99m}Tc-DTPA	—	GE > GE		(5)
Steak, bread, and ice cream	PEG	^{51}Cr-Cl$_3$	GE = GE		(8)
Saline	Phenol red	—	GE = GE		(7)
Milk	^{99m}Tc-SC	—	GE > GE		(9)
Chicken liver/ beef stew	—	^{99m}Tc-SC	GE > GE $\wedge$	$\wedge$	(13, 14)
Water	^{111}In-DTPA	—	GE = GE		(13, 14)
Water	Phenol red	—	GE $\geqq$ GE		This chapter
Corn oil/ dextrose	PEG	—	GE = GE		(12)
Chicken liver/ beef stew	—	^{99m}Tc-SC	GE $\geqq$ GE		(17)
Egg sandwich	—	^{99m}Tc-SC	GE $\geqq$ GE		(18)

parts. In the first 2 parts, I will briefly outline the reported findings for markers of liquids and solid emptying, while, in the last one, I will propose some conclusions based on these results.

1. Markers for Liquids

Radionuclide imaging was used to determine the emptying rate of ^{99m}Tc-DTPA (diethylene triamine pentaacetic acid) incorporated in either a liquid meal[3] (Ensure), cornflakes and milk,[4] or an egg salad sandwich.[3,5] As DTPA does not adhere firmly to solid particles, these three studies were mainly measuring emptying of the liquid phase of a mixed liquid and solid meal. In the first study, controls and patients were given a liquid meal and a mixed liquid and solid meal on two separate days.[3] In healthy controls, ^{99m}Tc-DTPA added to a liquid meal emptied slower than ^{99m}Tc-DTPA added to a mixed liquid and solid meal, while the opposite was observed in patients with reflux. As a result, the emptying of the ^{99m}Tc-DTPA added to the egg salad sandwich meal was slower in reflux patients whereas no difference was observed with ^{99m}Tc-DTPA added to the liquid meal (see Table 1). This observation was confirmed by using ^{99m}Tc-DTPA-tagged egg salad sandwich in a series of 100 patients, although there was a considerable overlap between normal subjects and patients.[5] Similar findings were reported in a series of 17 patients in which gastric emptying was measured using a single scintillation detector and a ^{51}Cr-tagged milk-protein liquid meal.[6] In contrast, this difference was not observed by other authors who measured gastric emptying either of cornflakes and milk tagged with ^{99m}Tc-DTPA using radionuclide imaging[4] or of saline using intragastric dye dilution technique with phenol red as a marker.[7] Similarly, gastric emptying of liquids was normal in reflux patients when determined by an intraduodenal dye dilution technique after a mixed solid-liquid meal.[8]

In infants with failure to thrive, pulmonary abnormalities, and severe gastroesophageal reflux, the emptying of a liquid meal tagged with ^{99m}Tc-sulfur colloid was significantly slower than in infants with reflux only and in adult controls.[9] This retarded gastric emptying in infants with malnutrition is difficult to interpret, however, because gastric emptying is also delayed in adults during starvation[10] and in anorexia nervosa patients,[11] two conditions that have similarities to infants evaluated in this study.

In another study, a meal containing corn oil and dextrose as well as a non-absorbable marker (PEG) was given to controls and patients with reflux and samples of the gastric contents were obtained at 15-min intervals for the subsequent 4 hours.[12] By measuring the concentration of PEG in the gastric contents, these authors evaluated concurrently the dilutional effect of gastric secretion as well as gastric emptying. Gastric emptying can be estimated using this technique because the same amount of gastric secretion being added to a small volume of gastric contents produces a greater dilution than when added to a large volume. As the concentration of PEG decreased similarly in both groups, the authors concluded that gastric emptying and secretion were not altered in patients with reflux, although opposite and simultaneous changes of both parameters could have yielded the same observation.

We have recently used a previously described phenol red dilution technique[2] to evaluate gastric emptying during fasting and after pentagastrin stimulation in 12 patients with gastroesophageal reflux. Mean fasting fractional emptying rate (i.e., the percentage of gastric contents emptied per min) was $12.0 \pm 2.1\%/min$ (mean $\pm$ SE), not significantly different from healthy controls ($8.8 \pm 1.5\%/min$). Similarly, no difference was observed after a 250 ml water load. In contrast, following pentagastrin stimulation, fractional emptying rate was significantly greater in reflux patients ($8.9 \pm 2.5\%/min$) compared to controls ($2.9 \pm 1.2\%/min$; $p < 0.05$). Patients were then divided in three groups based on their fasting fractional emptying rate (FER). Four patients had fasting FER within the range of mean ±2 SD of normal values. Fasting FER was less than normal in four patients and was greater than normal in four other patients. Following pentagastrin, FER was normal in six patients while it was accelerated in six others. Thus, 33% of patients with reflux appear to have a slower fasting emptying than normal controls, which is similar to what was observed after a liquid-solid meal. Furthermore, accelerated gastric emptying is observed in one-third of the patients basally and in 50% of them after pentagastrin stimulation. This acceleration of emptying of liquids could result from insufficient receptive relaxation of the stomach.

2. Markers for Solids

Emptying of both solids and liquids was evaluated in 37 patients with reflux and in healthy controls using ^{99m}Tc-sulfur colloid-tagged chicken livers and ^{111}In-DTPA.[13,14] In these studies, emptying of liquids was not significantly different in the two groups, but emptying of solids was significantly slower in 57% of the patients while it was faster in 5% of them. In those patients with a delay of gastric emptying, administration of metoclopramide was found to increase gastric emptying.[4,14-16]

These results have not been confirmed in two recent studies. Gastric emptying of chicken liver meal tagged *in vivo* with ^{99m}Tc-sulfur colloid was measured in a group of 33 refluxers and in 15 controls.[17] Gastric emptying of solids was not significantly different in those two groups, even when patients with reflux were separated into those with and those without erosive esophagitis. In fact, only two patients (6%) had abnormally slow gastric emptying. To investigate whether this variability of the results was related to the heterogeneity of the population of patients with gastroesophageal reflux, we have recently determined gastric emptying of a scrambled egg meal (tagged with ^{99m}Tc-sulfur colloid) in a more homogeneous population of refluxers, i.e., 14 patients with Barrett's esophagus.[18] Mean gastric emptying was not significantly different in Barrett's patients compared to controls. However, values obtained in five patients fell outside of the normal range set as the mean ±2 SD: two had slower emptying and three had accelerated emptying.

3. Comments

Based on these data, gastric emptying of saline, water, gastric juice, and other liquid meals does not appear to be significantly altered in patients with gastroesophageal reflux, whereas the liquid phase of an egg salad sandwich meal may empty more slowly than normal in certain of those patients. Similarly, emptying of the solid component of a mixed liquid and solid meal containing chicken liver appears to be delayed in 57% of patients with reflux in some series, but only in 6–14% in other series. The relevance of these observations is unclear. In fact, ^{99m}Tc does not appear to have been detected in the esophagus during studies in which radionuclide imaging was used, suggesting that reflux does not occur concurrently with delayed gastric emptying. This is especially surprising since, in almost all the above-mentioned studies, subjects lay supine under the gamma camera, which could have enhanced reflux.

The cause of an abnormal gastric emptying in some patients with reflux is unclear. Gastric emptying of liquids is thought to be regulated by the motility of the proximal stomach, while gastric emptying of solids depends principally on the distal stomach motor activity. In addition, the smooth muscle fibers forming the lower esophageal sphincter belong, in fact, to the third muscular layer of gastric wall[19] and this layer may play an important role in the adaptive relaxation of the proximal stomach. Therefore, since lower esophageal sphincter motility is thought to be defective in patients with reflux esophagitis, it would not be surprising if gastric motility was altered in those patients. So far, however, no study has evaluated the motility of the proximal stomach in patients with reflux. Motility of the distal stomach was evaluated manometrically in a group of 13 patients with reflux esophagitis and in nine age-matched controls.[4] On the average, the number of antral contractions and cumulative antral activity was reduced in patients with reflux, although 50% of them had values similar to those of controls. Metoclopramide enhanced these parameters in some, but not all, subjects in both normal and reflux patients.

In conclusion, gastric emptying and gastric motility may be reduced in some patients with gastroesophageal reflux while gastric emptying is accelerated in others; however, the relevance of these abnormalities to the pathogenesis of the disease is difficult to establish, especially because the treatment of gastric retention with metoclopramide also improves esophageal emptying.

Duodenogastric Reflux

Duodenogastric reflux has been reported in some patients with gastroesophageal reflux.[12,20] It may be damaging for two reasons: first, it increases the volume available for gastroesophageal reflux and, second, it adds detergents to the gastric contents (see section on Bile Salts and Bile Acids).

Evaluation of duodenogastric reflux in 32 patients with gastroesophageal reflux has been performed by using measurements of the intragastric concentration and output of bile acids in the fasting gastric juice.[20] Although these patients were diagnosed as having only symptomatic sliding hiatal hernia, most subjects were probably true gastroesophageal refluxers because they had heartburn with or without esophagitis and strictures. Mean bile acid output and concentration were significantly higher in the group of patients compared to healthy volunteers, although there was a considerable overlap of individual values. Concentrations and outputs of bile acids were not individual values. Concentrations and outputs of bile acids were not significantly affected by the presence or absence of strictures, heartburn, and esophagitis. A similar technique was used in a smaller group of 10 patients with gastroesophageal reflux, which were compared with 10 healthy controls.[12] ^{14}C-chenodeoxycholic acid was given orally on the night before the test and continuous aspiration of the gastric contents was performed the next morning during a one-hour fasting period. The concentration of ^{14}C in the gastric juice was similar in the two groups during the basal hour, but after a corn oil–dextrose meal, it was significantly higher in reflux patients.

These data, however, have not been confirmed by another group of investigators using an intraduodenal dye dilution technique. These authors found that the percentage of duodenal marker refluxing into the stomach was not significantly different in patients with gastroesophageal reflux compared with controls.

Gastric Fluid Output

To my knowledge, there is no published paper in which the volume of gastric fluid output was determined in patients with gastroesophageal reflux, although acid output may be increased (see Acid, below). In a study in which we measured gastric emptying and gastric secretion concurrently, fluid output was not significantly different in reflux patients and in healthy controls basally (1.5 ± 0.2 and 1.3 ± 0.2 ml/min, respectively), after a water load (1.9 ± 0.2 and 2.5 ± 0.3 ml/min), and after pentagastrin (5.9 ± 0.9 and 4.0 ± 0.3 ml/min). In patients with the Zollinger-Ellison syndrome, fluid hypersecretion is accompanied by acid hypersection and rapid gastric emptying,[2] suggesting that each of these three factors could play an important role in the reflux esophagitis that is often observed in these patients.

Composition of Gastric Juice

As stated earlier, the composition of gastric contents is the major factor that determines how damaging reflux will be. This composition depends on the relative amount and composition of three inputs: swallowed food, drinks, and medications, gastric secretion, and duodenogastric reflux.

Swallowed Food, Drinks, and Medications

Most foods and drinks dilute and buffer gastric acid although some soft drinks and spicy foods have a low pH. Thus, reflux occurring during the immediate postprandial period should be less damaging than reflux occurring at night, especially if there is gastric acid hypersecretion. Finally, medications such as aspirin could be damaging if the drug refluxes after being dissolved in the gastric contents.

Acid

Concentration of acid in the gastric contents is a major determinant of the severity of experimental esophagitis, although the presence of pepsin appears to play an important role.[21] In patients with gastroesophageal reflux, both cimetidine[22,23] and ranitidine[24] significantly decrease both the symptom frequency and severity as well as the use of antacids. Esophageal endoscopic appearance tends to be improved by both drugs, although the difference is not statistically significant.[22-24] Thus, even in the absence of gastric hypersecretion, reflux of pure gastric juice into the esophagus will result in esophagitis, especially if esophageal emptying is defective (see Chapter 2). If the acid concentration and output are increased, as is the case in the Zollinger-Ellison syndrome and in certain patients with duodenal ulcer disease, gastroesophageal reflux is extremely noxious.[25] A preliminary report suggests that acid output may be higher in some patients with reflux compared to healthy controls;[26] a prospective study is currently under way to confirm this potentially important observation. In our unpublished study of gastric emptying and gastric secretion, we found that acid output was slightly, but not significantly, greater in patients with reflux compared with controls basally (4.4 ± 0.8 vs. 3.2 ± 0.6 mEq/hr, respectively), following the water load (11.2 ± 2.0 vs. 7.5 ± 1.2 mEq/hr) and after stimulation with pentagastrin (41.7 ± 6.5 vs. 32.1 ± 3.6 mEq/hr). As fluid output was not significantly different in the two groups (see Gastric Fluid Output, above), acid concentration was also similar in both groups.

The role of acid concentration in the damage of the esophagus has been extensively explored using the perfused rabbit esophagus model developed by Chung et al.[27] In this model, the net rate of diffusion of H^+ out of the esophageal lumen, or H^+ flux, has been used as an index of the loss of the esophageal mucosal barrier, thus reflecting a damage to the esophagus. Using this technique, Chung et al found that the H^+ flux out of the esophagus was both concentration-dependent and time-dependent: significant H^+ flux was observed within one hour of exposure to concentrations of HCl > 80 mM, while a concentration of 20 mM was sufficient if exposure was sustained from more than 3 hours. These results have been subsequently confirmed and expanded by Harmon et al.[28] These authors found that during the first 30 minutes of exposure to acid, the diffusion rate of H^+ varied dramatically as a function of intragastric pH, increasing from 0.2 μEq/min at pH 2, to 3.5 μEq/min at pH 1. However, it should be remembered that pH 1 is lower than any physiological pH. Thus, a ten-fold increase of intra-esophageal concentration of HCl from 10 to 100 mM resulted in an immediate twenty-fold increase of the *diffusion rate*. By analogy with renal clearance, we can calculate the *transmural esophageal clearance* for H^+, expressed in μl/min, by dividing the rate of diffusion by the intra-esophageal H^+ concentration. This calculated *transmural clearance* is not to be confused with esophageal clearance in intact subjects and animals which is, in fact, esophageal emptying. *Transmural esophageal clearance* increases two-fold from 20 to 35 μl/min when intra-esophageal

H^+ concentration is increased ten-fold. However, the *diffusion rate* increases to 10 μEq/min when the exposure with 100 mM HCl solution is prolonged for 30 additional minutes, as compared to 0.1 μEq/min with 10 mM HCl solutions.[28] During this 30–60 minute time interval, therefore, the *calculated transmural clearance* for H^+ is 100 μl/min at pH 1, ten-fold greater than at pH 2 (10 μl/min).

The observations of Harmon et al were later confirmed by using the potential difference across the esophageal mucosa to evaluate the precise time course of the damage in the same rabbit esophagus model.[29] Furthermore, the extent of the damage caused by acid has been evaluated precisely using light and electron microscopy.[30]

Thus, the relative impermeability of the esophageal mucosa to acid appears to be only temporary, suggesting that the esophagus is damaged only if the gastric juice is too acid *and* if esophageal emptying of refluxed gastric juice is too slow.

Pepsin

As could be expected, the damage caused by acid is further enhanced by the presence of pepsin. A preliminary report suggests that pepsin output and concentration may be greater in some patients with reflux as compared with matched controls; however, the results of a prospective study currently under way will be needed before a final conclusion can be made.[26]

Because human gastric juice normally contains 1,500 to 2,500 units/ml and the porcine pepsin usually contains 2,500 to 3,500 units/mg at pH 1, concentration of pepsin used to reproduce physiological conditions should be 1 mg/ml or less. Using such concentrations, Lillemoe et al[31] observed that a significant dose-dependent increase of the H^+ *diffusion rate* was observed after 2 to 3 hours of exposure to 10 mM HCl solutions (pH 2). H^+ *diffusion rate* was not significantly affected by 0.1 mg pepsin/ml (2 μEq/min), but was increased to 5 μEq/min at 0.5 mg/ml and 8 μEq/min at 1 mg/ml.[28] Thus, the *transmural H^+ esophageal clearance* of the rabbit esophagus is approximately 80 μl/min during the first hour of exposure to 100 mM HCl solution without pepsin or during the third hour of exposure to 10 mM HCl solutions with 1 mg pepsin/ml. Furthermore, perfusion of pepsin solutions at pH 2 for 2 to 3 hours significantly and dose-dependently increases the absorption of tritiated water as well as the secretion of glucose and K^+, the appearance of hemoglobin and, as expected, the microscopic damage to the mucosa.[28]

Other Enzymes

It is unclear whether trypsin and amylase can cause esophageal damage under physiological and pathological conditions, although it would be expected that these pancreatic enzymes are inactivated by the low pH normally present in the stomach. This assumption is supported by the work of Lillemoe et al[31] who found that the addition of trypsin to the perfusion medium at pH 2 did not affect any of the parameters reflecting esophageal damage.

In contrast, these enzymes appear important in the genesis of esophagitis in patients with gastric anacidity and gastroesophageal reflux.[32] This also appears to be true in experimental alkaline esophagitis as indicated by the finding that sequential perfusion of the rabbit esophagus with pH 7.5 solutions containing trypsin followed by 10 mM HCl solutions caused a significant increase of hemoglobin flux as well as gross and microscopic damages, but no significant change of H^+ diffusion rate.[33,34]

Lipase is normally present not only in the duodenal juice, but may also be secreted by lingual glands and possibly by the stomach.[35] So far, however, the role of this enzyme in gastroesophageal reflux has not been explored.

Bile Salts and Bile Acids

Studies evaluating the role played by bile acids in reflux esophagitis are important and relevant, as indicated by the reported occurrence of duodenogastric reflux in certain patients with reflux esophagitis (see above).[19,20,36]

Studies performed at low pH have shown that the diffusion of H^+ out of the esophageal lumen is dramatically increased in the presence of bile acids both *in vitro*[37] and *in vivo*.[31,38] Potential difference (PD) is usually decreased, although an initial increase of PD was reported *in vitro*.[37] Interestingly, these effects are only present with taurochenodeoxycholic acid, but not with tauroursodeoxycholic acid.[39] This observation is clinically relevant because it would explain why one of the side effects of medical treatment of gallstones with chenodeoxycholic is dyspepsia; it also suggests that therapy with chenodeoxycholic acid treatment could be replaced by ursodeoxycholic acid when intolerance develops in the course of treatment. However, the increased permeability to H^+ is followed only by submucosal edema without mucosal disruption. This minimal damage is similar to that encountered with 10 mM HCl alone, a situation under which H^+ diffusion is significantly less.[31]

Under alkaline conditions, the effect of bile acids is more controversial. Early studies by Cross and Wangensteen demonstrate that bile salts and bile perfused at neutral pH produced extensive lesions of the mucosa.[40] In contrast, subsequent experiments indicate that pure bile causes only minimal damage of the esophageal mucosa.[33,34,41–43] Studies performed using a Ussing-type chamber preparation demonstrate that, at pH 7.4, sodium taurocholate has no effect on PD or on the resistance (R) across the rabbit esophageal mucosa. In contrast, the deconjugated bile salt sodium deoxycholate, which is highly insoluble at pH 2 because its pK_a is much greater than 2,[28] dramatically suppresses both PD and R at pH 7.4.[37] In the rabbit esophagus perfused *in situ*, sequential exposure to pH 7.5 solutions containing taurodeoxycholate followed by 10 mM HCl solutions causes a dramatic increase of water and H^+ loss through the mucosa as well as an increase in the flux of glucose and K^+ into the esophageal lumen. However, the pathologic injury score is not significantly increased.[33]

In conclusion, the potential role of bile components, per se, in causing macroscopic and histologic damage to the esophageal mucosa remains to be established. However, the available experimental studies demonstrate that bile salts and bile acids can break the esophageal mucosal barrier both in the presence and in the absence of acid. Therefore, these barrier-breaking properties are likely to enhance the damage caused by other agents such as acid, pepsin, and trypsin.

General Conclusions

The esophagus does not normally secrete acid, enzymes, or detergents; in addition, its mucosa has no natural protection against these digestive chemicals, which is in contrast to the gastric and intestinal mucosae. The defenses of the esophagus against noxious material reside in swallowed saliva and in its ability to prevent reflux and, if reflux occurs, to empty rapidly its contents. If these primary defenses are insufficient, esophageal damage will be primarily related to the composition of the gastroduodenal secretions and, possibly, to gastric motility.

As I have discussed in this chapter, the major factors causing damage to the esophagus appear to be acid and pepsin, or, under alkaline conditions, trypsin. In addition, duodenogastric reflux and the presence of bile in the esophagus probably play an important potentiating influence. The possible role played by disturbances of gastric motility remains controversial: delayed gastric emptying does not seem to be an important factor, as it is found only in some patients with reflux esophagitis. Furthermore, it appears to be significant only for solids and during the postprandial period and is not observed concurrently with detectable gastroesophageal reflux.

References

1. Ahtaridis G, Snape WJ Jr, Cohen S: Lower esophageal sphincter pressure as an index of gastroesophageal acid reflux. *Dig Dis Sci* 1981; 26: 993–998.
2. Dubois A, Van Eerdewegh P, Gardner JD: Gastric emptying and secretion in Zollinger-Ellison syndrome. *J Clin Invest* 1977; 59:255–263.
3. Ippoliti A, McCallum R, Sturdevant R: Gastric emptying in patients with gastroesophageal reflux. *Clin Res* 1976; 24:535A.
4. Behar J, Ramsby G: Gastric emptying and antral motility in reflux esophagitis. *Gastroenterology* 1978; 74:253–256.
5. McCallum RW, Berkowitz DM, Lerner E: Gastric emptying in patients with gastroesophageal reflux. *Gastroenterology* 1981; 80:285–291.
6. Baldi F, Corinaldesi R, Ferrarini F, Stanghellini V, Miglioli M, Barbara L: Gastric secretion and emptying of liquids in reflux esophagitis. *Dig Dis Sci* 1981; 26:886–889.
7. Csendes A, Henriquez A: Gastric emptying in patients with reflux esophagitis or benign strictures of the esophagus secondary to reflux compared to controls. *Scand J Gastroenterol* 1978; 13:205–207.
8. Coleman SL, Rees DW, Malagelada JR: Normal gastric function in reflux esophagitis. *Gastroenterology* 1979; 76:115A.
9. Hillemeier AC, Lange R, McCallum R, Seashore J, Gryboski J: Delayed gastric emptying in infants with gastroesophageal reflux. *J Pediatr* 1981; 98:190–193.
10. Keys A, Brozek J, Henschel A, et al: *The Biology of Human Starvation.* Minneapolis: University of Minnesota Press. 1950: 587–600.
11. Dubois A, Gross HA, Ebert MH, Castell DO: Altered gastric emptying and secretion in primary anorexia nervosa. *Gastroenterology* 1979; 77:319–323.
12. Kaye MD, Showalter JP: Pyloric incompetence in patients with symptomatic gastroesophageal reflux. *J Lab Clin Med* 1974; 83:198–206.
13. McCallum RW, Mensh R, Lange R: Definition of the gastric emptying abnormality present in gastroesophageal reflux patients. In Wienbeck M, ed. *Motility of the Digestive Tract.* New York: Raven Press, 1982: 355–362.
14. McCallum RW: The role of gastric emptying in gastroesophageal reflux disease. In: Dubois A, Castell DO, eds. *Esophageal and Gastric Emptying.* Boca Raton, FL: CRC Press. 1984: 121–128.
15. Fink SM, Lange RC, McCallum RW: Effect of metoclopramide on normal and delayed gastric emptying in gastroesophageal reflux patients. *Dig Dis Sci* 1983; 28:1057–1061.

16. McCallum RW, Fink SM, Lerner E, Berkowitz DM: Effects of metoclopramide and bethanechol on delayed gastric emptying present in gastroesophageal reflux patients. *Gastroenterology* 1983; 84:1573–1577.

17. Shay S, Eggli D, VanNostrand D, Johnson L: Gastric emptying of solid food in patients with gastroesophageal reflux. *Gastroenterology* 1985; 88:1582A.

18. Johnson DA, Winters C, Drane WE, Spurling TJ, Karvelis KC, Silverman ED, Cattau EL Jr, Chobanian SJ, Hacker JF, Dubois A: Solid phase gastric emptying in Barrett's esophagus. *Gastroenterology* 1985; 88:1434A.

19. Rayl JE, Balison JR, Thomas HF, et al: Combined radiographic, manometric and histologic localization of the canine lower esophageal sphincter. *J Surg Res* 1972; 13:307–314.

20. Stol DW, Murphy GM, Collis JL: Duodeno-gastric reflux and acid secretion in patients with symptomatic hiatal hernia. *Scand J Gastroenterol* 1973; 7:97–101.

21. Goldberg HI, Dodds WJ, Gee S, et al: Role of acids and pepsin in acute experimental esophagitis. *Gastroenterology* 1969; 56:223–230.

22. Behar J, Brand DL, Brown FC, Castell DO, Cohen S, Crossley RJ, Pope CE, II, Winans CS: Cimetidine in the treatment of symptomatic gastroesophageal reflux: a double-blind controlled trial. *Gastroenterology* 1978; 74:441–448.

23. Wesdorp E, Bartelsmann J, Pope K, Dekker W, Tytgat GN: Oral cimetidine in reflux esophagitis: A double-blind controlled trial. *Gastroenterology* 1978; 74:821–824.

24. Sherbaniuk R, Wensel R, Bailey R, Trautman A, Grace M, Kirdeikis L, Jewell P, Pare P, Levesque D, Farley A, Archambault A, Thomson ABR: Ranitidine in the treatment of symptomatic gastroesophageal reflux disease. *J Clin Gastroenterol* 1984; 6:9–15.

25. Richter JE, Pandol SJ, Castell DO, McCarthy DM: Gastroesophageal reflux disease in the Zollinger-Ellison syndrome. *Ann Intern Med* 1981; 95:37–43.

26. Coleman S, Hirschowitz BI: Studies of gastric secretion as a risk factor for esophagitis. *Gastroenterology* 1984; 86:1051A.

27. Chung RSK, Magri J, DenBesten L: Hydrogen ion transport in the rabbit esophagus. *Am J Physiol* 1975; 229:496–500.

28. Harmon JW, Johnson LF, Maydonovitch CL: Effects of acid and bile salts on the rabbit esophageal mucosa. *Dig Dis Sci* 1981; 26(1):65–72.

29. Orlando RC, Powell DW, Carney CN: Pathophysiology of acute acid injury in rabbit esophageal epithelium. *J Clin Invest* 1981; 68:286–293.

30. Carney CN, Orlando RC, Powell DW, Dotson MM: Morphologic alterations in early acid-induced epithelial injury of the rabbit esophagus. *Lab Invest* 1981; 45:198–208.

31. Lillemoe KD, Johnson LF, Harmon JW: Role of the components of the gastroduodenal contents in experimental acid esophagitis. *Surgery* 1982; 92:276–284.

32. Lambert R: Relative importance of biliary and pancreatic secretions in the genesis of esophagitis in rats. *Am J Dig Dis* 1962; 7:1026–1030.

33. Lillemoe KD, Johnson LF, Harmon JW: Alkaline esophagitis: A comparison of the ability of components of gastroduodenal contents to injure the rabbit esophagus. *Gastroenterology* 1983; 85:621–628.

34. Harmon JW, Lillemoe K, Johnson LF: Pathophysiology of acid and alkaline esophagitis in rabbit model. In Allen A, et al, eds. *Mechanisms of*

Mucosal Protection in the Upper Gastrointestinal Tract. New York: Raven Press. 1984: 81–89.

35. Hamosh M: Lingual and breast milk lipases. *Adv Pediatr* 1982; 29: 33–67.
36. Crumplin MKH, Stol DW, Murphy GM, Collins JL: The pattern of bile salt reflux and acid secretion in sliding hiatal hernia. *Br J Surg* 1974; 61:611–615.
37. Kivilaakso E, Fromm D, Silen W: Effect of bile salts and related compounds on isolated esophageal mucosa. *Surgery* 1980; 87:280–285.
38. Chung RSK, Johnson GM, DenBesten L: Effect of sodium taurocholate and ethanol on hydrogen ion absorption in rabbit esophagus. *Am J Dig Dis* 1977; 22:582–588.
39. Lillemoe KD, Kidder GW, Harmon JW, Gadacz TR, Johnson LF, et al: Tauroursodeoxycholic acid is less damaging that taurochenodeoxycholic acid to the gastric and esophageal mucosa. *Dig Dis Sci* 1983; 28:359–364.
40. Cross FS, Wangensteen OH: Role of bile and pancreatic juice in production of esophageal erosions and anemia. *Proc Soc Exp Biol Med* 1951; 77:862–866.
41. Redo SF, Barnes WA, Ortiz de la Sierra A: Perfusion of the canine esophagus with secretions of the upper gastrointestinal tract. *Ann Surg* 1959; 149:556–564.
42. Helsingen N: Oesophagitis following total gastrectomy. *Acta Chir Scand* 1961; 273(Suppl 1):1–21.
43. Henderson RD, Mugashe F, Jeejeebhoy KN, et al: The role of bile and acid in the production of esophagitis and the motor defect of esophagitis. *Ann Thorac Surg* 1972; 14:465–473.

DIAGNOSIS

6

Overview of Diagnostic Tests In Reflux Disease

Donald O. Castell, M.D.

Chapter Contents

From Castell DO, Wu WC, Ott DJ (eds): *Gastroesophageal Reflux Disease: Pathogenesis, Diagnosis, Therapy.* Mount Kisco, NY, Futura Publishing Co., Inc., 1985.

The patient who describes a recurring symptom of retrosternal burning, worse after eating and when lying down or bending over, and relieved by antacid ingestion has classical heartburn secondary to GE reflux. With this symptom complex, one could make a case for not requiring any additional diagnostic tests prior to beginning a course of anti-reflux therapy. Unfortunately, many patients do not describe such typical heartburn and may present as a diagnostic dilemma. This is particularly true of the patient with reflux symptoms without heartburn, such as hoarseness or chronic cough. In these patients, it may become quite important to establish a diagnosis of GE reflux disease prior to beginning a more specific therapeutic regimen. In addition, since GE reflux disease has a variety of manifestations, different types of diagnostic tests may be essential. By understanding the different kinds of information obtained with each of these tests, the physician can more clearly define the type of reflux disease present in each particular patient.[1] I have found it useful over the years to separate the potential tests of reflux into three categories: those indicating that *reflux is possible*, those identifying the *effects or results of reflux*, and those actually *measuring reflux*. Table 1 lists the various tests that fit into each of these categories.

**Table 1.
Diagnostic Tests for GE Reflux Disease**

Tests Indicating Possible Reflux

Presence of hiatal hernia
    Radiographic
    Endoscopic
LES Pressure

Tests Showing Effects or Results of Reflux

Acid perfusion (Bernstein) test
Endoscopy
Mucosal biopsy
Barium esophagram (double contrast)

Tests Measuring Actual Reflux

Barium esophagram
Standard acid reflux test
Gastroesophageal scintiscan
Prolonged pH monitoring

Tests Indicating Reflux Is Possible

The diagnostic tests included in this category should be considered as having very weak discriminating ability to diagnose or exclude reflux disease.

Hiatal Hernia

Although a hiatal hernia may well be found in the presence of reflux disease, a direct causal relationship between those two is quite doubtful. Significant reflux can and does occur in the absence of a demonstrable hiatal hernia and many individuals with a clear-cut hiatal hernia are asymptomatic and without evidence of reflux disease. This is discussed by Drs. Ott, Katz, and Wu in Chapter 3.

Lower Esophageal Sphincter (LES) Pressure

Although the level of LES pressure at any particular point is currently considered to be *the* major determinant of GE reflux, it is now well established that an isolated measurement of the LES pressure is not an important diagnostic discriminator of the presence or absence of significant reflux. In Chapter 8 Dr. Katz discusses the use of esophageal manometry in GE reflux disease.

Tests Indicating the Results of or Effects of Reflux

In most situations when a diagnosis of reflux disease is established clinically, it is done on the basis of observations made through the use of one of the tests in this category. It seems quite reasonable to conclude that significant reflux disease is present in a patient in whom a typical abnormality of the esophageal mucosa can be demonstrated. It also is appropriate to use this finding as a reasonable end point in diagnostic studies of patients with proposed GE reflux disease.

Acid Perfusion (Bernstein) Test

In our laboratory, we use the Bernstein test as a major discriminator in evaluation of patients with suspected reflux. This test detects the presence of acid sensitivity in the esophageal mucosa with an acceptable level of accuracy. It has been shown in different studies to have an overall sensitivity and specificity of approximately 80% each. If the patient's symptoms (heartburn, chest pain) can be reproduced by the instillation of acid into the mid-esophagus, a working diagnosis of reflux disease can be made and the patient treated appropriately. The acid perfusion test is reviewed by Dr. Richter in Chapter 9.

Esophagoscopy

Probably the most definite evidence of meaningful GE reflux disease is the clear demonstration of gross findings of esophagitis on endoscopy. Numerous recent studies have clarified the lack of specificity of simple erythema as a diagnostic discriminator, but the presence of erosions, friability, exudate, ulcers, or stricture allows a definitive diagnosis of esophageal injury secondary to reflux. Most likely, this is the test that is performed the vast majority of the time by the practicing gastroenterologist when seeking to make a diagnosis of GE reflux disease. It has been our practice to recommend the Bernstein test prior to, and instead of endoscopy, if possible, because of its greater simplicity and availability to even the non-gastroenterologist.[1] Drs. Wu and Geisinger discuss endoscopic findings in reflux in Chapter 10.

Esophageal Mucosal Biopsy

In the patient in whom endoscopy reveals equivocal findings (normal or erythema), mucosal biopsy may add significantly to the sensitivity of diagnostic procedures. Preferably, a suction biopsy should be obtained by passing the suction capsule adjacent to the endoscope and observing the site of biopsy.[2] This results in a larger piece of mucosa and allows better orientation of the specimen. An argument could be made for the lack of necessity for mucosal biopsy in patients who have clear-cut changes of esophagitis at the time of endoscopy. The one exception to this rule would be when looking for the diagnosis of Barrett's esophagus. In this situation, it becomes important to biopsy the mucosa in those patients with severe esophagitis in order to identify the abnormal columnar epithelium in this condition. Biopsy findings in GE reflux disease are discussed by Drs. Wu and Geisinger in Chapter 10.

Barium Esophagram

Through the use of a variety of radiographic techniques, including double contrast, examination of the esophageal mucosa becomes a very specific test for the changes of chronic GE reflux. The mucosal irregularities found by this method are considered to be quite specific for reflux esophagitis.[3] This test, however, does suffer from a lack of sensitivity, and is only likely to be positive when significant mucosal lesions are present. The use of barium studies in diagnosis of reflux is reviewed by Dr. Ott in Chapter 7.

Tests Measuring Actual Reflux

In those patients in whom a diagnosis of reflux disease is suspected but in whom evidence of esophageal injury is equivocal, a test which actually measures reflux may become important. It should be understood that these tests are usually not required in the majority of patients with reflux disease but rather in those in whom the diagnosis is questionable. In my experience, this has been particularly true in patients with some of the more unusual manifestations of reflux or patients with reflux disease without heartburn or esophagitis. Most representative of this group are either those patients with hoarseness or chronic pulmonary symptoms felt to be secondary to reflux, but without definite esophageal lesions, or some patients with unexplained chest pain.

Barium Esophagram

The demonstration of some barium reflux during radiographic studies of the upper GI tract is not terribly reliable because some degree of reflux can be seen at least intermittently in normal subjects, and many patients with GE reflux disease will not show barium reflux. The question is really one of degree. If the radiologist notes persistent or frequent reflux that is poorly cleared and fills much of the esophagus, then some degree of specificity can be placed on this finding. The potential for false positive and false negative results, however, makes the use of radiographic studies with barium of questionable value for determining the presence of reflux. Dr. Ott provides more perspective on barium studies in reflux disease in Chapter 7.

Standard Acid Reflux Test

The demonstration by an intra-esophageal pH probe of actual reflux of acid from the stomach during a series of maneuvers intended to increase intra-abdominal pressure has been advocated for a number of years as a critical test of actual reflux. As with the barium studies noted above, one has to be aware that at any particular time even normal individuals will have significant reflux, making this short-term study potentially unreliable because of occasional false positive results. In Chapter 11, Dr. Ravich reviews intra-esophageal pH testing in GE reflux.

Gastroesophageal Scintiscan

The use of radioisotopic material placed into the stomach has been advocated as a means to measure reflux in a semi-quantitative fashion. This test can be made more sensitive by attempting to induce reflux with increasing abdominal pressure by a binder. Although developed some years ago, scintigraphy has not gained wide popularity. One reason may be the requirement of specialized procedures in a radioisotope laboratory. Another difficulty may be the lack of reliability of this test. In our laboratory we have found that a number of patients with obvious reflux disease (Grade 3–4 esophagitis) will show a normal scintigraphic study during careful testing. Radioisotopic tests in reflux disease are discussed by Dr. Cowan in Chapter 12.

Prolonged pH Monitoring

In recent years prolonged pH monitoring has become the gold standard for measurement of actual reflux. This test seems to provide the most physiologic measurement of acid reflux, incorporating information obtained over an extended time period (overnight or 24 hours), following meals, and in varying body positions (upright vs. supine). It is difficult to make an accurate assessment of the sensitivity of this test, since it is generally accepted as the standard by which other diagnostic tests are compared. Prolonged pH monitoring is discussed in detail by Dr. Ravich in Chapter 11.

References

1. Richter JE, Castell DO: Gastroesophageal reflux. Pathogenesis, diagnosis, and therapy. *Ann Intern Med* 1982; 97:93–103.
2. Knuff TE, Benjamin SB, Worsham GF, Hancock JE, Castell DO: Histologic evaluation of chronic gastroesophageal reflux. *Dig Dis Sci* 1984; 29:194–201.
3. Ott DJ, Wu WC, Gelfand DW: Reflux esophagitis revisited: Prospective analysis of radiologic accuracy. *Gastrointest Radiol* 1981; 6:1–7.

7

Barium Esophagram

David J. Ott, M.D.

Chapter Contents

In recent years, the role of radiology in evaluating patients with suspected gastroesophageal reflux disease (GERD) has become better understood.[1] The barium esophagram, or more appropriately, the upper gastrointestinal series, has been used traditionally in the evaluation of patients with suspected gastroesophageal reflux and its complications. The method is capable of assessing for esophageal motor abnormalities, demonstrating gastroesophageal reflux, and showing the gross morphological changes of reflux esophagitis.

The upper gastrointestinal series is also an important screening method for differentiating between various upper gastrointestinal

From Castell DO, Wu WC, Ott DJ (eds): *Gastroesophageal Reflux Disease: Pathogenesis, Diagnosis, Therapy.* Mount Kisco, NY, Futura Publishing Co., Inc., 1985.

disorders that may mimic GERD clinically. Although heartburn and regurgitation are the typical symptoms of GERD, other esophageal disorders may present similarly. For example, esophageal motor disorders, such as diffuse esophageal spasm and achalasia, may cause chest pain and regurgitation, and esophageal neoplasms and lower esophageal rings may masquerade as peptic esophagitis.

The barium esophagram is considered the best means of diagnosing hiatal hernia, despite its controversial relationship to GERD. If appropriate radiographic techniques and criteria are used, the majority of patients with symptomatic GERD can be shown to have an accompanying hiatal hernia.[2-4] Conversely, most patients with hiatal hernia do not have endoscopic evidence of esophagitis, making hiatal hernia as an isolated finding a poor predictor of concomitant GERD (see Chapter 3).

This chapter reviews the radiographic techniques used to examine the esophagus that are pertinent to the evaluation of patients with suspected GERD. Specifically, the advantages and limitations of the barium esophagram for assessing esophageal motor abnormalities, gastroesophageal reflux, and reflux esophagitis will be discussed.

Radiographic Examination

In patients with suspected GERD, optimal radiographic evaluation of the esophagus depends on the use of a combination of examining techniques.[5-7] The full-column technique, mucosal relief technique, double-contrast technique, and a variety of motion-recording techniques are available to examine the esophagus radiographically. Each method has its advantages and limitations.

The full-column technique has been the conventional method used and simply requires filling the esophagus with a barium suspension (Figure 1). The patient is usually examined in the prone oblique position, while drinking barium rapidly through a straw. Esophageal motility is assessed in this position by observing individual swallows of barium traversing the entire length of the esophagus. Also, hiatal hernia, lower esophageal ring, and peptic stricture are best demonstrated with this method. A number of solid boluses, such as barium tablets, can be of further use to detect esophageal narrowing, particularly if the examination with fluid barium is unrevealing.[8] Mucosal surface abnormalities, however, will not be accurately detected with this method.

The mucosal relief technique is used to demonstrate the smooth, longitudinal folds of the collapsed esophagus when coated with a

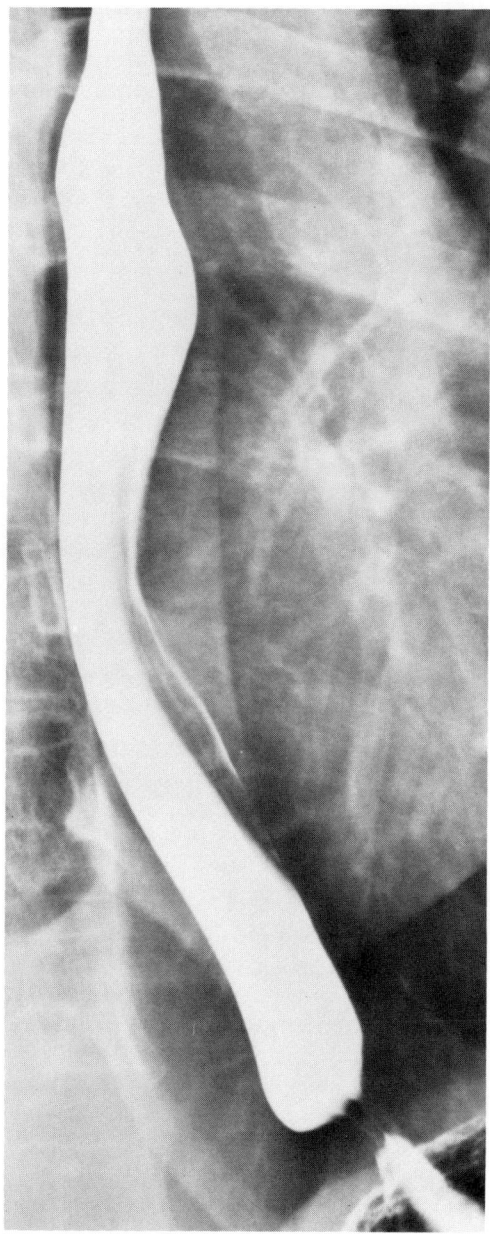

Figure 1: *Full-column view of the esophagus obtained with the patient in the prone position.*

dense barium suspension. Irregularity or thickening of these folds suggest esophagitis (Figure 2). Indeed, fold abnormality on the mucosal relief film may be the only radiographic finding in some pa-

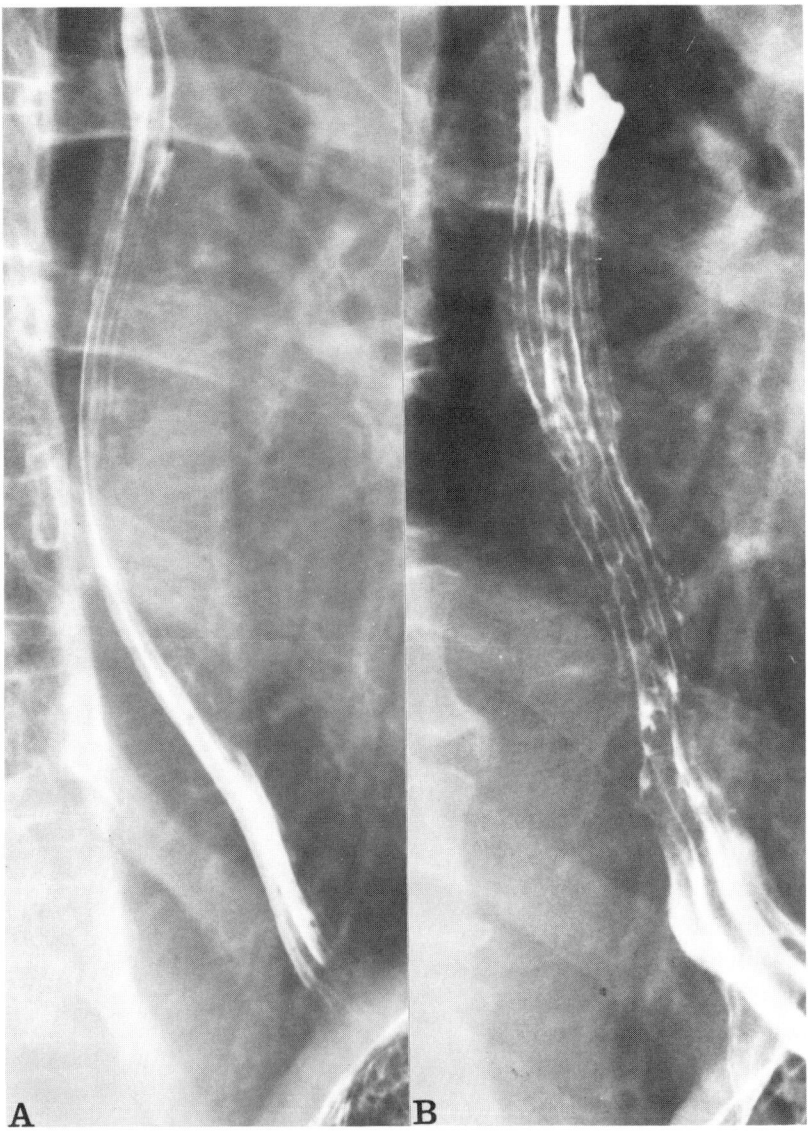

Figure 2: **A.** *Normal longitudinal folds of the collapsed esophagus on the mucosal relief film.* **B.** *Thickened, irregular folds in a patient with moderate esophagitis endoscopically.*

tients with GERD. On the other hand, lesions requiring maximal distension of the esophagus for their demonstration will not be seen with this technique.

The double-contrast technique requires coating of the esophageal surface with a dense barium suspension and distension of the organ with gas or air (Figure 3). The patient is most often examined standing in the left posterior oblique position. A gas-producing agent is swallowed with a small amount of water, immediately followed by rapid ingestion of high-density barium. This technique is easily incorporated into the routine double-contrast examination of the upper gastrointestinal tract.[9] The double-contrast method combines desirable effects of both the full-column and mucosal relief techniques by allowing for simultaneous examination of the distended esophagus and its mucosal surface. The main limitation of this technique is related to inadequate distension of the lower esophagus that may be seen in some patients.[10] As a result, hiatal hernias and lower esophageal narrowings may be missed with this method (Figure 4).

Motion recording techniques include fluoroscopic observation of the esophagus and various permanent recording methods, such as videotaping, cine recording, and spot-film cameras. These techniques are most useful for assessing esophageal motor abnormalities and for detection and quantitation of gastroesophageal reflux.

Evaluation of GERD

Currently, the major role of the barium esophagram in evaluating patients with suspected GERD appears to be in the detection of the gross morphologic changes resulting from reflux esophagitis. The radiographic examination can also assess for esophageal motor dysfunction and gastroesophageal reflux, although radionuclide scintiscanning may eventually prove more effective in these areas.[11-13]

Esophageal Motor Function

Abnormalities of esophageal motor function and volume clearance are fairly common in patients with GERD.[14-18] However, it may be difficult to decide whether these abnormalities predate and predispose to the development of reflux esophagitis, or whether they are a consequence of peptic inflammation. Radiologic imaging is not only capable of detecting the esophageal motor dysfunction that occasionally accompanies GERD, but may also be helpful in manag-

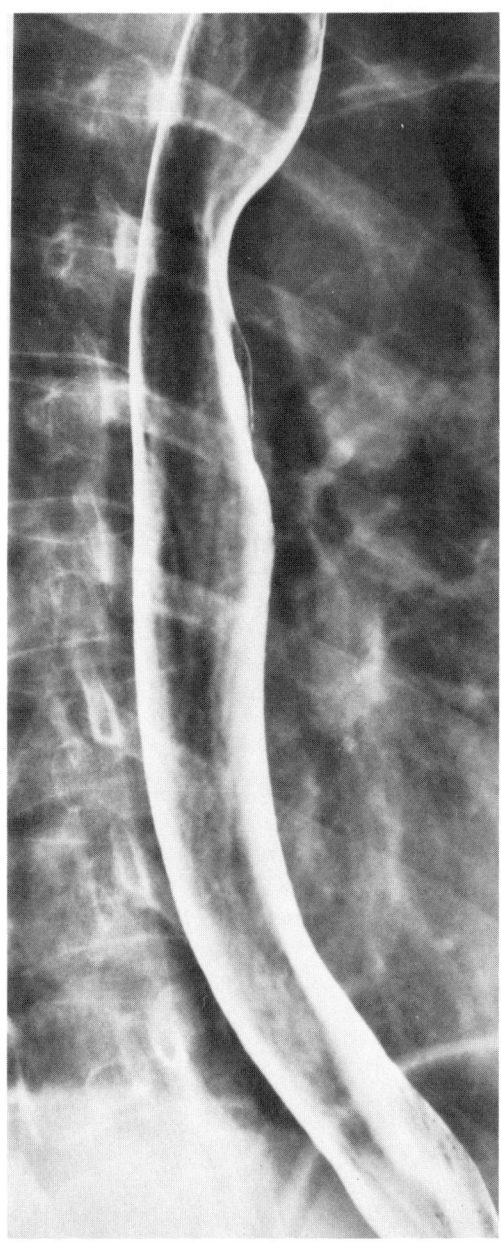

Figure 3: *Normal double-contrast appearance of the esophagus.*

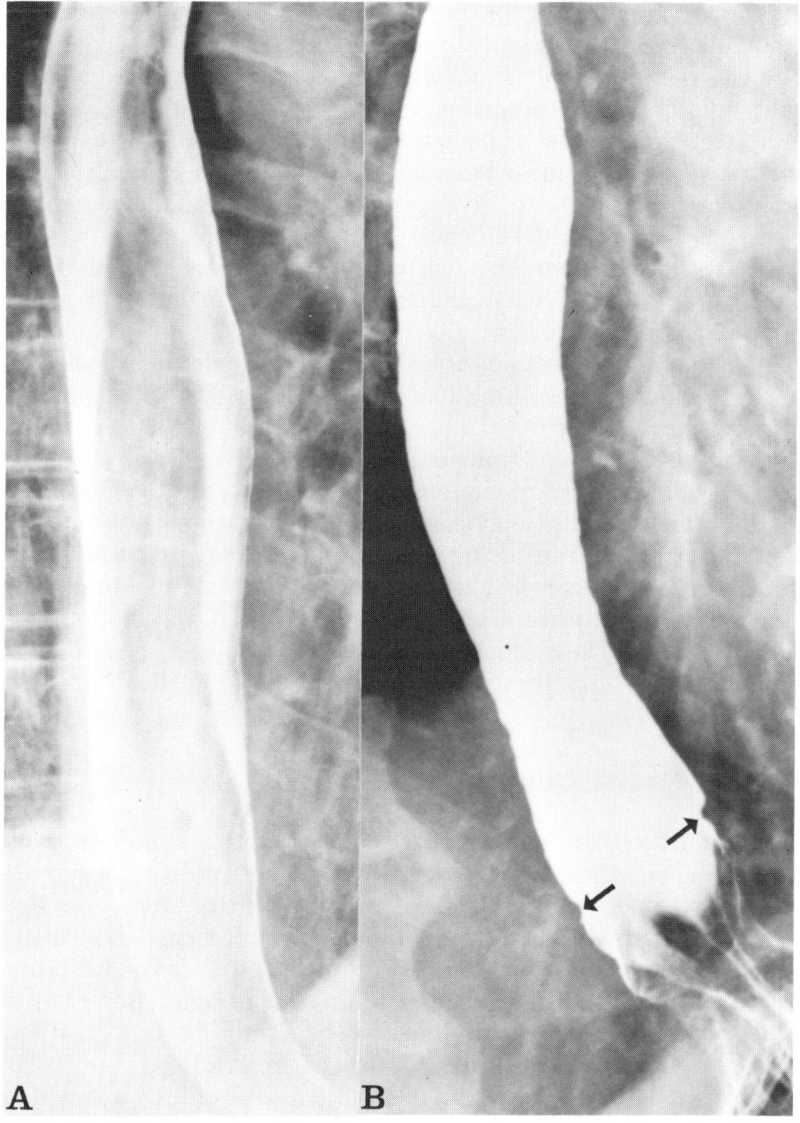

Figure 4: **A.** *Normal double-contrast view of the esophagus with the patient in the upright position. (Used with permission.[7])* **B.** *Full-column view of the distended esophagogastric region showing a lower esophageal mucosal ring (arrows) and hiatal hernia. (Used with permission.[7])*

ing patients by allowing for serial monitoring of esophageal function following medical or surgical therapy.

The barium esophagram with fluoroscopic observation compares favorably with esophageal manometry for evaluating primary motor function of the esophagus.[19] Esophageal motor disturbances that may occur secondarily in GERD include non-peristaltic contractions, incomplete or poor primary peristalsis, or even rarely aperistalsis.[20] Motor dysfunction from reflux esophagitis generally affects the lower half of the esophagus, where primary peristalsis may be disrupted and tertiary activity prominent in areas of active inflammation.

The radiologic examination also provides a relatively good estimate of esophageal volume clearance.[1,12] In a normal recumbent individual, a single peristaltic sequence usually clears nearly all of the swallowed barium from the esophagus. Occasionally, several swallows are required to completely empty the esophagus. Esophageal volume clearance may also be assessed when barium refluxes from the stomach, permitting evaluation of the effectiveness of secondary or subsequent primary peristalsis. Abnormal volume clearance typically accompanies the esophageal motor dysfunction seen in GERD.[12-14] Under these circumstances, poor esophageal volume clearance often portends a poor response to medical therapy.

Gastroesophageal Reflux

The demonstration of gastroesophageal reflux is an important finding in patients with suspected GERD because nearly half of those affected will not develop the gross morphological changes of reflux esophagitis.[21,22] Currently, 12–14 hour pH monitoring of the lower esophagus is the most sensitive means of detecting and quantitating gastroesophageal reflux.[23] The barium esophagram, however, is much less sensitive than prolonged pH monitoring for identifying gastroesophageal reflux. A major reason explaining this poorer radiographic sensitivity is the short observation time of only a few minutes generally available to assess for barium reflux fluoroscopically. Another contributing factor may be the higher specific gravity of barium, making it less prone to reflux than gastric juice.[24] Also, some symptomatic patients appear to reflux during random, transient relaxations of the lower esophageal sphincter rather than during prolonged sphincter hypotension.[14,25]

The radiographic demonstration of gastroesophageal reflux depends upon the fluoroscopic observation or recording of barium entering the esophagus from the stomach. The extent of reflux is noted by observing whether the retrograde flow of barium extends into the lower, middle, or upper third of the esophagus. Reflux of only small amounts of readily cleared barium into the lower esophagus is of questionable significance. Gastroesophageal reflux of barium may occur either spontaneously (free reflux) or during various provocative tests (stress reflux) that enhance its likelihood, such as the Valsalva maneuver. In addition, gastroesophageal reflux of barium may be sought while the patient swallows water, the so-called "water siphon test." When observed radiographically, the type, extent, and frequency of gastroesophageal reflux should be recorded, along with the effectiveness of the esophagus to clear the refluxed barium.

The value of the barium esophagram for demonstrating gastroesophageal reflux has been overemphasized, with reflux of barium observed in only 20–60% (33% average) of symptomatic patients (Table 1).[2,11,26–28] Although the use of provocative maneuvers may improve the radiographic demonstration of gastroesophageal reflux, the specificity of the resulting barium reflux is correspondingly reduced.[29,30] Thus, the absence of gastroesophageal reflux of barium can never be used to exclude GERD. Conversely, the occurrence of spontaneous, frequent, and extensive gastroesophageal reflux during the barium examination usually correlates well with the presence of reflux symptoms.[19,30,31]

A positive "water siphon test" is noted when barium refluxes into the esophagus while the patient is swallowing water.[32,33] A slightly greater percent of patients with GERD will demonstrate gastroesophageal reflux using this test when compared with the more standard radiographic methods. Unfortunately, swallowing relaxes

Table 1. Radiographic Detection of Gastroesophageal Reflux		
Author/Ref.	**Number**	**Sensitivity**
Battle et al/1973[26]	18/89	20%
Ott et al/1979[2]	10/40	25%
Velasco et al/1982[27]	20/53	38%
Fisher et al/1976[11]	15/30	50%
Rudd et al/1979[28]	15/25	60%
Totals	78/237	33%

the lower esophageal sphincter, thereby eliminating the pressure barrier that normally prevents gastroesophageal reflux, and adversely affecting the specificity of the "water siphon test." As a result, a substantial number of subjects without GERD will demonstrate reflux of at least small amounts of barium while performing this test, thus making it of questionable value for accurately separating symptomatic patients from unaffected individuals.[34-36]

Reflux Esophagitis

Patients with symptomatic GERD may exhibit a wide variety of surface appearances in the esophagus, ranging from a normal-looking esophageal mucosa to the gross morphologic changes of reflux esophagitis. Furthermore, some patients with GERD and normal esophageal endoscopy will show biopsy evidence of histologic esophagitis. Approximately 60% of those suffering from reflux disease will have abnormalities noted at endoscopy, and about two-thirds of those patients will show evidence of esophagitis radiographically.[4,37,38] Thus, the barium esophagram will demonstrate morphologic abnormalities in less than half of patients with GERD.

The more common structural abnormalities that may be seen radiographically in reflux esophagitis include mucosal and contour irregularity (Figure 5), longitudinal fold thickening (Figure 2), erosions and ulcerations (Figure 6), wall thickening (Figure 5) and segmental narrowing, particularly from stricture formation (Figure 7).[2,4,37-42] Pseudodiverticula (Figure 8), inflammatory polyps and pseudomasses, and esophagogastric fistualization may be observed less frequently.[43-47] Barrett's esophagus is suggested radiographically when focal esophagitis or stricture is separated from an accompanying hiatal hernia by a normal intervening segment of esophagus (Figure 9).[48-52] More recently, a reticulated mucosal pattern has been described in the columnar-lined esophagus using double-contrast technique.[53] The importance of this sign as an indicator of Barrett's esophagus, however, needs further investigation.

The reported specificity of the radiographic diagnosis of reflux esophagitis has been 86-93%.[2,4,37,38] Several reasons account for false positive interpretation of esophagitis on the barium esophagram. Borderline thickening of the longitudinal folds of the esophagus and transient irregularity of the esophageal margin due to non-specific motor activity are the most common causes of false positive error. An occasional problem is confusion between esophagitis and esophageal varices, both manifested by fold thickening. Finally, a lower esopha-

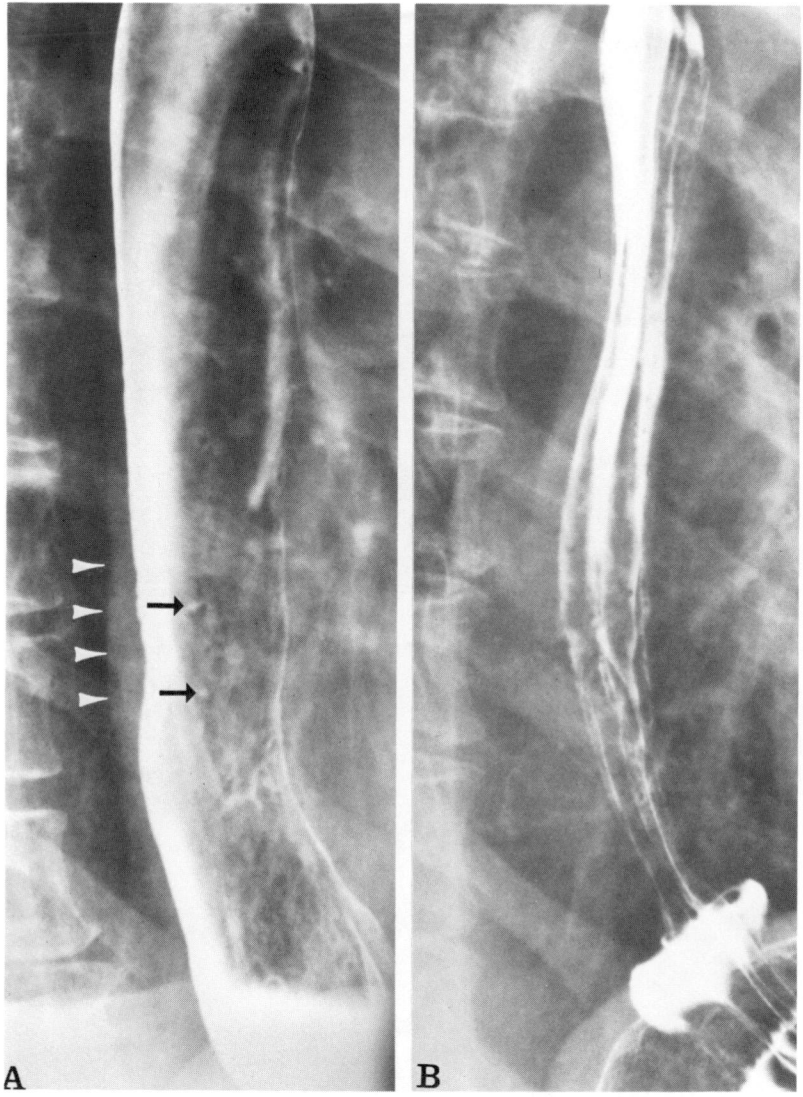

Figure 5: **A.** *Double-contrast film in a patient wih severe endoscopic esophagitis showing surface irregularity, erosions (arrows), and mild narrowing with wall thickening (arrowheads).* **B.** *Mucosal relief film in same patient demonstrating marked fold thickening and irregularity.*

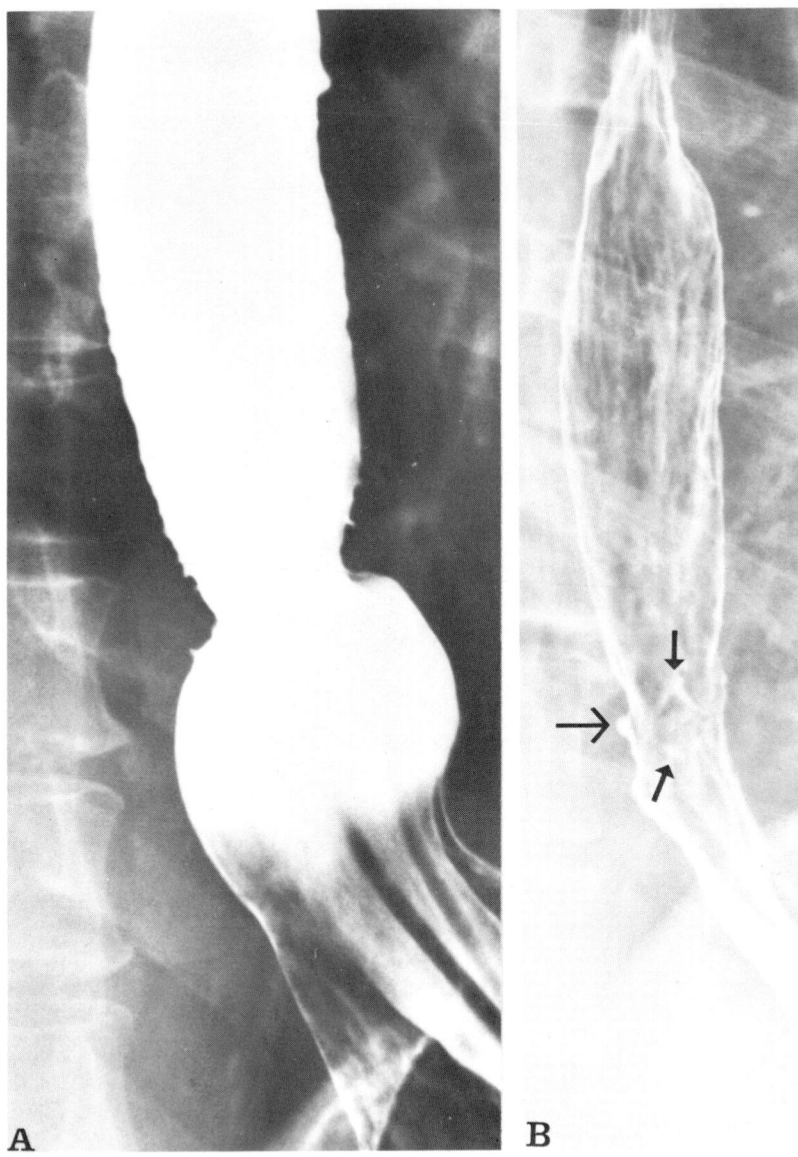

Figure 6: **A.** *Diffuse spiculation of the lower esophageal margins represent-ing ulceration endoscopically.* **B.** *Double-contrast view showing erosions, ulcerations, and scarring from esophagitis (arrows).*

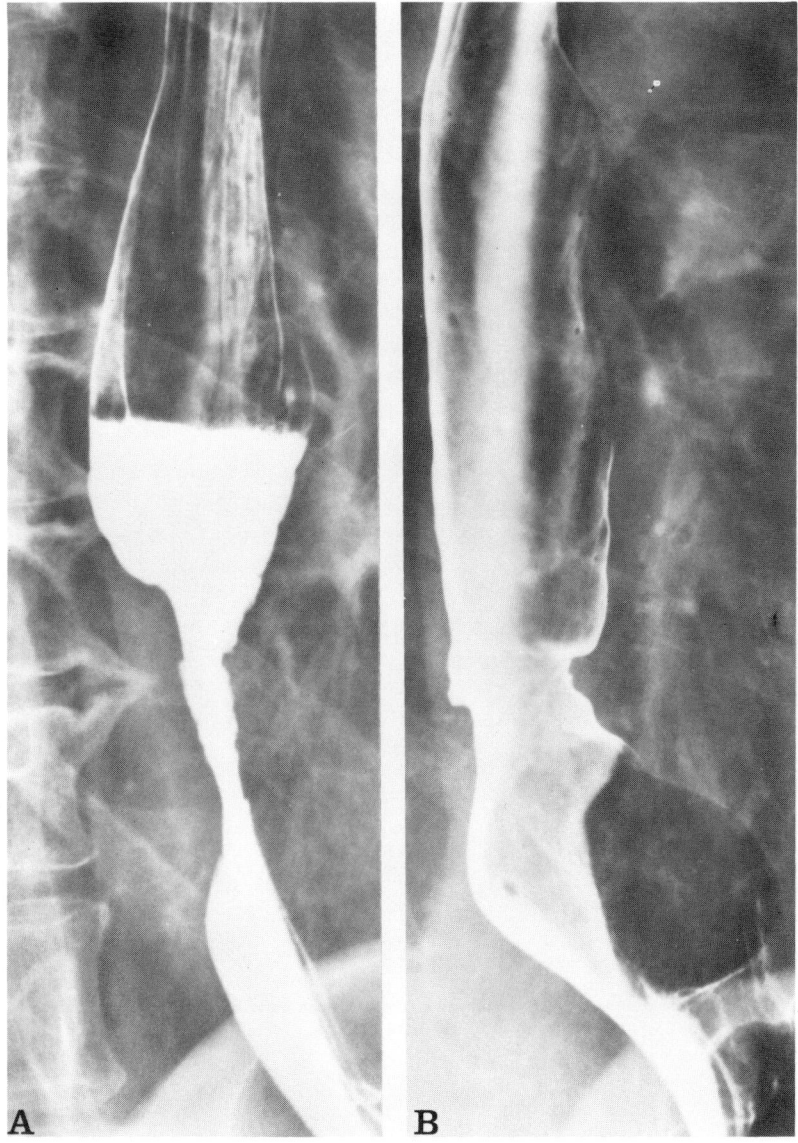

Figure 7: **A.** *Upright view of an irregular peptic stricture due to associated active esophagitis endoscopically.* **B.** *Smooth, eccentric peptic stricture on double-contrast examination.*

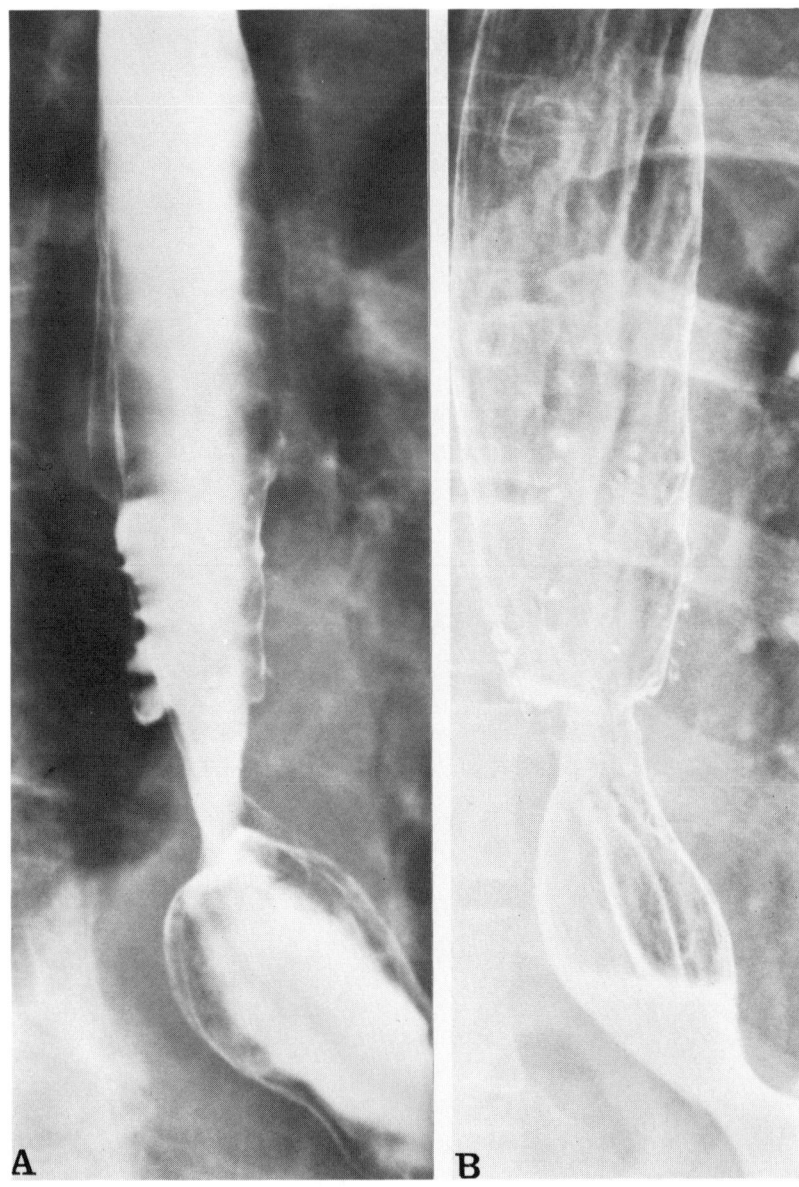

Figure 8: **A.** *Peptic stricture associated with multiple smooth outpouchings representing pseudodiverticula endoscopically.* **B.** *Peptic stricture with numerous small collections of barium. Differentiation between ulceration and pseudodiverticular formation is difficult.*

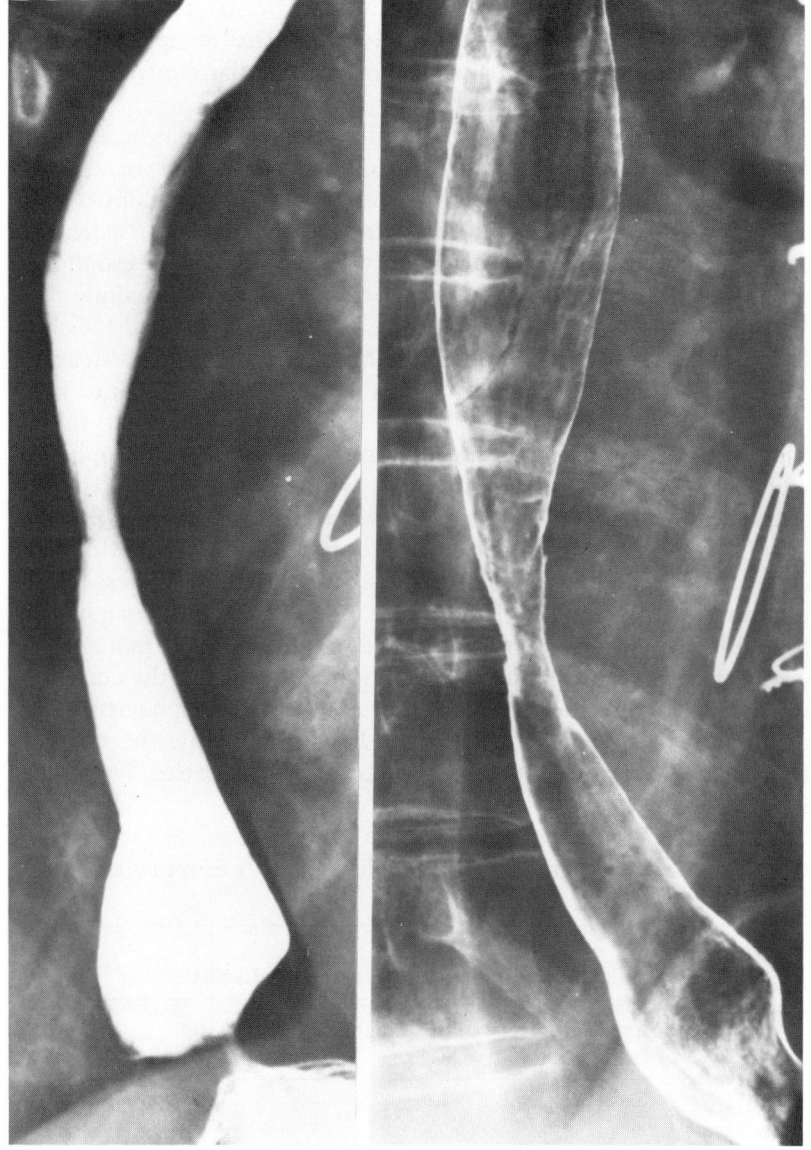

Figure 9: *Full-column and double-contrast views of a patient with Barrett's esophagus showing a mid-esophageal stricture.*

geal mucosal ring may mimic an annular peptic stricture. A mucosal ring is generally smooth, thin, and symmetric in appearance, in contrast to the usually broader and often irregular configuration of the annular peptic stricture.

The radiographic detection of reflux esophagitis has been shown to depend on the endoscopic severity of the disease. The signs used to diagnose esophagitis endoscopically include mucosal friability, exudation, erosions, ulceration, and stricture formation.[54,55] Although erythema has also been used as an endoscopic sign of esophageal inflammation, it appears to lack specificity when seen alone.[55-58] Various endoscopic grading systems have been described for classifying the severity of esophagitis; however, those classifications using fiberoptic instruments usually divide the disease into three grades.[2,4,37,38,59,60] Mild esophagitis is diagnosed when erythema, friability, and, in some cases, exudation are seen; moderate esophagitis when erosions and ulcerations occur; and severe esophagitis when marked ulceration or, most commonly, stricture formation is present.

The radiographic detection of esophagitis depends both on the endoscopic grade of the disease and on the thoroughness of the barium examination (Table 2, Figure 10).[4,37,38] In mild esophagitis, particularly manifested by only erythema and friability, radiographic detection has been generally poor. On the other hand, the combined sensitivity for diagnosing moderate and severe esophagitis radiographically has averaged 90–96%. Furthermore, in the category of peptic esophageal stricture, reported sensitivities have been 95–100%.[4,37,38,43]

A multiphasic approach using a combination of radiographic techniques is necessary to optimally detect reflux esophagitis. Radio-

Table 2.
Radiographic Detection of Reflux Esophagitis

Endoscopic Grade of Esophagitis	Radiographic Sensitivity*		
	SCT	DCT	Both
Mild	0–44%	0–35%	0–53%
Moderate	70–83%	55–93%	80–93%
Severe	80–95%	95–100%	100%
Totals	60–77%	60–80%	72–88%

SCT = Single-contrast techniques (full-column/mucosal relief)
DCT = Double-contrast technique
Both = Combined techniques
*Sensitivity ranges from three reports (4, 37, 38)

RADIOGRAPHIC DETECTION OF ESOPHAGITIS

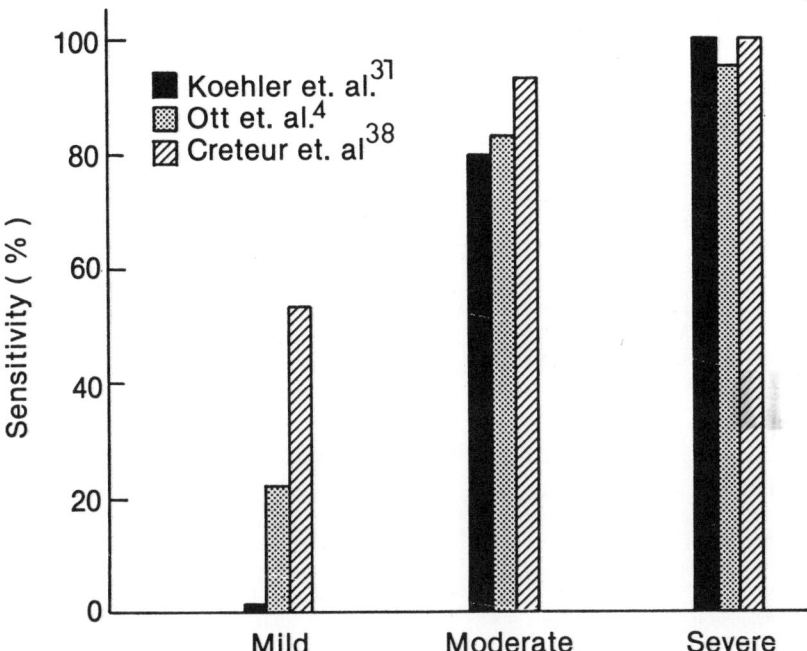

Figure 10: *Histogram comparing the radiographic detection of reflux esophagitis relative to the endoscopic grade of severity from three reported series.*

graphic sensitivities in all grades of endoscopic esophagitis have been 60–80% using single-contrast or double-contrast techniques alone, but have improved to 72–88% detection rates by combining techniques (Table 2, Figure 10). As a result, the recommended radiographic examination for evaluating patients with suspected reflux esophagitis should consist of upright double-contrast views, prone barium-filled views, and mucosal relief views of the esophagus.

Summary

The barium esophagram can serve an important role in evaluating patients with suspected GERD. Esophageal motor abnormalities, gastroesophageal reflux, and the gross morphologic changes of reflux esophagitis may be detected. Currently, the major role of the barium esophagram in GERD appears to be in the detection of endoscopic esophagitis because it will usually demonstrate the more severe forms of the disease that need to be accurately diagnosed.

References

1. Ott DJ, Dodds WJ, Wu WC, Gelfand DW, Hogan WJ, Stewart ET: Current status of radiology in evaluating for gastroesophageal reflux disease. *J Clin Gastroenterol* 1982; 4:365–372.
2. Ott DJ, Gelfand DW, Wu WC: Reflux esophagitis: radiographic and endoscopic correlation. *Radiology* 1979; 130:583–588.
3. Wright RA, Hurwitz AL: Relationship of hiatal hernia to endoscopically proved reflux esophagitis. *Dig Dis Sci* 1979; 24:311–313.
4. Ott DJ, Wu WC, Gelfand DW: Reflux esophagitis revisited: prospective analysis of radiologic accuracy. *Gastrointest Radiol* 1981; 6:1–7.
5. Gelfand DW, Ott DJ: Anatomy and technique in evaluating the esophagus. *Semin Roentgenol* 1981; 16:168–182.
6. Ott DJ, Gelfand DW, Wu WC: Sensitivity of single-contrast radiology in esophageal disease: a study of 240 patients with endoscopically verified abnormality. *Gastrointest Radiol* 1983; 8:105–110.
7. Ott DJ: Radiologic evaluation of the esophagus. In: Castell DO, Johnson LF, eds. *Esophageal Function in Health and Disease.* New York: Elsevier Biomedical, 1983: 211–235.
8. Wolf BS: Diagnostic tools in the study of the esophagus. Part IV. Roentgenology. In: Bockus HL, ed. *Gastroenterology* (Vol. 1), 3rd ed. Philadelphia: W.B. Saunders, 1974: 166–182.
9. Laufer I: *Double Contrast Gastrointestinal Radiology.* Philadelphia: W.B. Saunders, 1979: 59–77.
10. Balfe DM, Koehler RE, Weyman PJ, Baron RL, Reinus WR: Routine air-contrast esophagography during upper gastrointestinal examinations. *Radiology* 1981; 139:739–741.
11. Fisher RS, Malmud LS, Robert GS, Lobis IF: Gastroesophageal (GE) scintiscanning to detect and quantitate GE reflux. *Gastroenterology* 1976; 70:301–308.
12. Russell COH, Hill LD, Holmes III ER, Hull DA, Gannon R, Pope II CE: Radionuclide transit: a sensitive screening test for esophageal dysfunction. *Gastroenterology* 1981; 80:887–892.
13. McCallum RW: Radionuclide scanning in esophageal disease. *J Clin Gastroenterol* 1982; 4:67–70.
14. Dodds WJ, Hogan WJ, Helm JF, Dent J: Pathogenesis of reflux esophagitis. *Gastroenterology* 1981; 81:376–394.
15. Olsen AM, Schlegel JF: Motility disturbances caused by esophagitis. *J Thorac Cardiovasc Surg* 1965; 50:607–612.
16. Donner MW, Silbiger ML, Hookman P, Hendrix TR: Acid-barium swallows in the radiographic evaluation of clinical esophagitis. *Radiology* 1966; 87:220–225.
17. DeMeester TR, Johnson LF, Joseph GJ, Toscano MS, Hall AW, Skinner DB: Patterns of gastroesophageal reflux in health and disease. *Ann Surg* 1976; 184:459–469.
18. Russell COH, Pope II CE, Gannan RM, Allen FD, Velasco N, Hill LD:

Does surgery correct esophageal motor dysfunction in gastroesophageal reflux? *Ann Surg* 1981; 194:290–295.

19. Dodds WJ: Current concepts of esophageal motor function: Clinical implications for radiology. *AJR* 1977; 128:549–561.
20. Simeone JF, Burrell M, Toffler R, Smith GJW: Aperistalsis and esophagitis. *Radiology* 1977; 123:9–14.
21. Johnson LF, DeMeester TR, Haggitt RC: Endoscopic signs for gastroesophageal reflux objectively evaluated. *Gastrointest Endosc* 1976; 22:151–155.
22. Behar J, Biancani P, Sheahan DG: Evaluation of esophageal tests in the diagnosis of reflux esophagitis. *Gastroenterology* 1976; 71:9–15.
23. Johnson LF: 24-hour pH monitoring in the study of gastroesophageal reflux. *J Clin Gastroenterol* 1980; 2:387–399.
24. Lindell D, Sanmark S: Hiatal incompetence and gastro-oesophageal reflux. *Acta Radiol Diagn* 1979; 20:626–636.
25. Dodds WJ, Dent J, Hogan WJ, et al: Mechanisms of gastroesophageal reflux in patients with reflux esophagitis. *N Engl J Med* 1982; 307: 1547–1552.
26. Battle WS, Nyhus LM, Bombeck CT: Gastroesophageal reflux: Diagnosis and treatment. *Ann Surg* 1973; 177:560–564.
27. Velasco N, Pope CE, Gannan RM, Hill LD: Gastroesophageal scintigraphy for evaluation of gastroesophageal reflux and esophageal clearance (abstract). *Gastroenterology* 1982; 82:1204.
28. Rudd TG, Christie DL: Demonstration of gastroesophageal reflux in children by radionuclide gastroesophagography. *Radiology* 1979; 131: 483–486.
29. Vandervelde GM, Carlson HC: Esophageal reflux. *AJR* 1964; 92:989–993.
30. Wolf BS: Roentgenology of the esophagogastric region. In: Margulis AR, Burhenne HJ, eds. *Alimentary Tract Roentgenology* Vol. 1 (2nd ed). St. Louis: CV Mosby Co., 1973: 500–552.
31. Silverstein BD, Pope II CE: Role of diagnostic tests in esophageal evaluation. *Am J Surg* 1980; 139:744–748.
32. deCarvalho MM: Chirugie du syndrome hiato-oesophagien. *Arch Mal Appl Digest* 1951; 40:280–293.
33. Crummy AB: The water test in the evaluation of gastroesophageal reflux. *Radiology* 1966; 78:501–504.
34. Linsman JF: Gastroesophageal reflux elicited while drinking water (water siphonage test). *AJR* 1965; 94:325–332.
35. Donner MW, Margulies SI: Radiographic examination. In: Skinner DB, Belsey RHR, Hendrix TR, Zuidema GD, eds. *Gastroesophageal Reflux and Hiatal Hernia.* Boston: Little, Brown and Co., 1972: 59–85.
36. Blumhagen JD, Christie DL: Gastroesophageal reflux in children: Evaluation of the water siphon test. *Radiology* 1979; 131:345–349.
37. Koehler RE, Weyman PJ, Oakley HF: Single- and double-contrast techniques in esophagitis. *AJR* 1980; 135:15–19.
38. Creteur V, Thoeni RF, Federle MP, et al: The role of single and double-contrast radiography in the diagnosis of reflux esophagitis. *Radiology* 1983; 147:71–75.
39. Wolf BS, Marshak RH, Som ML, Winkelstein A: Peptic esophagitis, peptic ulcer of the esophagus and marginal esophagogastric ulceration. *Gastroenterology* 1955; 29:744–766.
40. Rabin MS, Schmaman IB: Radiological changes of reflux oesophagitis. *Clin Radiol* 1979; 30:187–191.

41. Kressel HY, Glick SN, Laufer I, Banner M: Radiologic features of esophagitis. *Gastrointest Radiol* 1981; 6:103–108.

42. McDermott P, Wallers KJ, Holden R, James WB: Double-contrast examination of the esophagus: The radiological changes of peptic oesophagitis. *Clin Radiol* 1982; 33:259–264.

43. Ott DJ, Gelfand DW, Lane TG, Wu WC: Radiologic detection and spectrum of appearances of peptic esophageal strictures. *J Clin Gastroenterol* 1982; 4:11–15.

44. Bleshman MH, Banner MP, Johnson RC, DeFord JW: The inflammatory esophagogastric polyp and fold. *Radiology* 1978; 128:589–593.

45. Rabin MS, Bremner CG, Botha JR: The reflux gastroesophageal polyp. *Am J Gastroenterol* 1980; 73:451–453.

46. Staples DC, Knodell RG, Johnson LF: Inflammatory pseudotumor of the esophagus. A complication of gastroesophageal reflux. *Gastrointest Endosc* 1978; 24:175–176.

47. Raymond JI, Khan AH, Cain LR, Ramin JE: Multiple esophagogastric fistulas resulting from reflux esophagitis. *Am J Gastroenterol* 1980; 73:430–433.

48. Cho KY, Hunter TB, Whitehouse WM: The columnar epithelial-lined lower esophagus and its association with adenocarcinoma of the esophagus. *Radiology* 1975; 115:563–568.

49. Robbins AH, Hermos JA, Schimmel EM, Friedlander DM, Messian RA: The columnar-lined esophagus—analysis of 26 cases. *Radiology* 1977; 123:1–7.

50. Robbins AH, Vincent ME, Saini M, Schimmel EM: Revised radiologic concepts of the Barrett esophagus. *Gastrointest Radiol* 1978; 3:377–381.

51. Mangla JC: Barrett's esophagus: an old entity rediscovered. *J Clin Gastroenterol* 1981; 3:347–356.

52. Bozymski EM, Herlihy KJ, Orlando RC: Barrett's esophagus. *Ann Int Med* 1982; 97:103–107.

53. Levine MS, Kressel HY, Caroline DF, Laufer I, Herlinger H, Thompson JJ: Barrett esophagus: Reticular pattern of the mucosa. *Radiology* 1983; 147:663–667.

54. Herrera AF: Endoscopic diagnosis of esophagitis. In: Bockus HL, ed. *Gastroenterology* (Vol. 1), 3rd ed. Philadelphia: W.B. Saunders, 1974: 271–274.

55. Pope II CE: Gastroesophageal reflux disease (reflux esophagitis). In: Sleisenger MH, Fordtran JS, eds. *Gastrointestinal Disease* (Vol. 1), 3rd ed. Philadelphia: W.B. Saunders, 1983: 449–476.

56. Trujillo NP, Boyce JR HW: Gastroscopic evaluation of the esophagogastric junctional area. *Gastrointest Endosc* 1967; 14:120–123.

57. Richter JE, Castell DO: Gastroesophageal reflux. Pathogenesis, diagnosis, and therapy. *Ann Int Med* 1982; 97:93–103.

58. Johnson LF, Moses FM: Endoscopic evaluation of esophageal disease. In: Castell DO, Johnson LF, eds. *Esophageal Function in Health and Disease.* New York: Elsevier Biomedical; 1983: 237–254.

59. Belsey RHR: Esophagoscopy. In: Skinner DB, Belsey RHR, Hendrix TR, Zuidema GD, eds. *Gastroesophageal Reflux and Hiatal Hernia.* Boston: Little, Brown and Co.; 1972: 107–118.

60. Behar J, Brand DL, Brown FC, et al: Cimetidine in the treatment of symptomatic gastroesophageal reflux. *Gastroenterology* 1978; 74:441–448.

8

Esophageal Manometry

Philip O. Katz, M.D., and
Donald O. Castell, M.D.

Chapter Contents

The development of infusion catheters and precise infusion systems, as well as standardization of manometry laboratories, has created a large increase in esophageal research over the last 20 years. Though of limited usefulness in the everyday diagnosis of reflux disease, the manometry laboratory may play a vital role in the diagnosis of the complex patient with atypical reflux symptoms—chest pain, excessive belching, nocturnal regurgitation, and asthma—and in those with "typical" symptoms who fail standard medical therapy. In addi-

From Castell DO, Wu WC, Ott DJ (eds): *Gastroesophageal Reflux Disease: Pathogenesis, Diagnosis, Therapy.* Mount Kisco, NY, Futura Publishing Co., Inc., 1985.

tion, manometry is very useful in evaluation of motility in patients with Barrett's esophagus, in confirming the diagnosis of scleroderma and should always be done to evaluate peristalsis prior to anti-reflux surgery.

Manometry has been and continues to be of major value in the area of esophageal research. Careful studies over the years have helped identify and characterize the lower esophageal sphincter (LES) and ascertain its possible role in the pathogenesis of reflux disease. Through pharmacologic manipulation of LES pressure and esophageal motility, investigators have been able to better clarify the role of diet, alcohol, cigarettes, and many drugs in the pathogenesis of gastroesophageal reflux, and to evaluate old and new therapy. Identification of the upper esophageal sphincter (UES) and its potential role in gastroesophageal reflux has been made possible by the use of manometric catheters.

This chapter will provide a brief overview of the development of manometry, discuss the changes in the esophageal body and in the UES, and their potential role in the pathogenesis of reflux disease. We will briefly review the techniques of measurement of the LES and its use in the clinical laboratory, and we will discuss the potential clinical applications of manometry in evaluation of the reflux patient.

Historical Perspective

Manometric studies were first performed by Kronecker and Meltzer in 1883 and 1884[1,2] using air-filled balloons and an external pressure transducer. Water-filled balloons were first used by Ingelfinger et al in 1940.[3] Because of the inaccuracy and delayed assessment of rapid pressure changes in the esophagus, these methods were not found clinically useful and were abandoned.

Studies with water-filled catheters first began in the 1950s and initiated development of the basic knowledge of the physiology and pathophysiology of esophageal motility. Fyke first identified the LES manometrically in 1956.[4] In the 1960s, the work of Pope,[5] Winans and Harris,[6] and Cohen and Harris[7] demonstrated that constantly perfused catheters with side openings allowed for more accurate quantitative pressure recordings, and demonstrated for the first time a difference between a competent and incompetent LES. Using these newer perfusion techniques, subsequent studies by Cohen and Harris showed excellent correlation between the LES pressure measurement and an assessment of LES strength. The latter was estimated by recording the force required to pull a 1 cm Teflon ball through the

LES.[7] The first quantitative recording of LES pressure using the rapid pull-through technique was done in 1972 by Waldeck.[8] Developed by Arndorfer et al[9] and Dodds et al,[10] the most widely used equipment includes low-compliance hydraulic capillary infusion systems with low, constant perfusion rates that allow quantitative measurements of both LES pressure and peristaltic pressure waves.

Lower Esophageal Sphincter

Although the pathogenesis of reflux disease is multifactorial, there is no doubt that the LES plays a role as an anti-reflux barrier. Unfortunately, since its identification manometrically by Fyke et al in 1956,[4] there has been considerable controversy as to the value of routine measurement of LES pressure in clinical practice.

With development of radially oriented infused catheters, investigators found asymmetry of the LES, with pressure higher on the left and posteriorly than in other directions. It is this asymmetry, coupled with differences in patient groups, recording techniques, and catheter assembly that makes it difficult to compare results of different studies. Because the sphincter is a dynamic barrier, day-to-day and hour-to-hour variation in pressure make interpretation of a single value difficult. Accurate sphincter pressure measurement may be technically difficult. Sphincter pressure is usually measured in one of two ways, each involved in pulling a series of 3–8 radially oriented recording orifices 1 centimeter apart from the stomach, across the sphincter into the esophageal body, and taking an average value as the LES pressure. This can be done with the station pull-through technique (SPT), in which the catheter is pulled through a series of stations 0.5–1 cm apart, pausing for 20–30 seconds at each station, until all orifices are in the body. The rapid pull-through (RPT) is a technique in which the patient suspends respiration and swallowing, and the catheter is rapidly pulled through the sphincter (at 1 cm per second). The RPT is performed faster, eliminates respiratory variation, allows quick location of the sphincter, and provides a clearer endpoint for measurement. It does not allow for assessment of sphincter relaxation and may be inaccurately measured if the patient performs a Valsalva maneuver or swallows during the pull-through. The SPT allows for assessment of relaxation but is subject to respiratory variation, observer scoring error, and demands patience on the part of the examiner. In our own laboratory we have found similar values using both methods[11] (Table 1) and use both techniques in each patient to gain as much information as possible about the LES pressure.

Table 1. Comparison of Lower Esophageal Sphincter Pressures Using SPT* and RPT+ (Values Obtained in 50 Normal Subjects)		
	Mean ± SD	Range
SPT (mmHg)	26.6 ± 10.8	(7.0−58.0)
RPT (mmHg)	27.8 ± 10.1	(7.0−55.0)

*SPT = station pullthrough technique
+RPT = rapid pullthough technique

The above information makes it easy to understand why there is large overlap in sphincter pressure between normals and those with reflux and why LES pressure is too insensitive in most cases to use as a routine test for diagnosis of reflux. Though patients with Barrett's esophagus and scleroderma have consistently low sphincter pressures, there is considerable overlap between the "usual" reflux patients and normals (See Figure 7, Chapter 3). In our own laboratory we feel that reliable discrimination of reflux can only be made at very low pressures (≤6 mmHg). Patients with pressures of 20−25 mmHg seem to have adequate protection against severe or frequent reflux in most clinical situations, but normal LES pressure should not be used as a single test to rule out reflux disease.

Esophageal Body

The manometric function of the esophageal body in reflux disease has not been extensively studied. In most cases esophageal clearing and peristalsis appear to be normal. Older studies using uninfused catheters demonstrated an increase in repetitive, simultaneous contractions, which seemed to cause ineffective esophageal emptying in a small percentage of reflux patients. Patients with severe, chronic, or refractory reflux may present a different picture from normals. An early study using infused catheters showed a decrease in primary peristalsis in about 20% of reflux patients with severe, chronic, and refractory reflux.[12]

Recent work has demonstrated decreased amplitude of contractions in the distal esophagus of reflux patients, and markedly decreased amplitude of distal contraction in patients with Barrett's esophagus as compared with both other reflux patients and normals[13] (Figure 1). In addition, acid-induced esophagitis in cats has been shown

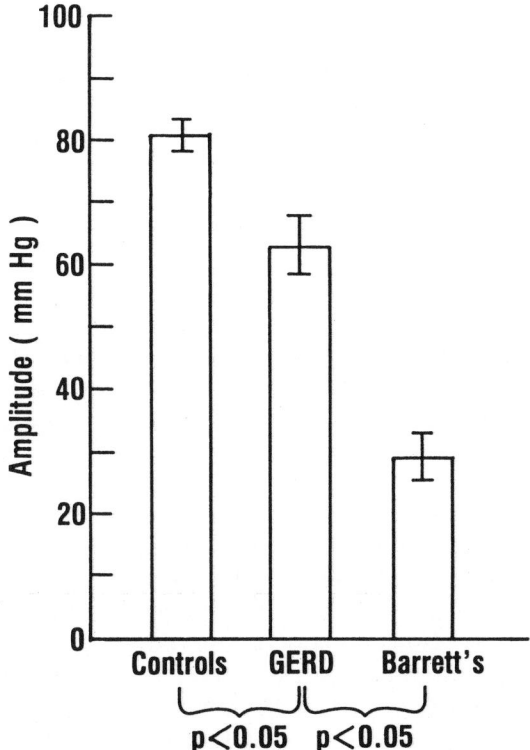

Figure 1: *Bar graph showing difference between mean distal amplitude in Barrett's, GERD and normal patients. GERD = gastroesophageal reflux disease.*

to result in decreased LES tone and decreased distal contraction amplitude.[14,15]

These and other studies have raised questions about the mechanism of reflux. Do abnormal pressures or increased reflux occur first? Are ineffective esophageal clearing mechanisms and resultant esophagitis responsible for an incompetent LES or vice versa? Though this issue remains to be resolved, it seems that abnormal peristalsis and decreased esophageal emptying, whether a primary or secondary disturbance, if present, creates the potential for a vicious cycle that may lead to more severe esophagitis.

Upper Esophageal Sphincter (UES)

Though not nearly as well studied, manometric examination of the UES has suggested a potential role for it in reflux disease. Consisting primarily of striated muscle, the UES is a high-pressure zone, ranging from 2.5 to 4.0 cm in length, residing between the 5th to 7th cervical vertebrae. Its nerve supply appears to be from the pharyngeal portions of the vagus nerve. It appears, as is the case with the LES, to be asymmetric, with the posterior and anterior pressures both considerably greater than lateral pressures. Peak anterior pressure occurs more proximally than posterior pressures. Like the LES, pressures can be measured by a pull-through technique, though accuracy is more difficult.

Because of the difficulty in accurate assessment of the UES, the amount of published information is small compared to study of the LES. Acid infusion in the upper esophagus just below the sphincter appears to have a stimulatory effect on the UES, causing a rise in pressure.[16] Saline infusion and balloon distension cause the same effect but to a lesser degree, suggesting that the UES operates as a barrier to reflux of esophageal contents and prevents aspiration and regurgitation. UES hypotension has been observed in patients with chronic reflux, who have spontaneous regurgitation of food into the pharynx. These same patients had a decreased response to acid infusion, suggesting a link between sphincter pressure and competence in the prevention of regurgitation. It must be mentioned, however, that most patients with reflux disease appear to have a normal and totally competent UES, and much more research is necessary before any definitive role of this sphincter in reflux disease can be postulated.

Role of Manometry in Evaluation of the Reflux Patient

What conclusions are reasonable from these observations? There is no question that a single isolated measurement of LES pressure, unless extremely low, is of limited usefulness in evaluation of patients with suspected reflux. Manometry can be uncomfortable for patients, is expensive, and requires special training to perform correctly. It is also clear that many patients with heartburn and suspected reflux will require no more than a thorough history and physical examination, and the addition of a barium swallow or upper gastrointestinal x-ray study, to rule out structural lesions and complications of reflux. Because most patients can be easily treated medically, there is but a small role for manometry in the routine evaluation of reflux disease.

It is the group of patients with atypical symptoms or those who fail to respond to medical therapy in whom more thorough evaluation may be needed to help confirm the diagnosis. Reflux may present as atypical chest pain about 10% of the time. Retrosternal burning may be caused by reflux, coronary artery disease, peptic ulcer disease, esophageal motility disorders, or biliary tract disease. Acid sensitivity (a positive Bernstein test) may be found in a small percentage of normals and in patients with cholelithiasis or after cholecystectomy. These patients usually require more extensive evaluation, which may include manometry.

Patients that have reflux associated with cigarettes or alcohol may present a problem for the clinician. This group will often demonstrate normal LES pressures and relaxation despite histologic and endoscopic esophagitis if studied during abstinence.[17] It might be useful to study these patients manometrically during smoking (or alcohol) and abstinence to see if changes in sphincter pressure can be documented. These patients should always be studied prior to antireflux surgery. If normal LES pressures are demonstrated, a further trial of abstinence and medical therapy may be indicated before surgery.

Some patients with chronic cough, pneumonitis, or asthma will have gastroesophageal reflux,[18] often with very few GI symptoms. Patients with recurrent pulmonary disease due to unknown etiology, particularly if symptoms occur predominantly at night, should have a thorough esophageal evaluation, with complete assessment of motility, LES pressure, and assessment of upper and lower sphincter relaxation (see Chapter 16). Intra-esophageal pH testing may also be helpful in these cases.

In the above examples manometry may prove useful. Sphincter pressures can be assessed, and if very low, a diagnosis of reflux can be supported. If high resting pressures are found, there is a low likelihood of significant reflux disease. Manometry can give information regarding peristaltic function and allows optimal placement of pH probes for intra-esophageal pH testing if desired.

Another group in whom manometry may prove useful in evaluation of reflux is in scleroderma patients. Esophageal involvement is frequent (70–80%) in these patients and symptoms may be misleading despite very low LES pressure and decreased amplitude of peristalsis in the lower esophagus.[19] In patients with suspected scleroderma, manometry may help confirm the diagnosis if the combination of very low LES pressure and weak-to-absent peristalsis in the distal esophagus is found. This manometric pattern becomes almost pathognomonic for scleroderma when combined with presence of a normal UES pressure and normal upper esophageal peristalsis. Manometry has been shown to be a more sensitive indication of esophageal involvement than conventional radiography.[20,21]

It is our feeling that all patients being considered for anti-reflux surgery should be evaluated manometrically. Rarely, an alternative diagnosis can be made. More importantly, preoperative manometry allows assessment of the adequacy of peristaltic pressures in the esophageal body. If the patient has severely disordered or weak peristalsis, a fundoplication may result in postoperative dysphagia, due to defective esophageal clearing. With the pre-operative information of weak peristalsis, the surgeon may wish to perform a "loose" fundoplication or postpone surgery until another trial of medical therapy can be completed.

Conclusion

At present, the major value of the manometry laboratory in gastroesophageal reflux appears to be in research. Work in the last 20 years has provided much insight into the pathogenesis of reflux disease and has allowed us to evaluate pharmacologic and environmental agents as causes of reflux, and to investigate numerous therapeutic modalities. Controversial issues still remain, so much work remains to be done.

There appears to be little use for manometry in everyday evaluation of reflux patients. This technique should be reserved for evaluation of the complex patient or the patient with suspected reflux who does not respond to medical therapy (Table 2).

Table 2. Indications for Manometry in GE Reflux Disease
1. Support diagnosis in the complex patient a. Atypical symptoms b. Failed medical therapy
2. Patients considered for anti-reflux surgery
3. Assess motility in known reflux/Barrett's patients
4. Evaluate possible scleroderma
5. Placement of pH probe

References

1. Kronecker H, Meltzer SJ: Der Schluckmechanismus, seine erregung und seine hemmung. *Arch Ges Anat Physiol Suppl* 1883; 7:328–332.
2. Meltzer SJ: Recent experimental contributions to the physiology of deglutition. *N Y Med J* 1894; 59:389.
3. Ingelfinger FJ, Abbot WO: Intubation studies of human small intestine: Diagnostic significance of motor disturbances. *Am J Dig Dis* 1940; 7:468–474.
4. Fyke FE, Code CF, Schlegel JF: The gastroesophageal sphincter in healthy human beings. *Gastroenterologia* (Basel) 1956; 86:135–150.
5. Pope CE: A dynamic test of sphincter strength: Its application to the lower esophageal sphincter. *Gastroenterology* 1967; 52:779–786.
6. Winans CHS, Harris LD: Quantitation of lower esophageal sphincter competence. *Gastroenterology* 1967; 52:773–778.
7. Cohen S, Harris LD: Lower esophageal sphincter pressure as an index of lower esophageal sphincter strength. *Gastroenterology* 1970; 58:157–162.
8. Waldeck F: A new procedure for functional analysis of the lower esophageal sphincter (LES). *Pflügers Arch* 1972; 335:74–84.
9. Arndorfer RC, Stef JJ, Dodds WJ, Lineham JH, Hogan WJ: Improved infusion system for intraluminal esophageal manometry. *Gastroenterology* 1977; 73:23–27.
10. Dodds WJ, Stef JJ, Arndorfer R, Linehan H, Hogan WJ: Improved infusion system for esophageal manometry. *Clin Res* 1974; 22:602 (abstract).
11. Nelson JL, Wu WC, Richter JE, Blackwell JN, Johns DN, Castell DO: What is normal esophageal motility? *Gastroenterology* 1983; 84:5:1258 (abstract).
12. Miller WN, Hogan WJ, Dodds WJ, et al: A comprehensive investigation of patients with symptoms of gastroesophageal reflux (GER). *Gastroenterology* 1974; 66:747 (abstract).
13. Knuff TE, Benjamin SB, Worsham F, Hancock JE, Castell DO: Histologic evaluation of chronic gastroesophageal reflux: An evaluation of biopsy methods and diagnostic criteria. *Dig Dis Sci* 1984; 29:194–201.
14. Eastwood GL, Castell DO, Higgs RH: Experimental esophagitis in cats impairs lower esophageal sphincter pressure. *Gastroenterology* 1974; 69:146–153.
15. Higgs RH, Castell DO, Eastwood GL: Studies on the mechanism of esophagitis induced lower esophageal sphincter hypotension in cats. *Gastroenterology* 1976; 71:51–56.
16. Gerhardt DC, Schuck TJ, Bordeaux RA, Winship DH: Human upper esophageal sphincter. Response to volume, osmotic and acid stimuli. *Gastroenterology* 1975; 75:268–274.
17. Johnson LF, Kikendall JW: Tests of esophageal function. In: Castell DO, Johnson LF, ed. *Esophageal Function in Health and Disease.* Elsevier Biomedical. 1983: 194.
18. Kjellen G, Brundin A, Tibbling L, Wranne B: Oesophageal function in asthmatics. *Eur J Resp Dis* 1981; 62:87–94.

19. Chobanian SJ, Castell DO: Esophageal abnormalities in systemic disease. *Esophageal Function in Health and Disease.* In: Castell DO, Johnson LF, ed. Elsevier Biomedical. 1983: 273–294.
20. Neschis M, Siegelman SS, Rotstein J, Parker JG: The esophagus in progressive systemic sclerosis. A manometric and radiologic correlation. *Am J Dig Dis* 1970; 15:443–447.
21. Saladin TA, French AB, Zarafonetis CJD, Pollard HM: Esophageal motor abnormalities in scleroderma and related diseases. *Am J Dig Dis* 1966; 11:522–535.

9

Acid Perfusion (Bernstein) Test

Joel E. Richter, M.D.

Chapter Contents

Instillation of acid into the esophagus to reproduce the symptoms of heartburn was first proposed as a test for gastroesophageal reflux disease by Bernstein and Baker in 1958.[1] Of all the esophageal function tests, none is more elegant in its simplicity of concept than the esophageal acid perfusion (Bernstein) test. The simplicity and accuracy of this test has made it a popular investigative tool. Today, 25 years after its introduction, the acid perfusion test still remains the best screening test for gastroesophageal reflux disease.

From Castell DO, Wu WC, Ott DJ (eds): *Gastroesophageal Reflux Disease: Pathogenesis, Diagnosis, Therapy.* Mount Kisco, NY, Futura Publishing Co., Inc., 1985.

Test Format

The acid perfusion test was developed because of the need for a reliable method for the reproduction of esophageal pain in order to differentiate it from angina pectoris. Since 1946, regurgitation of acid pepsin had been generally accepted as a factor in causing esophagitis.[2] Therefore, it seemed reasonable to presume that bathing the esophageal mucosa with an irritant such as acid might produce pain only when inflammation is present. Knowing of the inconsistent results of previous investigators who used small amounts of acid over short periods, Lionel Bernstein and Lyle Baker decided to prolong the administration of acid into the esophagus by use of a continuous infusion. The experience with such a test was the basis of their initial report in 1958.[1]

As originally described, the acid perfusion test was performed with the patient sitting upright in a chair with a nasogastric tube placed 30 to 35 cm from the nares. The tube was positioned over one shoulder and connected to the test solutions behind the patient so that changes in solutions could be made unknown to the subject. Normal saline (0.9% NaCl) was administered for a control period of 15 to 30 minutes at a rate of 100 to 120 drops (6 ml to 7.4 ml) per minute. The control solution was followed by a similar administration of the test solution, 0.1 N HCl. The acid was administered for a full 30 minutes, or until symptoms were produced. The test was considered positive if delivery of the 0.1 N HCl solution elicited pain or burning consistent with the patients' subjective complaints. Transient, momentary symptoms were disregarded. A positive test elicited symptoms that were persistent and usually progressive in severity as long as the administration of acid was continued.

The location of the patient's pain and burning was considered to be critical in the original description of the acid perfusion test. Prior balloon distension studies had indicated that midline pain and burning extending above the level of the xiphoid should not be considered to be of gastric, duodenal, or small bowel origin, and therefore was presumably of esophageal origin.[1] Less classic symptoms could originate from the stomach, and further differentiating tests were required. Rapid disappearance of symptoms within one or two minutes after cessation of acid infusion and/or antacid administration was interpreted as confirming an esophageal origin of the symptoms. Repetitive reproduction and relief of symptoms by small amounts of acid and antacids further supported the diagnosis. Occasionally, atypical pain initiated by esophageal acid administration persisted for an hour or more despite cessation of acid and ingestion of antacids. In such uncommon cases, the patients were restudied on the following day with a tube placed in the stomach and 0.1 N HCl delivered at the same rate as into the esophagus. If this maneuver did not cause pain, but a repeat esophageal test immediately thereafter elicited the symptoms, the esophageal origin of the symptoms were accepted.

Over the subsequent years, the acid perfusion test has been modified by different investigators, but its basic components and simplicity prevail. With few exceptions,[3,4] the test is initiated by the perfusion of isotonic saline, but the duration of the perfusion may range from 5 to 30 minutes and the volume of instilled saline varies. Acid concentrations are the same, but the total volume of HCl (30 ml to 300 ml), the perfusion rate (3 ml to 7.5 ml per minute) and duration of infusion (10 to 30 minutes) have varied. The test is frequently done in the supine position in order to monitor esophageal motility during the acid perfusion. Recently, it has also become common practice to include relief of acid-induced symptoms by normal saline as a criterion for a positive acid perfusion test,[5,6] although this was not part of the original test.

Sensitivity and Specificity

The initial report by Bernstein and Baker stated that 19 of 22 patients with gastroesophageal reflux had a positive test, whereas 20 of 21 controls had a negative test resulting in a study sensitivity of 86% and specificity of 95%.[1] Over the last 25 years, subsequent studies have continued to find a high degree of clinical correlation. As summarized in Table 1, a review of seven series[1,3-5,7-9] which included control subjects found a sensitivity ranging between 42% and 100% and a specificity between 50% and 100%. Combining the total patients in these individual studies reveals that the acid perfusion test can be expected to have an overall sensitivity of 77% and specificity of 86%. Benz and associates[9] concluded that the acid perfusion test showed the greatest degree of correlation with reflux symptoms compared with other standard esophageal tests, including the acid reflux test, measurement of lower esophageal sphincter pressure, and the acid barium swallow. The relationship between endoscopic esophagitis and a positive acid perfusion test is questionable. Battle[3] reported an excellent correlation with the degree of esophagitis. Only 33% of patients with grade 1 esophagitis had a positive acid perfusion test while 75% with grade 4 esophagitis had a positive test. Other investigators[7,8,10,11] have failed to find any significant relationship between esophagitis and a positive response

Table 1.
Acid Perfusion Test (A Summary of
Published Clinical Experiences*)

Author/Ref	Patients with GERD (%+)		Controls (%+)		Sensitivity (%)	Specificity (%)
Bernstein[1]	19/22	(86)	1/21	(5)	86	95
Siegel[7]	25/25	(100)	0/25	(0)	100	100
Bennett[8]	28/29	(97)	6/15	(40)	97	60
Benz[9]	29/29	(100)	3/21	(14)	100	86
Battle[3]	37/89	(42)	0/24	(0)	42	100
Behar[5]	68/77	(88)	3/20	(15)	88	85
Breen[4]	23/27	(85)	7/14	(50)	85	50
Total	229/298	(77)	20/140	(14)	77	86

*Only studies with control subjects

to acid perfusion. Thus the acid perfusion test assesses esophageal acid sensitivity only and is not a test for esophagitis. Attempts to modify the test by increasing the infusion rate or administering the study in the supine position have not increased its sensitivity. Several groups[4,8] have observed that reflux patients usually become symptomatic early in the course of acid infusion, frequently within 7 to 15 minutes, whereas false positive studies are characterized by later symptoms. A shorter acid perfusion time may increase the specificity of the acid perfusion test to near 100%, but will also markedly decrease its sensitivity.

The failure to include certain components of gastric contents (pepsin, bile, pancreatic enzymes) in the perfusate may account for some of the negative results in subjects with symptoms of gastroesophageal reflux disease. Animal and human experiments have confirmed that bile and pepsin may further intensify the damaging effect of hydrogen ions on the esophageal mucosal barrier.[12,13] Some patients have symptoms that cannot be provoked by acid, but which are reproduced by perfusion with alkali.[14] False negative results also may occur in some patients with severe hemorrhagic esophagitis[5] or distal esophageal strictures.[15] False positive results are seen in approximately 15% of asymptomatic subjects. A preliminary report suggests these subjects may have abnormal nocturnal acid clearance.[16] Others have reported false positive tests in patients with duodenal ulcers associated with gastritis.[17]

Etiology of Symptoms

Pain in reflux esophagitis may be associated with alteration of both the motility and acidity of the esophagus, yet the causal relationship of these changes has not been established. Pain may result from several factors: contact of acid with the damaged esophageal mucosa, increased muscular activity, or a combination, i.e., acid-induced muscle spasm.

Siegel and Hendrix[7] found that motility changes accompanied pain in patients with a positive acid perfusion test. All 25 patients with histologic evidence of gastroesophageal reflux disease had an abnormal motility study during acid infusion, characterized by either increased amplitude and duration, simultaneous or spontaneous contractions, or increased esophageal tone. Only four asymptomatic control subjects had an abnormal motility study; two with acid alone and two with both acid and saline. Other investigators[18,19] using similar manometric equipment could not demonstrate any consistent relationship between pain and motility abnormalities. Atkinson and Bennett[18] found that acid perfusion increased the incidence of nonperistaltic contractions, but this correlated with pain in only 4 of 28 patients with a positive acid perfusion test. They also noted that sodium bicarbonate decreased pain without altering esophageal motility while anti-cholinergic drugs inhibited motor activity but did not significantly decrease the pain sensation. Tuttle et al[19] failed to find any motility abnormalities in reflux patients during either acid perfusion tests or spontaneous reflux episodes. Acid and saline infusions in the supine position did increase intra-esophageal pressures, but this was attributed to the volume of the liquid rather than any specific chemical properties of the solutions. Tuttle concluded that differences in techniques could account for the differences in reported findings. Siegel and Hendrix studied their patients in the supine position, while the other investigations were done in the sitting position. In the upright patient, it seems possible that infused fluids flow rapidly into the stomach without a sufficient volume remaining in the esophagus to produce detectable distension and possibly motor abnormalities. Conversely, in subjects examined while supine, accumulation of infused fluids might reasonably be expected to cause a higher elevation in intra-esophageal pressures and thereby produce esophageal distension and motility abnormalities.

Recent studies with modern low compliance, low volume pneumohydraulic perfusion systems have also failed to define any relationship between esophageal motility abnormalities and the production of pain with intra-esophageal acid. In our laboratory, we have studied 17 reflux patients with endoscopic esophagitis and a positive pain response to acid perfusion and 17 age-matched controls with a negative acid perfusion study.[20] In neither group were any significant changes observed in amplitude or duration of esophageal contractions during acid perfusion (Figure 1). A significant decrease in velocity was observed in both groups during acid infusion probably as a result of increased intra-esophageal fluid volume. Simultaneous contractions were not noted, while three patients and two control subjects had repetitive contractions during acid perfusion. Venturatos and colleagues,[21] in a similar study, reported that acid infusion had no significant effect on amplitude or velocity of peristaltic contractions, and did not increase the incidence of tertiary or simultaneous contractions in control and reflux subjects. Acid perfusion did, however, result in increased duration of peristaltic contractions, but the change was similar in both studied groups.

Considering all of the studies discussed above, the majority of evidence suggests that the symptoms of a positive acid perfusion test are not the result of an acid-induced esophageal motility disorder. Gastroesophageal reflux certainly *may* cause esophageal motility

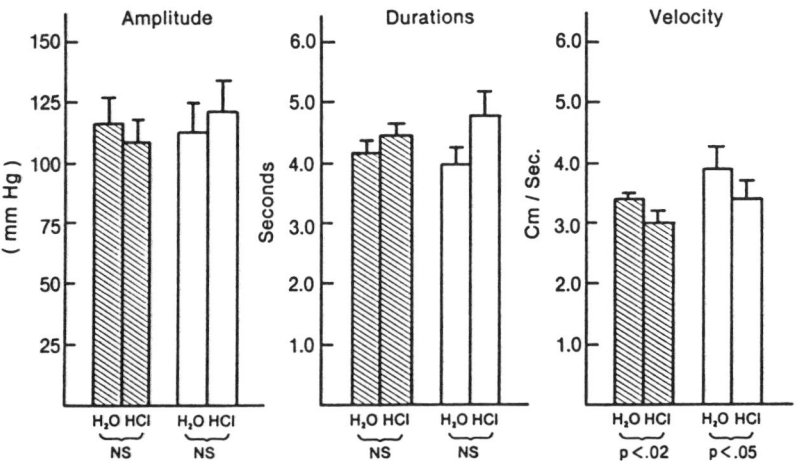

Figure 1: *Changes in mean distal amplitude, duration, and velocity of peristaltic contractions in 17 control subjects and 17 reflux patients during water and acid perfusion. Shaded bars represent reflux patients and open bars represent the control group. Each bar represents $\bar{x} \pm$ SEM. Acid perfusion did not significantly change distal amplitude or duration in either group. Acid perfusion significantly slows velocity of peristaltic contractions in both groups to a similar degree.*

disorders—especially diffuse spasm—but it is an uncommon clinical association.[22]

Intra-esophageal acid, therefore, appears to be the precipitating stimulus for the heartburn and pain during the acid perfusion test. It has become common practice to include relief of acid-induced symptoms by normal saline as a criterion for a positive acid perfusion test.[5,6] This clinical adage has been questioned by a recent study by Winnan and colleagues.[23] They report that 52% of patients with reflux esophagitis and acid-induced heartburn did not obtain relief by cessation of acid and institution of a saline infusion. Relief of pain was also not dependent on either elevation of esophageal pH above 4 or the use of antacids (Figure 2). This study suggests that once hydrogen ions have penetrated the surface epithelium, the degree of pain relief may be a complex phenomenon involving a patient's tolerance of heartburn and pain, the efficiency of the esophageal clearance mechanism, and the sensory nerve thresholds beneath the superficial

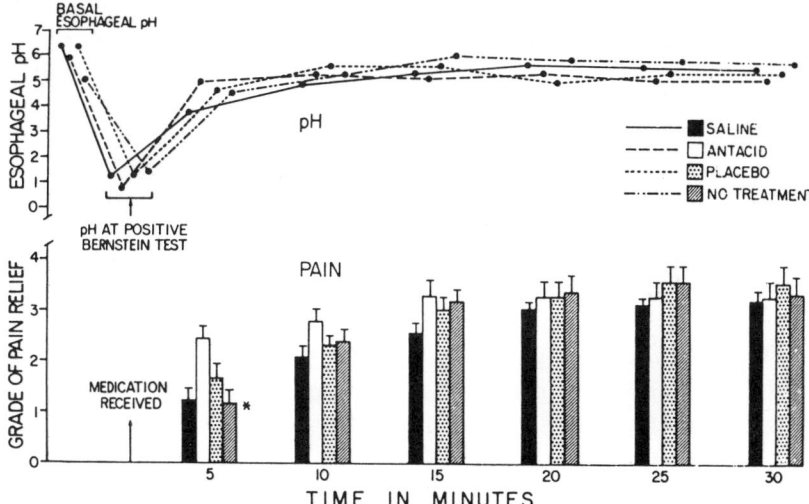

Figure 2: *Esophageal pH and chest pain relief (mean ± SEM) observed in six patients who received an esophageal saline infusion, ingested 30 cc of either antacid or an antacid-placebo, or had no treatment for a positive Bernstein test. Esophageal pH was recorded basally and during the induction of chest pain by acid infusion. The grade of relief of the chest pain and the corresponding esophageal pH are represented at 5-min intervals for 30 min after the treatments were administered. Asterisk (*) refers to 5-min period when antacid resulted in significantly better relief than no treatment. Reproduced by permission from Winnan GR, Meyer CT, McCallum RW: A reappraisal of criteria for the interpretation of the Bernstein test.* Ann Intern Med *1982; 96:320–322.*

layers of esophageal mucosa.[24] Thus, whereas reproduction of pain and heartburn by acid perfusion may be a reliable test, the relief of pain is not.

Clinical Application

It must be remembered that the acid perfusion test only demonstrates the sensitivity of the distal esophagus to acid. It is not a test for esophagitis and does not actually measure acid reflux. The test is designed to deliberately produce a symptom (heartburn, pain) known to be esophageal in origin that the patient can compare with symptoms he or she experiences spontaneously. If the acid perfusion test is positive particularly early in the infusion, one can be certain that the symptoms are esophageal in origin. A negative test, however, does not exonerate the esophagus.

Overall, the acid perfusion test is the best screening study to determine if thoracic symptoms are the result of gastroesophageal reflux disease. Patients with classic reflux symptoms do not routinely need an acid perfusion test. After an upper gastrointestinal series to exclude complicated reflux disease and peptic ulcers, treatment could be initiated with simple lifestyle modifications and antacids. The acid perfusion test should, however, be the first investigative test in patients who do not respond to simple medical therapy or in whom the diagnosis of reflux disease is not clear.[25] The acid perfusion test is particularly useful in patients with multiple or atypical chest symptoms. These individuals present to the gastroenterologist frequently after an extensive negative cardiac work-up including coronary angiography. Despite negative tests, these patients still often fear their symptoms represent an evasive form of angina pectoris. In these cases, the reproduction of symptoms during intra-esophageal acid perfusion can be both diagnostic and therapeutic. In our laboratory, we therefore combine the acid perfusion test with other provocative studies during our evaluation of non-cardiac chest pain. The acid perfusion test has been positive in approximately 10% of these patients in whom provocative testing elicited their atypical symptoms.[26] Similar results have been reported by other laboratories.[27,28]

The simplicity and safety of the acid perfusion tests makes it particularly applicable to the physician with a busy clinical practice. The test is essentially without hazards. Acid perfusion does not induce esophagitis or produce bleeding. A positive test is no more harmful than a spontaneous episode of reflux. The test is simple, rapid, does not require special equipment, and can be easily administered in the office without special personnel and with minimal patient discomfort. The high degree of sensitivity and specificity of the acid perfusion test combined with its practicality and low cost currently make it the ideal screening test for gastroesophageal reflux disease.

References

1. Bernstein LM, Baker LA: A clinical test for esophagitis. *Gastroenterology* 1958; 34:760–781.
2. Allison PR: Peptic ulcer of the esophagus. *J Thorac Surg* 1946; 15: 308–315.
3. Battle WS, Nyhus LM, Bombeck GT: Gastroesophageal reflux: Diagnosis and treatment. *Ann Surg* 1973; 177:560–565.
4. Breen KJ, Whelan G: The diagnosis of reflux oesophagitis: An evaluation of five investigative procedures. *Aust NZ J Surg* 1978; 49:156–161.
5. Behar J, Biancani P, Sheahan DG: Evaluation of esophageal tests in the diagnosis of reflux esophagitis. *Gastroenterology* 1976; 71:9–15.
6. Fisher RS, Cohen S: Gastroesophageal reflux. *Med Clin North Am* 1978; 62(1):3–20.
7. Siegel CI, Hendrix TR: Esophageal motor abnormalities induced by acid perfusion in patients with heartburn. *JCI* 1963; 42:686–695.
8. Bennett JR, Atkinson M: Oesophageal acid perfusion in the diagnosis of precordial pain. *Lancet* 1966; 2:1150–1152.
9. Benz LJ, Hootkin LA, Marguiles S, Donner MW, Cauthorne RT, Hendrix TR: A comparison of clinical measurements of gastroesophageal reflux. *Gastroenterology* 1972; 62:1–5.
10. Skinner DB, Booth DJ: Assessment of distal esophageal function in patients with hiatal hernia and/or gastroesophageal reflux. *Ann Surg* 1970; 172:627–637.
11. Clark J, Moosa AR, Skinner DB: Pitfalls in the performance and interpretation of esophageal function tests. *Surg Clin North Am* 1976; 56(1): 29–37.
12. Safaie–Shirazi S, DenBesten L, Zike WL: Effect of bile salts on the ionic permeability of the esophageal mucosa and their role in the production of esophagitis. *Gastroenterology* 1975; 68:722–733.
13. Lillemoe KD, Johnson LF, Harmon JW: Role of the components of the gastroduodenal contents in experimental acid esophagitis. *Surgery* 1982; 92:276–284.
14. Pellegrini CA, DeMeester TR, Wernly JA, Johnson LF, Skinner DB: Alkaline gastroesophageal reflux. *Am J Surg* 1978; 135:177–184.
15. Volpicelli NA, Bedine MS, Hendrix TR: Absence of acid sensitivity in patients with benign peptic esophageal strictures. *Gastroenterology* 1975; 68:A-150/1007.
16. Orr WC, Robinson WG, Johnson LF: Esophageal mucosal sensitivity in asymptomatic controls. *Gastroenterology* 1983; 84(2):1266A.

17. Moraes–Filho JP, Bettarello A: Lack of specificity of the acid perfusion test in duodenal ulcer patients. *Dig Dis Sci* 1974; 19:785–790.
18. Atkinson M, Bennett JR: Relationship between motor changes and pain during esophageal acid perfusion. *Am J Dig Dis* 1968; 13:346–350.
19. Tuttle SG, Rufin F, Bettarello A: The physiology of heartburn. *Ann Intern Med* 1961; 55:292–300.
20. Richter JE, Johns DN, Wu WC, Castell DO: Are esophageal motility abnormalities produced during intraesophageal acid perfusion (Bernstein) test? *Clin Res* 1983; 31:837A.
21. Venturatos SG, Burns TW, Neighbors BT: Gastroesophageal reflux: Are motility changes related to symptoms? *Gastroenterology* 1983; 84(2): 1342A.
22. Swamy N: Esophageal spasm: Clinical and manometric response to nitroglycerine and long acting nitrates. *Gastroenterology* 1977; 72: 23–27.
23. Winnan GR, Meyer CT, McCallum RW: Interpretation of the Bernstein test: A reappraisal of criteria. *Ann Intern Med* 1982; 96:320–322.
24. Hookman P, Siegel CI, Hendrix TR: Failure of oxethazaine to alter acid-induced esophageal pain. *Am J Dig Dis* 1966; 11:811–813.
25. Richter JE, Castell DO: Gastroesophageal reflux: Pathogenesis, diagnosis and treatment. *Ann Intern Med* 1982; 97:93–103.
26. Wu WC, Hackshaw BT, Richter JE, Castell DO: Esophageal manometry with provocative testing in patients with non-cardiac chest pain. *Gastroenterology* 1984; 86:1303A.
27. Brand DL, Martin D, Pope CE II: Esophageal manometrics in patients with angina-like chest pain. *Dig Dis Sci* 1977; 24:300–304.
28. Alban Davies H, Jones DB, Rhoades J: Esophageal angina as the cause of chest pain. *JAMA* 1982; 248:2274–2278.

10

Endoscopy and Biopsy

Kim R. Geisinger, M.D., * *and*
Wallace C. Wu, M.B., B.S.

Chapter Contents

*Dr. Geisinger is an American Cancer Society Junior Faculty Clinical Fellow.

From Castell DO, Wu WC, Ott DJ (eds): *Gastroesophageal Reflux Disease: Pathogenesis, Diagnosis, Therapy.* Mount Kisco, NY, Futura Publishing Co., Inc., 1985.

Fiberoptic endoscopy and barium esophagram are probably the most widely used diagnostic techniques in the diagnosis and management of gastroesophageal reflux disease (GERD). Unfortunately, significant limitations exist when endoscopy is used alone. The sensitivity and specificity of the examination can be improved considerably if esophageal biopsies are routinely performed. This chapter will discuss the use, limitation, and role of fiberoptic endoscopy and esophageal biopsies in GERD.

Endoscopy

Introduction

Barium esophagram, endoscopy, and esophageal biopsy are the only methods available to detect directly esophageal mucosal injury. Since most patients with symptoms of GERD do not have significant mucosal injury, endoscopy is clearly not indicated in all patients. Endoscopy is worthwhile in patients with atypical symptoms or non-cardiac chest pain, when complications of GERD are suspected, prior to proposed anti-reflux surgery, and to exclude other lesions of the esophagus, stomach, and duodenum.

Instrumentation

Any modern fiberoptic panendoscope will provide satisfactory visualization of the esophageal mucosa. However, if biopsies are to be performed, instruments with biopsy channels less than 2.8 mm in diameter should be avoided. Larger channels will allow biopsies of adequate size for pathological interpretations.

Current trends with endoscopic equipment are to make the diameter of the endoscope smaller, meanwhile maintaining the other capabilities of the instrument. These "skinny" endoscopes improve patient tolerance, minimize the amount of premedication needed, and facilitate outpatient endoscopy, without the use of sedation. Although not proven, these small caliber instruments may be less sensitive than the standard panendoscopes in the detection of esophageal strictures and lower esophageal rings. It is certainly conceivable that a 7.8 mm instrument can pass through a 10 mm peptic stricture without detecting any signs of obstruction. The absence of endoscopic evidence of esophagitis with some esophageal strictures makes their detection by the "skinny" instruments even more difficult.

Therefore, if small caliber panendoscopes are used, the endoscopic information must be correlated with the clinical history and barium esophagram before the diagnosis of peptic esophageal stricture secondary to GERD is excluded.

Endoscopy in GERD

Most patients with classic symptoms of GERD will not require endoscopy. However, in combination with esophageal biopsies, endoscopy can be an extremely useful tool in the diagnosis and management of patients with complicated GERD. Endoscopy is very useful in excluding other lesions of the esophagus, stomach, and duodenum that mimic GERD. It is also indicated in patients with suspected complications of GERD, such as erosive esophagitis, stricture formation, and Barrett's esophagus. Herpes and monilial esophagitis are being diagnosed with increasing frequency, particularly in immunosuppressed patients. Endoscopy with biopsy, cytology, and cultures are critical in differentiating these conditions from reflux esophagitis. Selected patients with non-cardiac chest pain may also require endoscopy to elucidate the cause of their symptoms. Furthermore, it is indicated to rule out neoplastic disease in patients with peptic stricture and Barrett's esophagus. Patients who have not responded to standard medical therapy and are being considered for surgical treatment should undergo both endoscopy and manometry.

The role of hiatal hernia in the pathogenesis of GERD is controversial and is discussed in Chapter 3. Most authorities consider that its role is permissive since GERD is rare in the absence of a hiatal hernia. Therefore, it may be important to demonstrate the presence or absence of hiatal hernia. Endoscopically, a hiatal hernia is diagnosed when the gastroesophageal junction is 2 cm or more above the diaphragmatic opening.[1,2] Johnson et al noted that the endoscopic presence of hiatal hernia alone correlated poorly with abnormal pH reflux testing. However, if its presence is combined with endoscopic esophagitis or a patulous diaphragmatic hiatus, the correlation is excellent.[2]

It has been stated that the presence of spontaneous reflux of gastric contents in a well sedated patient during an endoscopic examination is always pathological.[1] Unfortunately, this has never been documented. Johnson et al[2], however, had noted that a patulous diaphragmatic opening in association with a hiatal hernia or endoscopic evidence of esophagitis may be associated with GERD. They defined a patulous opening by the following criteria: (a) the proximal stomach could be viewed through the hiatus from the distal esophagus (antegrade view), or (b) when retrograde flexion of the instrument during gastroscopy showed a patulous diaphragmatic hiatus around the endoscope (retrograde view).

A number of endoscopic criteria have been proposed in the diagnosis of reflux esophagitis. Unfortunately, some of these signs are not well defined, and many are also subject to intra- and interobserver variation. Because of the difficulties with these diagnostic criteria, especially in early or minimal esophagitis, endoscopy is relatively insensitive in the evaluation of GERD. In fact, only 54% of patients with reflux documented by pH reflux studies have mucosal abnormalities endoscopically.[2] Fortunately, except in patients who smoke heavily, endoscopic esophagitis is quite specific for GERD.

Normal esophageal mucosa has a pinkish, pearly-white color, which contrasts with the salmon color of gastric mucosa. Therefore, the gastroesophageal mucosal junction is usually sharply defined and minimally irregular. It should not be more than 2 cm above the diaphragmatic hiatus; otherwise a hiatal hernia is present. Occasionally, the junction may be detected in the esophageal body, which should raise the possibility of Barrett's esophagus. An irregular and indistinct squamocolumnar junction is regarded by some to be an early, reliable objective finding in GERD.[1,3]

In the normal esophagus, there is usually a pattern of fine, tiny, linearly arranged blood vessels extending up to 3 cm above the GE junction in close proximity to each other. Proximal to this area, vessels are less numerous and tend to be less prominent. Loss of this fine vascular pattern is considered by some as one of the earliest endoscopic signs of GERD.[1,4,5] This is presumably due to edema of the mucosa obscuring the normal vascular pattern. This mechanism may also account for the indistinct GE junction described above. However, Johnson and Sladen independently found both signs to be poor criteria for esophagitis.[2,6] Erythema of the esophageal mucosa is affected by the types of instrument and light source used and is therefore a very unreliable sign of esophagitis.

Friability and granularity of the esophageal mucosa are probably less subject to observer variation than all the other early signs of esophagitis. Therefore, it is not surprising that all patients with these findings in one series had abnormal results in either a standard acid reflux test or an abnormal 24-hour pH monitoring.[2] In another report, nodularity was found in 15 of 57 patients with GERD and in none of the 10 controls.[4] However, granularity and nodularity of the lower esophagus need to be distinguished from glycogenic acanthosis, which does not appear to be related to GERD.

Erosions on the esophageal surface may be linear or punctate in appearance. They are characterized by a white center of adherent mucus surrounded by a red halo, and are considered as pathognomonic of GERD.[1] However, erosions have been found in some heavy cigarette smokers without evidence of reflux.[2] Erosions from GERD also need to be differentiated from those in monilial esophagitis. In general, monilial erosions have a more extensive mucous coating and tend to extend more proximally. Biopsy and cytology may be required to differentiate the two.

Esophageal ulcers are usually seen as white areas of variable shape and size with borders of erythema. It may be difficult to differentiate them from an erosion. Its presence not only signifies severe esophagitis but also raises the possibility of complications of GERD such as stricture and Barrett's esophagus. Again, biopsy, cytology, and cultures may be required to exclude neoplastic disease and infectious esophagitis.

Peptic esophageal stricture and Barrett's esophagus are discussed more fully in Chapters 16 and 17 of this monograph, respectively. Since neoplasm needs to be excluded in these patients, endoscopy and biopsy play an important role in the diagnosis and management of these patients with complications of GERD.

Endoscopy is clearly a useful tool in the diagnosis, management, and follow-up of selected patients with GERD. It is particularly useful in excluding other diseases that may mimic GERD and its complications. Unfortunately, since a significant number of patients with reflux may have normal endoscopy, and since more endoscopic signs of early esophagitis remain unsubstantiated and subject to observer bias, its role in the routine work-up and management of all patients with GERD remains limited.

Endoscopic Biopsy

Since Ismail-Beigi et al published their histologic criteria for gastroesophageal reflux using suction biopsies obtained with the Rubin tube,[7] it has been generally accepted that biopsies must be performed by this method to use their criteria. Unfortunately, this equipment is not widely available. Using it also involves the passage of another instrument in addition to the endoscope. Hence, most esophageal biopsies are still performed with the pinch biopsy forceps through the endoscope. These biopsies are then usually processed in the routine manner and without orientation. They provide minimal information except in advanced esophagitis. Johnson et al first evaluated pinch biopsies mounted on gel foam to assist with orientation.[8] They found these biopsies to be satisfactory. Subsequently, three studies comparing both techniques have shown suction biopsies to be clearly superior.[9-11] This is not surprising since suction biopsy provides more tissue for pathological interpretation. In our own experience, pinch biopsies are satisfactory provided that they are oriented and processed properly. All illustrations in this chapter are from oriented pinch biopsies performed through the standard endoscope. Therefore, oriented pinch biopsies still have a role in the diagnosis of GERD.

Pathology of GERD

Introduction

For more than a decade, a controversy has revolved about the histopathologic criteria for the diagnosis of reflux esophagitis in biopsy specimens. This debate has, for the most part, weighed the merits of inflammatory cell infiltrates versus reactive epithelial changes as to their reliability and sensitivity as markers of acid-induced esophageal injury. Several factors have contributed to this lack of agreement. First, the clinical parameters used to determine whether or not an individual has gastroesophageal reflux have demonstrated significant variation among the published studies. The spectrum has ranged from symptoms of heartburn to the use of 24-hour intra-esophageal pH monitoring to document reflux. The methods by which the biopsies have been evaluated have also differed. In some investigations, the alterations in the esophageal mucosa have been meticulously quantitated with ocular micrometers and other means and the measurements subjected to statistical analyses. In others, the simpler yet more subjective "visual" estimation of pathologic changes has been utilized. The numbers and sites of biopsies have also shown considerable heterogeneity. Even the histologic appearance of the normal esophagus has been questioned (Figure 1).[12]

Histology of Acute Reflux Esophagitis

Inflammatory Cell Infiltrates

The presence of various types of inflammatory cells, especially segmented leukocytes, in the mucosa was the major criterion used to

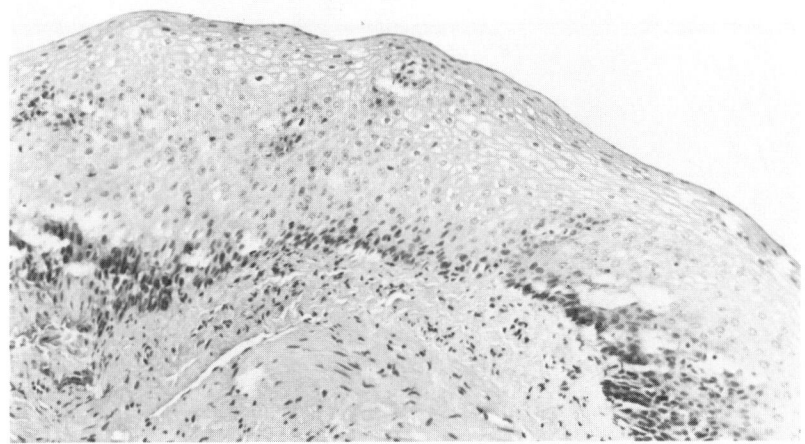

Figure 1: *The normal stratified squamous epithelium of the esophagus matures in an orderly fashion with the basal cells confined to the deepest layer and is without inflammation (× 100).*

define esophagitis in early studies, such as Palmer's communication.[13] Yardley stated that the presence of acute inflammatory cell infiltrates was a rather specific yet insensitive indicator of reflux esophagitis.[14] This was confirmed by Behar and Sheahan who reported the presence of neutrophils in 5% and 40% of patients with mild and severe esophagitis, respectively, but their absence in normal controls.[15] However, neither report specifically stated whether such infiltrates were within the squamous epithelium, the underlying lamina propria, or both. Seefeld and colleagues claimed that granulocytic infiltrates of the lamina propria were the most prominent alteration of esophagitis, being present solely in those with disease;[16] however, only 29% with reflux had such infiltrates. Ismail-Beigi et al found neutrophils in the lamina propria of 16% of their reflux patients, but none in controls.[7] Recently, it has been stated that the presence of acute and chronic inflammatory cells of all types in the lamina propria of the esophagus should be considered as normal and that the only significant exudative finding on biopsy is segmented white blood cells within the stratified squamous epithelium.[17] Thus, according to this declaration the interpretation of the earlier reports' data concerning inflammatory infiltrates may not be valid.

Goldman and his co-workers have championed intra-epithelial eosinophils as a rather sensitive and specific marker for esophagitis (Figure 2).[17,18] In their study of children with reflux, 39% had these elements within their esophageal epithelium, but the normal children

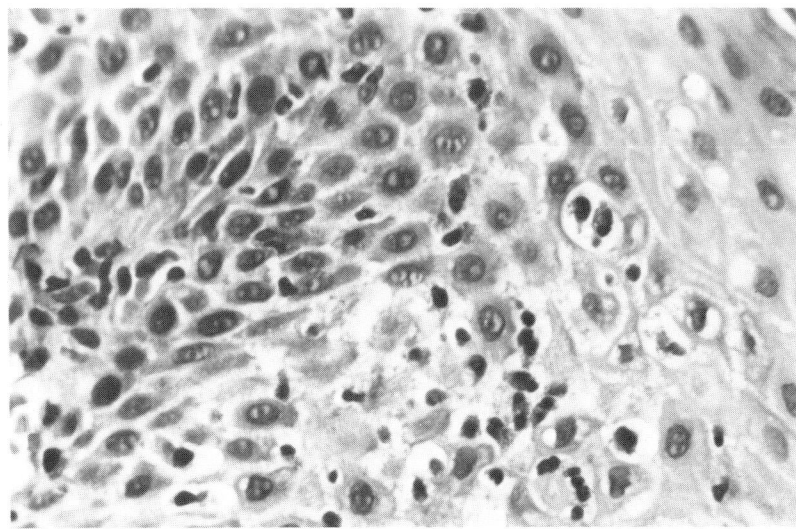

Figure 2: *Numerous segmented leukocytes, predominately eosinophils, are scattered throughout the epithelium (× 400).*

did not.[18] Neutrophils coexisted in the epithelium in slightly more than one-fourth of these children and were present in two of the patients who did not have intra-epithelial eosinophils. This tissue marker is valuable for several reasons. It does not require that a significant volume of lamina propria be included in the biopsy specimen, making the more commonly used pinch biopsies essentially as adequate as the larger suction biopsies for this interpretation. Furthermore, optimal orientation of the specimen prior to sectioning for histology is much less crucial. This criterion is also applicable to the diagnosis of reflux in adults, although no systematic investigation has been reported in older patients. Unfortunately, it is not highly sensitive, being present in less than half of reflux patients, and in some cases numerous histologic sections need to be examined for their detection. If this diagnostic criterion is expanded to include both neutrophils and/or eosinophils within the epithelium, increased sensitivity would result. This should allow for a histologic confirmation of reflux esophagitis in a larger percentage of patients and with fewer sections required per patient.

Reactive Epithelial Changes

In 1970, Ismail-Beigi et al published the results of their investigation of the histologic features of reflux esophagitis.[7] Their conclusions proclaimed that the changes in the squamous epithelium itself, rather than the inflammatory cell infiltrates, were the key to the diagnosis of this condition. The two major alterations were hyperplasia of the basal cells resulting in a thickening of this cellular zone and elongation of the vascular connective tissue papillae so that the lamina propria extended to within a few epithelial cell layers of the lumen. They stated that both the hyperplasia and the elongation may be due to an accelerated rate of exfoliation of squamous cells. In a subsequent study, they found that these changes occurred with a patchy distribution and were located anywhere from 2–8 cm proximal to the lower esophageal sphincter.[19]

Basal cells are characterized by a lack of differentiation, having a scanty rim of basophilic cytoplasm surrounding the nucleus. Their cytoplasm lacks significant quantities of glycogen and thus can be differentiated histochemically from the overlying, more mature squamous cells.[17] In the normal esophagus, Ismail-Beigi et al reported the basal cell zone to comprise less than 15% of the total epithelial thickness;[7] in contrast (average) 30% of the epithelium consisted of the basal cell zone in their patients with reflux (Figure 3).[7] These findings have been confirmed by several other groups.[5,8,15,18] Behar and Sheahan reported a slight increase in the mitotic activity of basal

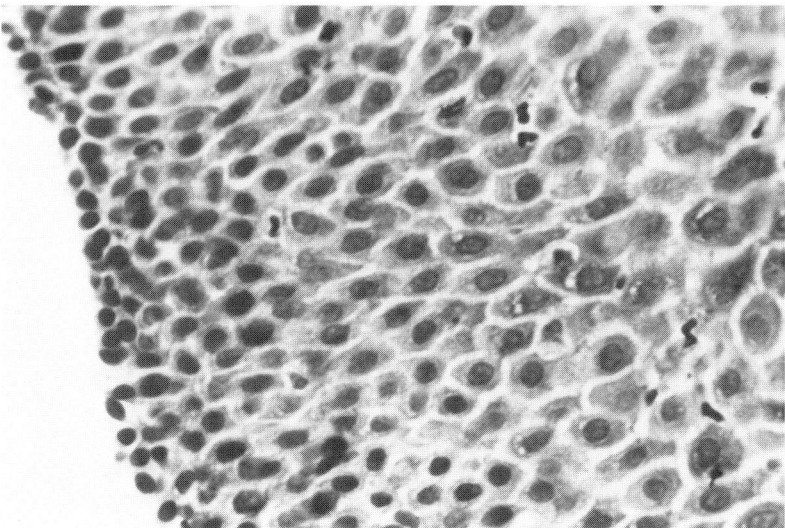

Figure 3: *Basal cell hyperplasia is prominent in this section of inflamed esophageal epithelium with its deepest portion at the left of the photomicrograph (× 400).*

cells with reflux.[15] Thus, when the basal cell zone exceeds 15% or 20% of the epithelium, hyperplasia exists.

The companion to this hyperplasia is the lengthening of the papillae. Ismail-Beigi and co-workers reported that in the normal esophagus, the connective tissue in the lamina propria never penetrates the epithelium to more than two-thirds of its total thickness.[7] Although most would agree that this increased papillary length occurs, others have used different cut-off points (Figures 4−6). Behar and Sheahan, Winter et al, and Kobayaski and Kasugai claimed elongation exists when the papillae extend for more than one-half of the epithelial thickness.[3,15,18] Seefeld et al and Johnson et al used 60% as their upper limit of normal.[7,16] These last two groups were among those utilizing the most quantitative approaches to this histomorphometric analysis. These studies were based on histologic materials in which the plane of sectioning was perpendicular to the mucosa. Most workers claim the need for such optimal orientation for this evaluation, requiring at least a minimum number of papillae be exposed along their entire length. Kobayaski and Kasugai, however, claimed that less perfectly oriented sections could also be used, as they believed that the connective tissue papillae increased in number as well as in length. As a result, horizontal sections reveal this ingrowth of new capillaries into the epithelium as increased numbers of papillary profiles.[14] After constructing imaginary lines perpen-

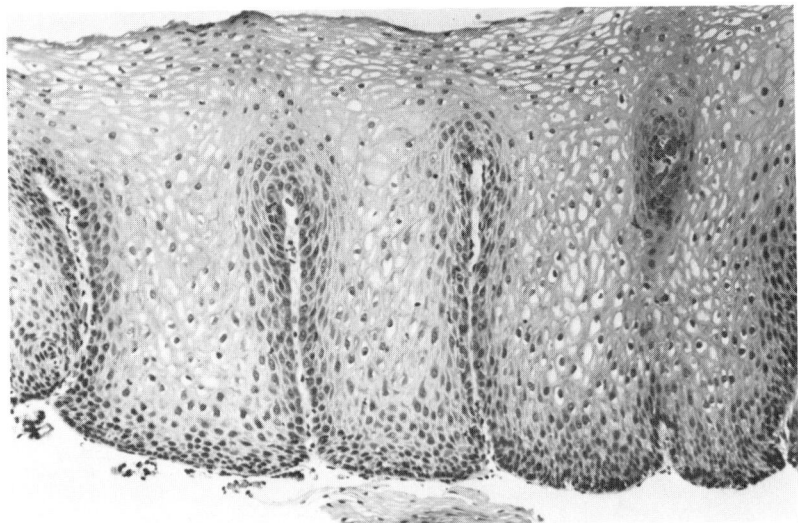

Figure 4: *Papillomatosis is readily evident in this case of reflux esophagitis. Note the lack of inflammatory infiltrates (× 100).*

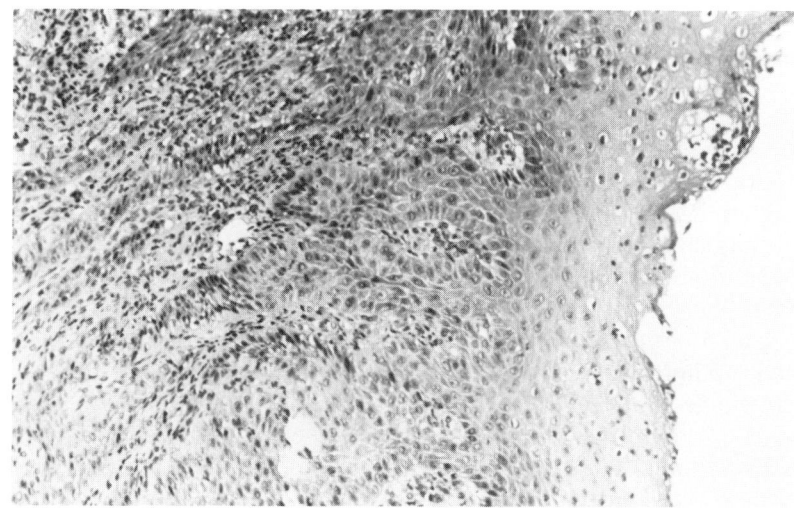

Figure 5: *Infiltration by leukocytes, papillomatosis, and basal cell hyperplasia are all present in this biopsy specimen from a patient with gastroesophageal reflux (× 100).*

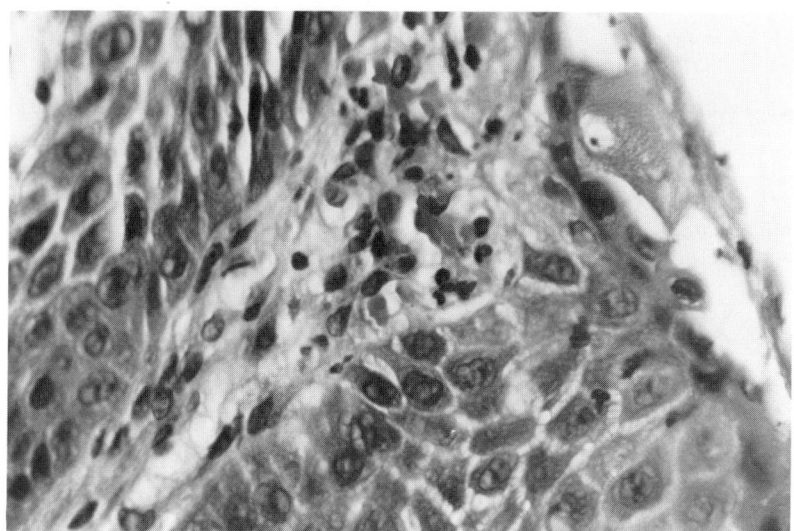

Figure 6: *This vascular connective tissue papilla is separated from the esophageal lumen (upper right hand corner) by a thin layer of epithelial cells (× 400).*

dicular to the epithelium's basement membrane, the profiles were observed; overlapping of the connective tissue papillae on any of these imaginary lines was construed as evidence of reflux esophagitis (Figure 7). In the practical setting, this tenet is useful and does correlate with clinical parameters of esophagitis. Yardley agreed that the number of papillae was increased in reflux esophagitis.[14] Ismail-Beigi et al did not believe this was true.[7]

Johnson et al defined reflux by what is probably the most sensitive and specific assay: intra-esophageal monitoring of pH for 24 hours.[8] They found a direct correlation between papillary height and both a 24-hour pH score and the percentage of time the pH was less than 4. Their relative basal cell hyperplasia also correlated with the percentage of time below pH 4. The overall thickness of the squamous epithelium was the same between their 31 controls and 69 reflux patients. The longer than normal papillae were associated with thinner than normal suprapapillary epithelium in their reflux patients. They hypothesized that the acid-induced injury stimulated a more rapid desquamation which, in turn, provoked a compensatory hyperplasia of the basal cells and thus, elongation of the papillae. Yardley, in addition, suggested that the elongation also may result from a direct proliferation of the lamina propria as papillae.[14]

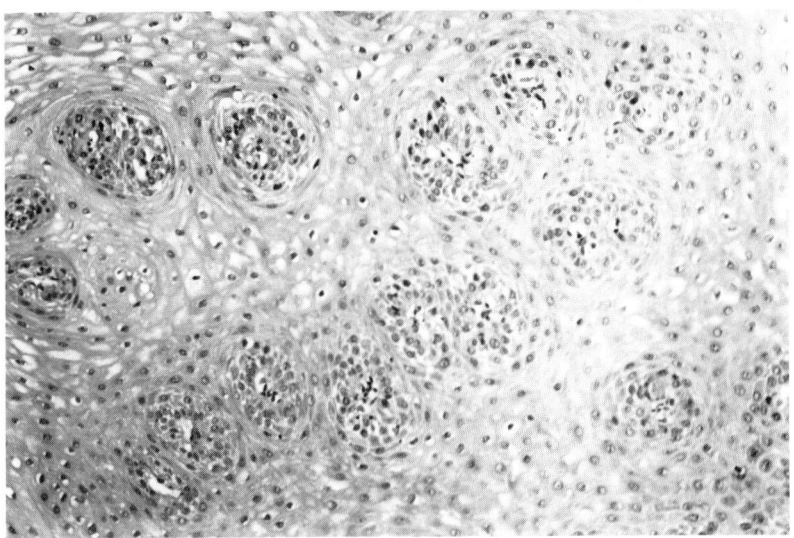

Figure 7: *A greatly increased number of profiles of papillae, as well as a sprinkling of inflammatory cells, are detected in this horizontal section of mucosa (× 100).*

Although the evidence is strongly supportive that these reactive epithelial changes are characteristic of reflux esophagitis, some investigators are not in total agreement. Seefeld et al, for example, compared 24 patients with reflux with 20 controls and found no statistically significant differences in epithelial measurements between the two groups.[16] In addition, they could not demonstrate a correlation between any single epithelial measurement and any function test. However, they did not include long-term intra-esophageal pH measurements in their battery of clinical exams. Weinstein and his co-workers reported the results of their esophageal studies in 19 asymptomatic subjects.[12] Most of them had multiple biopsies taken from the distal 10 cm of the esophagus. When the histologic criteria published by Ismail-Beigi et al[19] were applied to these specimens, nearly 75% of the subjects had at least one biopsy that could be considered abnormal and 27% had three or more abnormal biopsies. Three of the subjects had an abnormal manometry study and two others had a positive infusion test. Yet, their inclusion in the data did not significantly affect the overall statistics. Three-fourths of the abnormal biopsies were located in the distal 2.5 cm of the esophagus. They concluded that their results negated the criteria of Ismail-Beigi et al, at least for biopsies taken from the distal-most portions of the esophagus. However, as recently stated by Fink et al, Weinstein's investigation did not incorporate pH reflux tests and thus did not exclude the possibility of subclinical reflux in their subjects.[10]

Microvascular Alterations

Geboes and colleagues have presented what they believe is a very early histologic feature of reflux esophagitis, namely changes in the superficial vascular supply.[5] In addition to the previously described inflammatory cell infiltrates and reactive epithelial alterations, they detailed changes that included dilatation of the capillaries of the superficial portions of the elongated papillae of lamina propria (Figure 8). In some instances, these vessels lost portions of their endothelial lining, a finding that they confirmed ultrastructurally. As a result, pools of blood were separated by only a few epithelial cell layers from the lumen of the esophagus. Erythrocytes were shown at least focally to contact directly squamous epithelial cells. Furthermore, the number of capillaries in the epithelium was increased.[5] Eight years earlier Yardley had called attention to changes in the blood vessels, referring to this last feature as "vascularized epithelium".[14] Geboes et al detected these changes in 83% of their reflux

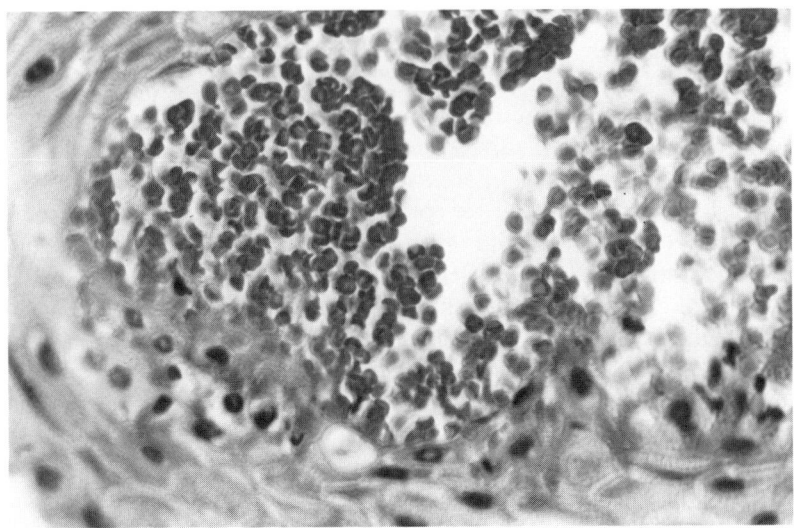

Figure 8: *This greatly distended superficial capillary has lost its endo-thelium, resulting in direct contact of the blood vessel with the squamous epithelium (× 400).*

patients and in only 10% of their controls. They claimed that these vascular phenomena are more closely associated with the endoscopic appearance of the esophageal mucosa in early or mild esophagitis than are the hyperplastic changes of the epithelium. Goldman and Antonioli confirmed this distension and congestion of small blood vessels in the elongated papillae, especially near the luminal surface, as an early alteration in esophagitis.[17] In conjunction with this were focal microhemorrhages. They commented that although endoscopy itself can induce dilatation of blood vessels, it is restricted to the deeper portion of the mucosa in most cases. Thus, properly oriented specimens would be important in the evaluation of this element. They questioned whether or not this vascular dilatation extended the diagnostic specificity more than papillary elongation alone.

Histology of Chronic Reflux Changes

Erosion and Peptic Ulcer

In distinct contrast to the ongoing discussions concerning the alterations in acute and mild esophagitis, the pathologic changes associated with long-standing reflux are agreed upon by all. Denudation of the mucosa may occur to varying depths. When only the more superficial layers of squamous cells are eliminated, the entity is referred to as erosion. When the full thickness of the mucosa including the muscularis mucosae is destroyed by the reflux of gastric contents, an ulcer results. Histologically, these may be indistinguishable from the typical peptic ulcer of the stomach and duodenum. The granulation tissue in the base of the ulcer develops into scar, which may occupy broad zones of submucosa. When the ulcers heal, the submucosal fibrotic reaction persists. According to Sandry, the epithelium that comes to cover the healing ulcer is usually glandular but may be squamous in nature.[20]

Barrett's Esophagus

The most distinctive histologic modification is glandular metaplasia or Barrett's esophagus that may occur in more than 10% of all patients with chronic reflux (Figure 9).[21] The morphologic forms of columnar epithelium that may occur were well defined in the report of Paull et al.[22] They showed that three patterns of metaplasia could be discerned in different patients. A fundic-type epithelium complete

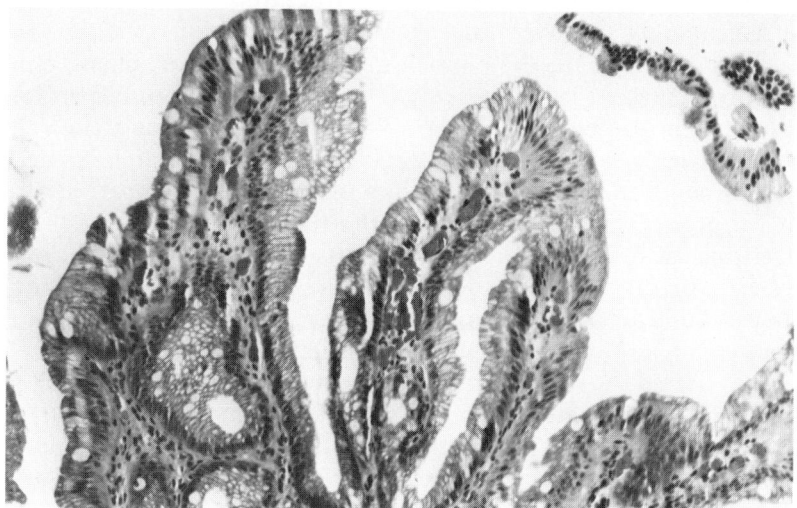

Figure 9: *The villous architecture and alternating goblet cells and absorptive-like cells partially replace the squamous epithelium in this case of Barrett's esophagus (× 100).*

with chief cells and parietal cells with varying degrees of atrophy was found in 5 of their 11 subjects. An epithelium resembling that found in the cardia was detected in 4 patients and was termed junctional-type. They referred to the most common type of columnar epithelium as specialized. This variant, which was present in all but 2 patients, was characterized by a villous-like architecture, mucous glands, and goblet cells. The majority of patients had more than one of these types of glandular mucosa. In these situations, a distinct topographical order was discovered. The fundic-type was always the most distally located in the esophagus and the specialized (intestine-like) assumed the most proximal position. Similar findings were described in a very recent large study of children.[23] However, the relative frequency of the different morphologic patterns differed from that of Paull et al; the fundic epithelium was the most common type detected.

The association of adenocarcinoma and Barrett's esophagus is widely recognized, accounting for the vast majority of primary esophageal adenocarcinomas.[17,21,24] As might be expected, dysplastic changes in the glandular epithelium precede the development of these malignant neoplasms. Kalish et al discovered dysplasia in the glandular mucosa adjacent to adenocarcinomas arising within a Barrett's esophagus in 96% of their cases.[24] Most of these carcinomas produced acid mucosubstances, suggesting their development in the specialized (intestine-like) columnar epithelium.

Fortunately, these terminal events are unusual and rather easy to diagnose histologically. The much more common early changes in reflux may present more difficulty in their recognition. In part, at least, this is the consequence of diverging opinions as to which morphologic features constitute the incipient alterations in esophagitis. In addition, individual patients may actually respond differently to gastroesophageal reflux in that inflammatory infiltrates may constitute the first change in some patients, whereas epithelial hyperplasia or modification in the vasculature may be the earliest in others. Various combinations of these changes are frequently present in patients who come to biopsy. It is this constellation of histologic findings that in the proper clinical setting may be diagnosed as reflux esophagitis. When one or more of these elements are lacking for a given patient, an interpretation of changes consistent with reflux esophagitis may still be rendered with a great deal of certainty.

References

1. Morrissey JF: Endoscopic evaluation of gastroesophageal sphincter dysfunction. *South Med J* 1978; 71:56−61.
2. Johnson LF, DeMeester TR, Haggitt RC: Endoscopic signs for gastroesophageal reflux objectively evaluated. *Gastrointest Endosc* 1976; 22:151−155.
3. Kobayashi S, Kasugai T: Endoscopic and biopsy criteria for the diagnosis of esophagitis with a fiberoptic esophagoscope. *Dig Dis Sci* 1974; 19:345−352.
4. Hattori K, Winans CS, Archer F, Kirsner JB: Endoscopic diagnosis of esophageal inflammation. *Gastrointest Endosc* 1974; 20:102−104.
5. Geboes K, Desmet V, Vantrappen G, Mebis J: Vascular changes in the esophageal mucosa: An early histologic sign of esophagitis. *Gastrointest Endosc* 1980; 26:29−32.
6. Sladen GE, Riddell RH, Willoughby JMT: Oesophagoscopy, biopsy, and acid perfusion test in diagnosis of "reflux oesophagitis." *Br Med J* 1975; 1:71−76.
7. Ismail-Beigi F, Horton PF, Pope CE: Histological consequences of gastroesophageal reflux in man. *Gastroenterology* 1970; 58:163−174.
8. Johnson LF, DeMeester TR, Haggitt RC: Esophageal epithelial response to gastroesophageal reflux. *Dig Dis Sci* 1978; 23:498−509.
9. Komorowski RA, Leinicke JA: Comparison of fiberoptic endoscope and Quinton tube esophageal biopsies in esophagitis. *Gastrointest Endosc* 1978; 24:154−155.
10. Fink SM, Barwick KW, Winchenbach CL, DeLuca V, McCallum RW: Reassessment of esophageal histology in normal subjects; a comparison of suction and endoscopic techniques. *J Clin Gastroenterol* 1983; 5:177−183.
11. Knuff TE, Benjamin SB, Worsham F, Hancock JE, Castell DO: Histologic evaluation of chronic gastroesophageal reflux. An evaluation of biopsy methods and diagnostic criteria. *Dig Dis Sci* 1984; 29:194−201.
12. Weinstein WM, Goboch ER, Bowes KL: The normal human esophageal mucosa; a histologic reappraisal. *Gastroenterology* 1975; 68:40−44.
13. Palmer ED: Subacute erosive ("peptic") esophagitis. *Arch Pathol* 1955; 59:51−57.
14. Yardley JH: Biopsy findings in low-grade reflux esophagitis. In: Skinner DB, Belsey RH, Hendrix TR, Zuidema GD, eds. *Gastroesophageal Reflux and Hiatal Hernia*. Boston: Little, Brown and Co., 1972; 52−58.
15. Behar J, Sheahan DC: Histologic abnormalities in reflux esophagitis. *Arch Pathol* 1975; 99:387−391.
16. Seefeld U, Krejs GJ, Siebenmann RE, Blum AL: Esophageal histology of gastroesophageal reflux. Morphometric findings in suction biopsies. *Am J Dig Dis* 1977; 22:956−964.
17. Goldman H, Antonioli DA: Mucosal biopsy of the esophagus, stomach, and proximal duodenum. *Hum Pathol* 1982; 13:423−448.
18. Winter HS, Madara JL, Stafford RJ, Grand RJ, Quinlah J-E, Goldman H: Intraepithelial eosinophils: A new diagnostic criterion for reflux esophagitis. *Gastroenterology* 1982; 83:818−823.

19. Ismail-Beigi F, Pope GE: Distribution of the histological changes of gastroesophageal reflux in the distal esophagus of man. *Gastroenterology* 1974; 66:1109–1113.
20. Sandry RJ: Pathology of reflux esophagitis. In: Skinner DB, Belsey RH, Hendrix TR, Zuidema GD, eds. *Gastroesophageal Reflux and Hiatal Hernia*. Boston: Little, Brown and Co., 1972: 43–52.
21. Naef AP, Savary M, Ozzello L: Columnar-lined lower esophagus: An acquired lesion with malignant predispostion. *J Thorac Cardiovasc Surg* 1975; 70:826–835.
22. Paull A, Trier JS, Dalton MD, Camp RC, Loeb P, Goyal RK: The histologic spectrum of Barrett's esophagitis. *N Engl J Med* 1976; 295:476–480.
23. Dahms BB, Rothstein FC: Barrett's esophagus in children: A consequence of chronic gastroesophageal reflux. *Gastroenterology* 1984; 86:318–323.
24. Kalish RJ, Clancy PE, Orringer MB, Appelman HD: A clinical, epidemiologic and morphologic comparison between adenocarcinomas arising in Barrett's esophageal mucosa and in the gastric cardia. *Gastroenterology* 1984; 86:461–467.

11

The pH Probe in the Evaluation of Gastroesophageal Reflux Disease

William J. Ravich, M.D.

Chapter Contents

The pH probe is a key instrument in the evaluation of gastroesophageal reflux disease (GERD). It forms the basis of a number of tests used for clinical diagnosis. In addition, it has served as an important research tool in the investigation of this disorder. This chapter reviews the application of pH probe technology to the diagnosis and treatment of GERD, as well as its contribution to our current understanding of its pathophysiology.

The ideal pH electrode should be of small caliber to improve

From Castell DO, Wu WC, Ott DJ (eds): *Gastroesophageal Reflux Disease: Pathogenesis, Diagnosis, Therapy.* Mount Kisco, NY, Futura Publishing Co., Inc., 1985.

patient tolerance and to avoid effects on esophageal motility. Though flexible, some degree of stiffness of the connecting wire is necessary to maintain the proper location in the esophagus despite alterations in patient position and pressure gradients. It should be rapidly responsive to changes in pH over the ranges confronted in the esophagus and stomach (pH 1 – 8). For prolonged recordings, calibration drift must be minimal. Once in place, the probe must not be damaged by contact with bodily fluids, and should be durable to withstand sterilization procedures, or sufficiently inexpensive to be disposable. Finally, especially for prolonged recordings, the connections between the probe and pH meter, as well as reference electrode and patient, must be secure to avoid artifactual changes in the recordings that may be difficult to distinguish from actual reflux episodes.

The ideal probe is probably not yet commercially available. The glass electrode represents the industry standard. New small caliber microelectrodes improve patient comfort, an especially important feature in prolonged studies. Glass electrodes, however, are easily damaged by minor trauma.

Recently, antimony electrodes have become available. These are less susceptible to damage, but may be less accurate at low pH due to oxidation in an acid environment.[1] Glass radiotelemetry capsules—available in Europe—have internal reference electrodes.[2] Although well tolerated by patients, the capsule is tethered by string or suture material and may change position in the esophagus during the study. Also, the relatively large size of the capsule theoretically could alter esophageal motility.

Diagnostic Tests

The acid reflux test (ART) was introduced for clinical use in 1958.[3] With various modifications, it remains one of the basic clinical laboratory tests for the diagnosis of reflux disease. The acid clearance test—though no longer in general clinical use—remains a valuable research tool. Continuous pH monitoring (CpHM) is now considered the best method for diagnosing GERD, and has proven to be a powerful tool for the investigation of its pathophysiology.

Acid Reflux Test (ART)

Technique

The ART is a short duration laboratory test for the evaluation of the competence (or incompetence) of the anti-reflux barrier. The test is performed in the fasting subject, usually after instillation of 300 cc of dilute (0.1 N) HCl into the stomach to assure acidification and adequate intragastric pressure. The probe is placed 5 cm above the proximal margin of the manometrically defined lower esophageal sphincter (LES). Alternative methods for probe localization are less reliable and should not be used. A reflux episode is generally defined as a drop in pH to less than 4.

The patient is studied while at rest and during various provocative maneuvers intended to stress the anti-reflux barrier. In some laboratories, the test is performed before and after acid instillation. It is reasonably assumed that patients who reflux without additional intragastric volume have a weaker anti-reflux barrier than those refluxing after instillation of acid. It is also claimed that patients refluxing during the period of rest are more susceptible to reflux than those refluxing with maneuvers only. While these assumptions may be logical, the acid reflux test is inherently non-quantitative, and the grading of reflux by this test has not been substantiated. We have occasionally seen patients who reflux during a 10-minute recording at rest but fail to reflux during provocative maneuvers.

In an attempt to assure comparability of results, Kantrowitz et al[4] suggested a standardized protocol for the performance of ART— "Standard Acid Reflux Test" or "SART." This protocol calls for brief periods of evaluation in four different positions (supine, right and left lateral, and 20 degree head down) and during five different maneuvers (quiet respiration, deep breathing, Valsalva and Muller manuevers, and coughing). In a subsequent study, the same laboratory found that one or two transient reflux episodes could be detected in as many as 26% of asymptomatic controls, and suggested three or more episodes, or the presence of a prolonged drop in pH, as criteria for a positive test. This produced false positive result in only 2.2% of control subjects.[5]

Diagnosis

In Skinner's study, only 54% of patients thought to have symptoms due to reflux were found to meet the strict criteria for positive tests described above.[5] Using an identical protocol, DeMeester and Johnson[6] found that 80% of patients with severe reflux symptoms had a positive SART, but the test was substantially less sensitive in patients with mild to moderate symptoms. In addition, they found a 20% false positive rate in a small group of subjects without symptoms suggestive of reflux.

Other studies, using different patient populations, modified test protocols, and alternative criteria for the interpretation of an abnormal study, have demonstrated variable results with a true-positive rate ranging from 82% to 100%, and a false positive rate of from 5% to 37%.[7-10] In a study aimed at defining an optimal combination of studies for diagnosing GERD, the ART in association with esophageal mucosal biopsy gave the most specific results without impairing the sensitivity of either test.[8] However, this conclusion depends on the relatively high true-positive rates detected with each test individually—rates that are higher than those found using the same techniques elsewhere.

Until the advent of CpHM, the ART was probably the best available test for the objective diagnosis of GERD, more sensitive than either barium swallow[7] or gastroesophageal scintiscan.[11]

Acid Clearance Test (ACT)

Technique

In 1968, Booth described a test for the evaluation of esophageal acid clearance.[12] The test involved infusion of a 15 cc bolus of 0.1 N HCl 5 cm above a pH probe placed in the distal esophagus. The patient is instructed to swallow, either ad libitum or at defined intervals (usually of 30 seconds duration). The acid clearance time is defined as the number of swallows required to raise the esophageal pH above 5. Normal individuals cleared the esophagus by approximately 10 to 12 swallows.[12,13] Patients with reflux vary considerably, some emptying with 12 swallows, while others may fail to clear even after 40 swallows.

Diagnosis

In the initial studies, the ACT was found to clearly discriminate between asymptomatic controls and patients with typical reflux symptoms.[12] However, subsequent studies from the same and different laboratories[5,13] showed that as many as 50% of refluxers have normal tests. In addition, repeated study of the same normal subject on different days demonstrated substantial variation of results with one study lying outside the originally defined normal limits.[14] False positive results would be expected in patients with disorders of esophageal motility other than GERD, a group in whom confirmation of reflux as a possible underlying factor would be important. Because of the high incidence of false negative results, the ACT is of limited use for the diagnosis of GERD. Recently, it has been largely replaced as a means of documenting impaired esophageal clearance by esophageal scintigraphy, which is better tolerated and provides more quantitative information. However, the ACT remains a useful tool for the investigation of GERD and the mechanisms of acid clearance after reflux occurs.

Continuous pH Monitoring (CpHM)

Technique

The performance of prolonged pH recordings requires relatively few equipment adjustments. The probe is placed in a manner identical to that used in the ART. By attaching the pH meter to a strip chart recorder, a permanent record of pH over time is obtained. Placing the entire recording system on a movable cart at the patient's bedside permits assessment of reflux for 24 hours or more. Since acid is not infused into the stomach, reflux of endogenously secreted gastric acid is detected. The patient is permitted to eat, drink, and sleep. The study therefore evaluates reflux as it occurs under near-physiologic conditions. After the discomfort of tube placement, patients are generally able to tolerate the long periods of intubation with minimal discomfort. The patient maintains a diary of chronological events, such as the time of eating and sleeping and the time at which symptoms occur, for subsequent correlation with reflux activity.

Certain dietary and drug restrictions are placed on the patient during the study. A diet excluding foods with pH less than 5 is used to avoid confusion between acidic material moving down the esophagus and refluxing gastric contents moving up. A surprising number of foods, especially liquids, are acidic and must be avoided. Leafy vegetables and stringy food can produce a sensation of food wrapping around the probe—a potentially distressing situation—and should be avoided as well.

Foods and medication that alter gastric acid production or esophageal motility are also prohibited during the study. Caffeine-containing foods, smooth muscle relaxants, anti-cholinergic agents, sedatives, smoking, and alcohol should therefore be restricted.

For the initial study, drugs used for the treatment of GERD should be stopped at least 48 hours before the start of the test. If necessary, antacids may be continued until the night prior to the study. A major advantage of CpHM is the ability to objectively and quantitatively assess the effect of treatment on reflux. For this purpose, additional studies may be performed with any one or combination of therapeutic measures, and compared with the initial study.

CpHM is generally performed on inpatients because of the bulky equipment required. The study periods extend from 15 to 24 hours and should include periods after meals and during sleep. As with the ART, a reflux event is usually defined as a drop in pH to less than 4, and analysis includes the total number of individual reflux episodes, the mean duration of reflux episodes, and the longest reflux episode. The tracing can be separately analyzed for periods after meals and during sleep. A composite pH scoring system has been proposed using six different measurements of reflux.[15] What measure of reflux severity is best, however, has not been clearly established.

In the earliest comprehensive application of this technique as a diagnostic test,[15] asymptomatic controls were found to reflux for less than 4.2% of the entire 24-hour recording period. Normal individuals refluxed less than 6.3% of the time while in the upright position during the day, and less than 1.2% of the time while recumbent at night.

The test combines features of an acid reflux test, acid sensitivity test, and acid clearance test. Aside from detecting and quantitating the duration of contact between gastric acid and esophageal mucosa, temporal correlation of reflux events with symptoms occurring during pH monitoring permit confirmation of reflux as their cause. In addition, the time required to clear the esophagus of refluxed acid can be a measure of acid clearance. In one study, the mean duration of reflux episodes correlated well with results of the acid clearance test.[13]

The major limitations of CpHM include the requirement for hospitalization dictated by equipment size, and the long, tedious hours required to calculate and analyze the data. Depending on the amount of detail desired, manual data analysis may require one to four hours. To alleviate this problem, rapid computerized analysis has been developed to evaluate data using conventional pH monitoring equipment.[16]

Recently, a number of centers have reported development of portable systems for CpHM using either cassette- or microprocessor-based technology permitting computerized data handling.[17–19] These devices permit outpatient CpHM with rapid data analysis, necessary for the broad clinical application of CpHM. Portable pH monitor systems are now commercially available.

Diagnosis

CpHM is considered to be the best single test for the diagnosis of GERD. Johnson and DeMeester found that 84% of patients with a clinical diagnosis of GERD had composite 24-hour pH score significantly exceeding that found in normal controls.[15] Based on other studies used for the diagnosis of GERD, they concluded that most patients with suspected GERD and negative CpHM had other disorders symptomatically mimicking reflux disease. Because of the lack of any other definitive test for evaluating GERD, the validity of this conclusion and the actual accuracy of CpHM is difficult to confirm. Causes for false negative results include possible daily variation in the severity of reflux in individual patients and absence of sufficient gastric acid secretion.

Acidic gastric contents are required for the detection of acid reflux. Initial introduction of the probe into the stomach to determine the pH of the gastric contents is usually sufficient to confirm the presence of sufficient acid. Failure to detect gastric pH less than 4 suggests inadequate acid production, precluding the performance of CpHM. This limits evaluation in patients with previous gastric surgery and those with substantial duodenogastric reflux capable of neutralizing gastric acid.

The use of CpHM for the diagnosis of "alkaline reflux" has been proposed, but this application has certain theoretical and practical problems that may substantially limit its use. The appropriate criterion for detection of "alkaline reflux" is a source of concern. The proposal that a pH greater than 7 be used to represent a reflux event may be too close to normal esophageal pH values, which may reach 6.8.[20] Calibration drift or other artifactual changes may also be misinterpreted as alkaline reflux using this criterion.

On the other hand, a considerable amount of duodenogastric reflux may occur before gastric pH is raised above 7. Bile staining of gastric contents is frequently noted during routine upper endoscopy for non-reflux conditions. The pH of these contents is rarely above 7. Duodenogastric regurgitation may therefore neutralize gastric contents to pH above 4, but fail to increase pH above 7 to permit the detection of "alkaline reflux."

Another possible objection to the diagnosis of "alkaline reflux" is more conceptual than practical. Alkaline solutions at pH similar to those found in the duodenum are not damaging to the esophageal mucosa. Rather, it is the bile and trypsin content of the duodenum that is potentially damaging to the esophagus.[21,22] Esophageal damage secondary to bile and trypsin is independent of pH. In light of the frequent finding of bile staining of gastric contents, a certain degree of "bile reflux" may be responsible for esophageal damage in many patients with GERD.

CpHM has provided some insight into the development of a number of clinical presentations and endoscopic findings related to reflux. The severity of reflux has been found to correlate with symptom severity[23] and with the frequency[15] and degree of histological reactive changes.[24] Anti-reflux surgery which normalized the results of CpHM was found to result in improvement in reactive changes in five patients.[24]

Forty-six percent of 50 patients presenting with angina-like chest pain as their predominant presenting symptom, but with normal coronary angiograms, were found to have abnormal CpHM.[25] Of those with abnormal pH monitoring, 91% responded symptomatically to medical or surgical therapy for reflux over a two- to three-year follow-up. All 12 patients who had pain during CpHM associated with an episode of reflux responded to therapy.

In a study of 22 patients with Barrett's esophagus, 21 had abnormal CpHM, the one exception being a patient with previous gastric surgery for peptic ulcer disease. Quantitation of reflux severity also suggested that patients with Barrett's esophagus have more severe reflux than those with reflux esophagitis without Barrett's esophagus.[26]

CpHM has been used as a means of confirming reflux as a cause of pulmonary symptoms.[27,28] It plays an important role in children who often do not sense, or are too young to communicate, reflux symptoms. Pulmonary complications, such as recurrent infections, asthma, or sudden apnea are potential sequelae of GERD in childhood.[29,30]

Insights into the Pathophysiology of GERD

Physiologic Reflux

While most people experience occasional symptoms of reflux, such as heartburn, CpHM has shown that most normal individuals reflux daily.[9,31,32] Characteristically, "physiologic reflux" tends to occur after meals and decreases in frequency over time (Figure 1). Such episodes of post-prandial reflux tend to be of short duration, with rapid clearance of the refluxed material. Reflux during sleep, however, is an infrequent event in normal controls. This suggests that the anti-reflux barrier is more effective in the recumbent position, although it is equally likely that the causes of reflux are exaggerated after meals. Not unexpectedly, most reflux events are not appreciated by normal subjects.

A study using combined continuous manometric and pH techniques suggested that reflux occurring in normal individuals is us-

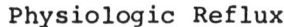

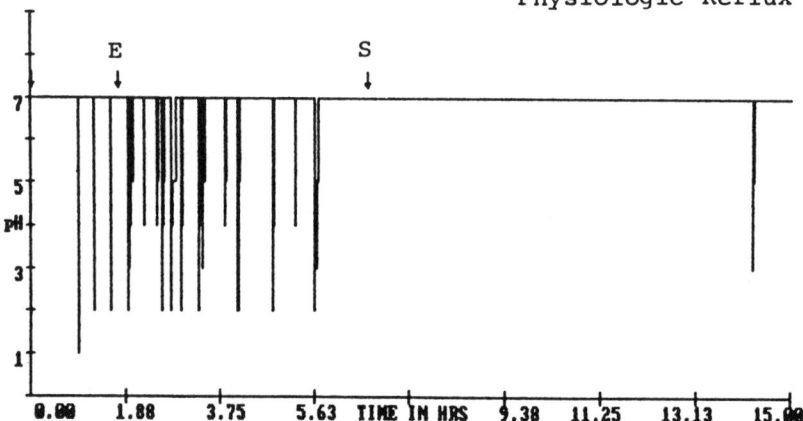

Figure 1: *Normal "physiologic" reflux. The tracing shows numerous reflux episodes (ph ≤ 4) of short duration. Little reflux occurred while supine at night. Percentage of time with pH less than or equal to 4 = 1.3% of total recording. Percentage of time with pH less than or equal to 4 = 3.3% for 4-hour period after eating. Digitalized recording using microprocessor-based portable system. Arrows at top represent patient indicator button use. (E = eating; S = supine).*

ually associated with transient episodes of LES relaxation unassociated with swallowing.[33] While such transient relaxations of the LES could occur at any time, their frequency increased dramatically in the three-hour period following eating. About 93% of transient LES relaxations occurring post-prandially were associated with reflux, while transient LES relaxations occurring at other times were associated with evidence of reflux in only 69%. Overall, 98% of reflux episodes in normal individuals were associated with relaxation of the LES. Though LES pressure varied during the course of the study period, reflux did not appear to relate to such fluctuations. One fault with this study is that subjects remained recumbent during the entire recording period. It is possible that reflux in normal individuals in the upright position after meals may not occur by the same mechanism.

Pathologic Reflux

If normal individuals reflux, what characterizes "pathologic" reflux? DeMeester et al[9] have shown that reflux is not simply a matter of degree (Figure 2). They found that all refluxers are not alike, and that there are different patterns of "pathologic reflux." The

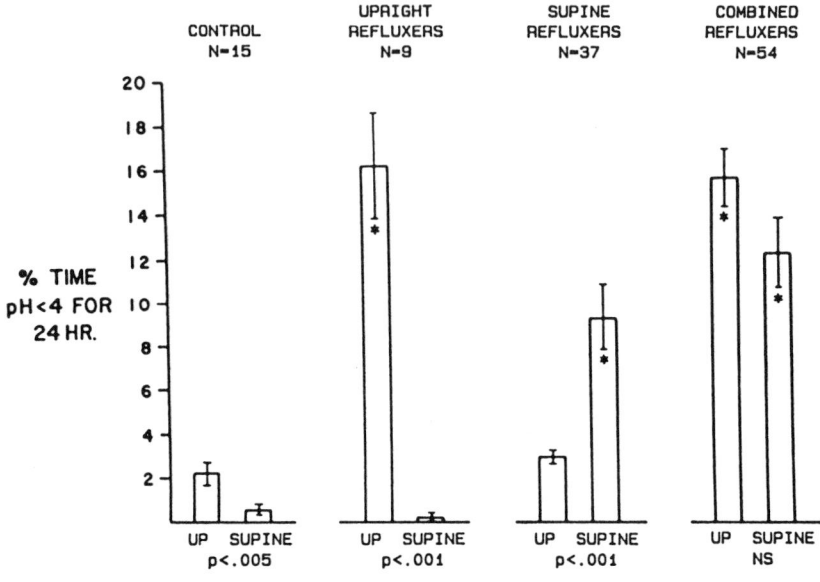

Figure 2: *The results of 24-hour pH monitoring of the distal esophagus in 15 asymptomatic subjects and 100 patients with reflux symptoms (Reproduced from DeMeester et al:* Annals of Surgery 1976: 184:459–469 *with permission of author and publisher.)*

most common pattern involved increased reflux both in the upright position during the day and in the supine position at night ("combined refluxers"). Overall, 54% of the symptomatic patients demonstrated this combined pattern. However, 37% of the patients had abnormal reflux only in the supine position at night ("supine refluxers"). During the day in the upright position, these patients had normal amounts of reflux. In addition, 9% of refluxers had an abnormal reflux pattern in which increased amounts of reflux occurred during the day in the upright position ("upright refluxers"). In these patients, reflux occurring at night was no more severe than that found in normal individuals.

The underlying reason for these different patterns of reflux is unclear. However, DeMeester et al[9] suggested that the mechanism of reflux in "upright refluxers" may be different from that in "supine refluxers" or "combined refluxers." They based this impression on the increased frequency of symptoms of the "gas bloat" syndrome after anti-reflux surgery in upright refluxers, and postulated that these patients had aerophagia as an underlying cause of symptoms.

However, they indicated that symptoms were unreliable in predicting the reflux pattern. They also remarked on the decreased frequency of complications of reflux, such as gross esophagitis and stricture formation in upright refluxers, as compared with those with other reflux patterns. The finding that patients with abnormal nocturnal reflux are at increased risk for the development of esophagitis has been confirmed by others.[34]

Reflux occurring during the day tends to be concentrated in the post-prandial period, as in normal controls. What distinguishes pathologic post-prandial reflux is its increased frequency and the delayed clearance once reflux occurs. Abnormal reflux occurring at night is far less frequent than that occurring in the upright position after meals. However, once reflux occurs, clearance in the supine position during sleep is slow, and the esophageal lumen remains acidic for prolonged periods of time (Figure 3).

The mechanism of reflux in ten patients with endoscopically confirmed reflux esophagitis, using combined continuous manometric and pH monitoring techniques, has been compared with that obtained in ten normal controls.[35] Whereas in normals 94% of reflux episodes were associated with transient relaxation of the LES, only 65% of the episodes in patients with GERD were associated with LES relaxation. Of the other reflux episodes in reflux patients, approxi-

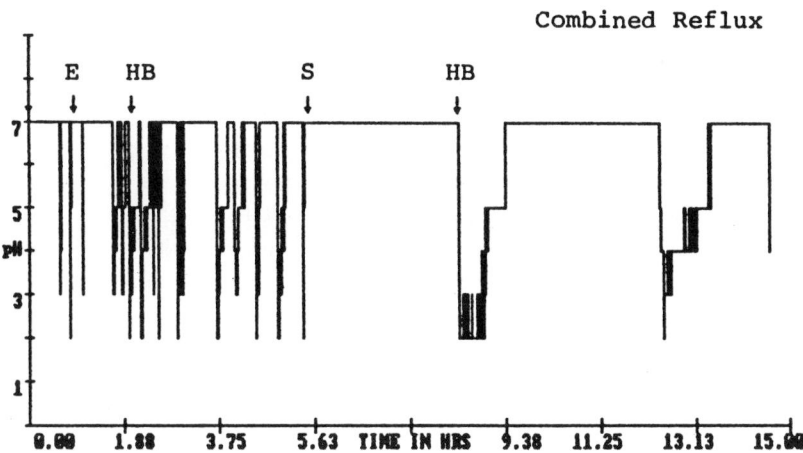

Figure 3: *Abnormal (pathologic) reflux. The tracing, performed on the same instrument as in Figure 1, shows more frequent and prolonged reflux episodes in the post-prandial period than normal. Episodes of nighttime reflux are characteristically less frequent than in the post-prandial period, but are cleared poorly. (E = eating; S = supine; HB = heartburn).*

mately half were due to a sudden increase in intragastric pressure, while the rest occurred spontaneously without sudden changes in LES or in intragastric pressure. As with the previously described report from the same laboratory,[33] the performance of the studies entirely with the subjects recumbent requires caution in extrapolating the results to reflux occurring in the upright position after meals. In addition, no information on the mechanism of reflux in purely "upright refluxers" is available, as the use of patients with relatively severe endoscopic esophagitis probably excluded those with this reflux pattern.

Anti-reflux Barrier

For over two decades, many have argued over the relative importance of the normal anatomic configuration of the esophagogastric junction and the pressure of the LES in preventing gastroesophageal reflux. The recognition that GERD can occur in the absence of hiatal hernia, and that hiatal hernia can exist without GERD discredited those supporting the importance of anatomy.[36] However, substantial overlap in LES pressure between symptomatic refluxers and asymptomatic controls also undermined those emphasizing the role of the LES.[8] Despite an interesting study showing that the amount of intragastric volume necessary to overcome the anti-reflux barrier as detected by a modified ART correlated reasonably well with LES pressure,[10] studies using CpHM have convincingly shown that a moderately low LES pressure alone is not always associated with abnormal reflux, and that occasional patients with high LES pressures in excess of 30 mmHg can reflux abnormally.[37]

Studies utilizing CpHM provide support for both sides of the dispute. The presence of a hiatal hernia, confirmed by both endoscopic and x-ray criteria, was significantly associated with both increased frequency of reflux in upright and supine positions, and an increased mean duration of reflux in the recumbent position.[24] In another study,[37] the frequency of reflux was inversely correlated with the manometrically determined length of the intraabdominal segment of esophagus. Whereas 81% of patients with less than 1 cm of abdominal esophagus had abnormal reflux by CpHM, the frequency of abnormal studies declined with increasing abdominal length, until with over 3 cm of abdominal esophagus, only 38% had abnormal CpHM. In the same study, LES pressure also correlated inversely with the frequency of an abnormal CpHM. While 83% of patients with LES pressure of 0 to 5 mmHg had abnormal reflux, only 18% of those with LES pressures of greater than 30 mmHg were found to reflux. On the basis of this study it appears that both factors—the length of abdominal esophagus and LES pressure—correlate independently with the likelihood of documenting reflux by CpHM.

Acid Clearance

Esophageal damage results largely from the duration of time that the mucosa is exposed to noxious gastric contents. This is not only a result of the severity of reflux, but also involves the ability of the esophagus to rid itself of gastric material once reflux has occurred. Mechanisms of esophageal clearance are therefore important in the pathophysiology of reflux disease. The acid clearance test indicates that patients with reflux frequently have impaired esophageal clearance.[5,13] Whether impaired clearance is part of a motor disorder underlying reflux disease, or is entirely a consequence of reflux-induced damage remains unclear. Regardless, impaired clearance would be expected to exaggerate the severity of reflux damage.

Clearance during an ACT occurs in a step-wise fashion in response to each swallow, with little if any change in pH between swallows.[13,33,38] The decreased frequency of swallowing during sleep is a major factor in the typically prolonged episodes of acid exposure that occur during sleep, as is the loss of gravitational effect in returning refluxed material back to the stomach.

Though it has been assumed that acid clearance occurred by peristaltic activity stripping the esophagus of any contents, Helm et al[38] have demonstrated the critical role that saliva plays in acid clearance. Oral aspiration of saliva obliterates the step-wise pattern of acid clearance in normal individuals, while the use of oral lozenges and bethanechol, which stimulate salivation, improve acid clearance.

Orr et al[39] found that acid infused into the esophagus was cleared equally well by reflux patients and normal controls in the recumbent position, both while awake or asleep. Clearance was delayed in both groups during sleep. Arousal results in improved esophageal clearance. This effect of arousal probably reflects an increase in frequency of swallowing occurring in the aroused individual.[33] Acid infusion can cause arousal, which probably is a protective reflex to clear refluxed gastric contents, but the latency period between acid infusion and arousal was significantly greater in reflux patients.[39]

Treatment of GERD

Because of the essentially qualitative nature of most tests used to document reflux, no objective means were available for measuring the effect of therapy on reflux until the introduction of CpHM. Johnson and DeMeester, in their original article on 24-hour pH recordings, recognized the potential value of CpHM for evaluating therapy.[15] Though the effect of a variety of therapeutic measures on GERD is known, it is surprising that after ten years, more data are not available on the use of CpHM to monitor therapy.

DeMeester and Johnson showed that Nissen fundoplication could normalize the results of CpHM,[9] a finding confirmed by others.[40] CpHM would be an appropriate means of objectively assessing the comparative effectiveness of other anti-reflux surgical procedures. Meaningful studies, however, may be too difficult to conduct because of the preference of individual surgeons for different techniques and of the difficulty in performing the various operations on comparable patient populations.

Elevation of the head of the bed—a time-honored part of empirical treatment regimens—has been shown to significantly decrease nighttime reflux occurring in the recumbent position.[41,42] This effect appeared to be primarily due to improved esophageal emptying, as measured by the mean duration of acid reflux.[42] While this probably was in part due to the effect of gravity on returning reflux material to the stomach, it is equally likely that elevation of the head of the bed decreases the volume of material refluxed, thereby shortening the time required to subsequently clear the esophagus. Thus, the beneficial effect of bed elevation may depend on one or both of these explanations.

Bethanechol was shown to significantly decrease the severity of reflux during recumbent periods, but surprisingly had no effect on upright reflux.[42] As with elevation of the head of the bed, this response appeared to be due predominantly to a decrease in the mean duration of acid reflux, rather than to a decrease in the number of reflux episodes. Adjustment of the dose from the usual 25 mg four times a day to a single 25 mg dose before sleep was equally effective in decreasing the severity of recumbent reflux. The combination of elevation of the head of the bed and bethanechol was more effective than either alone.

Only scattered reports are available on the effect of other treatment modalities. One study showed that cimetidine significantly decreased reflux severity[43] while another demonstrated that it significantly decreased the number of reflux episodes but had no effect on the total acid exposure time of the esophagus.[44] Gaviscon was found to decrease reflux severity in one study,[45] but not in another.[42]

Some caution is necessary when evaluating the effects of therapeutic intervention by CpHM. The lack of reproducible data may affect direct comparison of results of individual studies before and after treatment. In our experience, reflux severity in GERD may vary considerably from day to day. Such variations may be misinterpreted as supporting a beneficial effect where none exists, or may mask such an effect when present.

A decrease in reflux severity should not be misinterpreted to indicate that no reflux is taking place. It is now appreciated that acid is not the only agent in the stomach capable of producing esophageal injury. To the extent that pH-independent noxious agents, such as bile acids and trypsin, are responsible for symptoms or esophageal mucosa damage in GERD, the alteration of gastric pH by antacids or H_2 blockers may decrease reflux as detected by CpHM, but not necessarily alter the volume of material being refluxed. This might explain why the use of therapy directed against gastric acidity alone is often ineffectual in improving histologic evidence of reflux damage.

Similarly, if a drug that increases pH is found to be equal at decreasing acid reflux to one that exclusively acts on the LES, they may still not be equally effective in the treatment of GERD. The drug affecting the LES decreases the reflux of all possible noxious materials, while the other drug leaves the bile and trypsin unaffected.

Conclusion

pH probe technology forms the basis of a number of important tests for the evaluation of gastroesophageal reflux disease. Aside from their importance for diagnosis, innovative use of these tests has had a major impact on the rapid increase in knowledge about the pathophysiology of reflux in health and disease.

Until recently, continuous pH monitoring has been primarily an investigative tool available in a few research centers. The need to hospitalize patients and the time required for the analysis of recordings severely limited its application as a clinical test. With the development of portable continuous pH monitors and computerized data analysis programs, the stage is set for the broad clinical application of continuous pH monitoring in gastroesophageal reflux disease.

References

1. Meldrum SJ, Watson BW, Riddle HC, Brown RL, Sladen GE: pH profile of gut as measured by radiotelemetry capsule. *Br Med J* 1972; 2:104–106.
2. Branicki FJ, Evans DF, Ogilvie AL, Atkinson M, Hardcastle JD: The assessment of gastro-oesophageal reflux using a portable radiotelemetry system. In: Weinbeck M, ed. *Motility and the Digestive Tract*. New York: Raven Press 1982: 279–286.
3. Tuttle SG, Grossman MI: Detection of gastroesophageal reflux by simultaneous measurements of intraluminal pressures and pH. *Proc Soc Exp Biol Med* 1958; 98:225–227.
4. Kantrowitz PA, Corson JG, Fleischli DJ, Skinner DB: Measurement of gastroesophageal reflux. *Gastroenterology* 1968: 56:666–673.
5. Skinner BD, Booth DJ: Assessment of distal esophageal function in patients with hiatal hernia and/or gastroesophageal reflux. *Ann Surg* 1970; 172:627–637.
6. DeMeester TR, Johnson LF: The evaluation of objective measurements of gastroesophageal reflux and their contribution to patient management. *Surg Clin North Am* 1976; 56:39–53.
7. Benz LJ, Hootkin LA, Margulies S, Donner MW, Cauthorne RT, Hendrix TR: A comparison of clinical measurements of gastroesophageal reflux. *Gastroenterology* 1972; 62:1–5.
8. Behar J, Biancani P, Sheahan DG: Evaluation of esophageal tests in the diagnosis of reflux esophagitis. *Gastroenterology* 1976; 71:9–15.
9. DeMeester TR, Johnson LF, Joseph GJ, Toscano MS, Hall AW, Skinner DB: Patterns of gastroesophageal reflux in health and disease. *Ann Surg* 1976; 184:459–470.
10. Ahtaridis G, Snape WJ, Cohen S: Lower esophageal sphincter pressure as an index of gastroesophageal acid reflux. *Dig Dis Sci* 1981; 26;993–998.
11. Fisher RS, Malmuc LS, Roberts GS, Lobis IF: Gastroesophageal (GE) scintiscanning to detect and quantitate GE reflux. *Gastroenterology* 1976; 70:301–308.
12. Booth DJ, Kemmerer WT, Skinner DB: Acid clearing from the distal esophagus. *Arch Surg* 1968; 96:731–734.
13. Stanciu C, Bennett JR: Oesophageal acid clearing: One factor in the production of reflux esophagitis. *Gut* 1974; 15:852–857.
14. Boesby S: Continuous oesophageal pH recordings and acid-clearing tests. *Scand J Gastroenterol* 1977; 12:245–247.
15. Johnson LF, DeMeester TR: Twenty-four hour monitoring of the distal esophagus. *Am J Gastroenterology* 1974; 62:325–332.
16. Troxell RB, Kohn SR, Gray JE, Welch RW, Harloe ED, Goyal RK: A computer-assisted technique for twenty-four hour esophageal monitoring. *Dig Dis Sci* 1982; 27:1057–1062.
17. Weiser HS, Lepsihn G, Mueller-Lissner SA, Pace S, Blum AL, Siewert R: Reflux characteristics of healthy volunteer examined by long-term-pH-metry. In: Weinbeck M, ed. *Motility of the Digestive Tract*. New York: Raven Press. 1982: 287–292.
18. Vantrappen G, Servaes J, Janssens J, Peeters T: Twenty-four hour esophageal pH- and pressure recording in outpatients. In: Weinbeck M, ed. *Motility of the Digestive Tract*. New York: Raven Press. 1982: 293–298.

19. Johannes RS, Ravich WJ, Schneider W, Massey JT, Johns RJ, Hendrix TR: A continuous portable intraesophageal pH monitoring system. In: *Proceedings of the Seventh Annual Symposium of Computer Applications in Medical Care.* Silver Spring, MD: IEEE Computer Society Press. 1983: 911–917.

20. Pellegrini CA, DeMeester TR, Wernly JA, Johnson LF, Skinner DB: Alkaline gastroesophageal reflux. *Am J Surg* 1978; 135:177–183.

21. Harmon JW, Johnson LF, Maydonovitch CL: Effects of acid in bile salts in the rabbit esophageal mucosa. *Dig Dis Sci* 1981; 26:65–72.

22. Lillemoe KD, Johnson LF, Harmond JW: Role of the components of gastroduodenal contents in experimental acid esophagitis. *Surgery* 1982; 92:276–284.

23. Little AG, DeMeester TR, Kirchner PJ, O'Sullivan GC, Skinner DB: Pathogenesis of esophagitis in patients with gastroesophageal reflux. *Surgery* 1980; 80:101–107.

24. Johnson LF, DeMeester TR, Haggitt RC: Esophageal epithelial response to gastroesophageal reflux: A quantitative study. *Am J Dig Dis* 1978; 23:498–509.

25. DeMeester TR, O'Sullivan GC, Bermudez G, Midell AI, Cimochowiski GE, O'Drobinck J: Esophageal function in patients with angina-like chest pain and normal coronary angiograms. *Ann Surg* 1982; 196: 488–497.

26. Iascone C, DeMeester TR, Little AG, Skinner DB: Barrett's esophagus: Functional assessment, proposed pathogenesis, and surgical treatment. *Arch Surg* 1983; 118:543–549.

27. Pellegrini CA, DeMeester TR, Johnson LF, Skinner DB: Gastroesophageal reflux in pulmonary aspiration: Incidence, functional abnormality and results of surgical therapy. *Surgery* 1979; 36:110–119.

28. Chernow B, Johnson LF, Yanowitz WR, Castell DO: Pulmonary aspiration as a consequence of gastroesophageal reflux: A diagnostic approach. *Dig Dis Sci* 1979; 24:839–844.

29. Herbst JJ: Gastroesophageal reflux and pulmonary disease. *Pediatrics* 1981; 68:132–134.

30. Jolley SG, Herbst JJ, Johnson DG, Matlak ME, Book LS: Esophageal pH Monitoring during sleep identifies children with respiratory symptoms from gastroesophageal reflux. *Gastroenterology* 1981; 20:1501–1506.

31. Pattrick FG: Investigation of gastroesophageal reflux in various positions with a 2-lumen pH electrode. *Gut* 1970; 11:659–667.

32. Kaye MD: Post-prandial gastroesophageal reflux in healthy people. *Gut* 1977; 18:709–712.

33. Dent J, Dodds WJ, Freedman RH, Sekiguchi T, Hogan WJ, Arndorfer RC, Petrie DJ: Mechanism of gastroesophageal reflux in recumbent asymptomatic human subjects. *J Clin Invest* 1980; 65:256–267.

34. Atkinson M, VanGelder A: Esophageal intraluminal pH recording in the assessment of gastroesophageal reflux and its consequences. *Am J Dig Dis* 1977; 22:365–370.

35. Dodds WJ, Dent J, Hogan WJ, Helm JF, Hauser R, Patel G, Egide MS: Mechanisms of gastroesophageal reflux in patients with reflux esophagitis. *N Engl J Med* 1982; 307:1547–1552.

36. Cohen S, Harris LD: Does hiatus hernia affect competence of the gastroesophageal sphincter? *N Engl J Med* 1971; 284:1053–1056.

37. DeMeester TR, Wernly JA, Bryant GH, Little AG, Skinner DB: Clinical

and in vitro analysis of determinants of gastroesophageal competence: A study of the principles of anti-reflux surgery. *Am J Surg* 1979; 137:39−45.

38. Helm JF, Dodds WJ, Riedel DR, Teeter BC, Hogan WJ, Arndorfer RC: Determinants of esophageal acid clearance in normal subjects. *Gastroenterology* 1983; 85:607−612.

39. Orr WC, Robinson MG, Johnson LF: Acid clearance during sleep in the pathogenesis of reflux esophagitis. *Dig Dis Sci* 1981; 26:423−427.

40. Godall RJR, Temple JG: Effect of Nissen fundoplication on competence of the gastrooesophageal junction. *Gut* 1980; 21:607−613.

41. Stanciu C, Hoare RC, Bennett JR: Correlation between manometric and pH tests for gastroesophageal reflux. *Gut* 1977; 18:536−540.

42. Johnson LF, DeMeester TR: Evaluation of elevation of the head of the bed, bethanechol and antacid foam tablet in gastroesophageal reflux. *Dig Dis Sci* 1981; 26:673−680.

43. Aprill N, Echrich J, Wang C, Klementschitsch P, DeMeester TR, Winans C: Quantitative reduction of gastroesophageal acid reflux by cimetidine. *Gastroenterology* 1979; 76:1092.

44. Bennett JR, Buckton G, Morten HD: Cimetidine in gastroesophageal reflux. *Digestion* 1983; 26:166−172.

45. Stanciu C, Bennett JR: Alginate/antacid in the reduction of gastroesophageal reflux. *Lancet* 1974; 1:109−111.

12

Gastroesophageal Scintigraphy

Robert J. Cowan, M.D.

Chapter Contents

Nuclear medicine techniques offer several advantages for the investigation of functional abnormalities of the esophagus and stomach. Radioisotopes can be incorporated into foodstuff with minimal alteration in the physiologic character of the material; the ingested radiolabeled material can be readily detected, and images of its progress can be generated; the information obtained can be quantitated allow-

From Castell DO, Wu WC, Ott DJ (eds): *Gastroesophageal Reflux Disease: Pathogenesis, Diagnosis, Therapy.* Mount Kisco, NY, Futura Publishing Co., Inc., 1985.

ing calculation of various indices and transit times; and continuous monitoring of the patient can be performed without increasing the radiation exposure.

Such procedures are still in the evolutionary phase, but a number have been introduced for evaluation of areas related to gastroesophageal reflux disease. These include demonstration and quantification of the degree of reflux, evaluation of gastric emptying of ingested material, and investigation of esophageal transit. Each of these areas will be covered through a survey of the current state of development of the technique and review of its application in relation to gastroesophageal reflux.

Gastroesophageal Reflux

Findings in Adults

A radionuclide technique for evaluation of gastrointestinal reflux in adults was initially reported by Drs. Fisher, Malmud, and others from Temple University, and most of the reports to date in adults have come from this insitiution.[1] Their method, which has become the most widely used "standard" technique, utilized a nonabsorbable radionuclide marker, technetium sulfur colloid, in 300 uCi doses administered in water or acidified orange juice in a volume of 300 ml. Serial images (30-second intervals) with a gamma camera were used to search for reflux of radioactivity into the esophagus. Their initial technique utilized a double lumen tube for administration of the radiopharmaceutical, and this was left in place throughout the data collection period. However, comparative studies with and without the tube delivery showed no significant difference, and this was discarded in later studies. Patients were imaged supine to encourage reflux, and both spontaneous and induced reflux were evaluated through the use of an abdominal binder inflated to increasingly higher pressures (Figure 1). In their earlier reports, a maximum pressure of 35 mm of mercury was used, but this was later modified and extended up to 100 mm.[2] Their preliminary results indicated a 90% sensitivity in patients with positive acid reflux tests and a false positive rate of 10% in normal controls.

Quantitation was achieved through a computer interfaced to the gamma camera which allowed determination of counts within regions of interest corresponding to stomach, esophagus, and background areas (Figure 2).

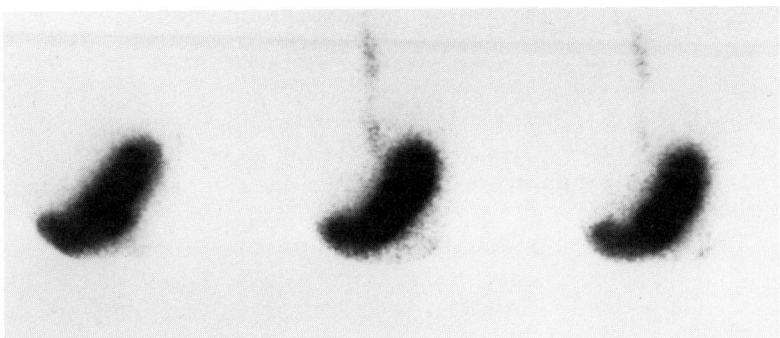

Figure 1: *Esophageal activity indicating gastroesophageal reflux is not present on the first image but does appear after inflation of the abdominal binder to 25 and 50 mmHg.*

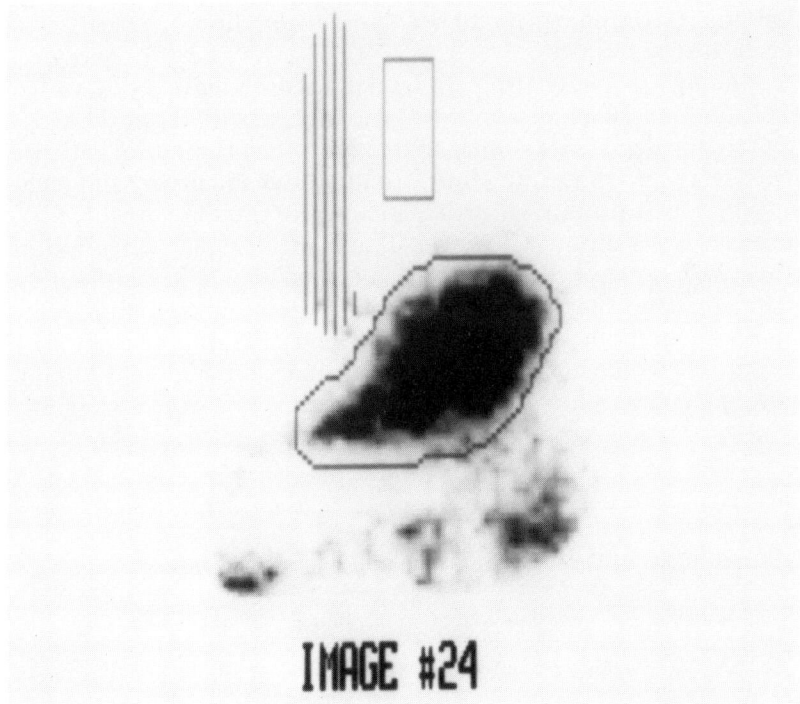

Figure 2: *Typical region of interest placement over esophagus, stomach, and background area for calculation of gastroesophageal reflux index.*

$$\text{GER Index} = \frac{\text{Esophageal counts} - \text{Background counts}}{\text{Gastric counts}} \times 100$$

Indices above 4% were considered abnormal. Other groups have used lower limits or have relied mainly on visual identification of reflux on the images. Computer manipulation was also used to enhance image contrast.

The Temple group extended their study[3] to evaluate criteria for selection of patients for anti-reflux surgery and suggested that a GER index greater than 10% would be useful in choosing patients for whom operative intervention might be appropriate. They also recommended utilization of the test to evaluate patients with typical "heartburn" and non-specific chest pain. An additional application was the evaluation of various forms of pharmacologic and antacid therapy.[4]

It was pointed out soon after the initial description of the technique that both amount of reflux and rapidity of subsequent esophageal clearance of the reflux influenced the GER index, and that a more appropriate terminology might be a "measure of the esophageal exposure to gastric refluxate."[5]

Findings in adults from other laboratories have been varied (Table 1). Velasco, et al[7] confirmed the high sensitivity of the technique, reporting results similar to that with the pH probe in patients with severe and moderate clinical reflux after modifying the technique by substituting a Valsalva maneuver for the abdominal binder. Hoffman and Vansant,[6] however, found inconsistent detection of reflux, with positive tests in only 4 (14%) of 29 patients with reflux documented by other techniques. This group also found a similar low sensitivity for the acid reflux test. Variable results were also noted by McCallum[8] who mentioned relatively infrequent demonstration of gastroesophageal reflux in patients with reflux who were undergoing

Table 1. Sensitivity of Detection of Gastroesophageal Reflux in Adults						
Author/Ref.	Radionuclide		Barium		Acid Reflux	
Fisher[1]	27/30	(90%)	15/30	(50%)	30/30	(100%)
Hoffman[6]	4/29	(14%)	—		4/29	(14%)
Velasco[7]	40/54	(74%)	20/53	(38%)	38/49	(78%)
Totals	71/113	(63%)	35/83	(42%)	72/108	(67%)

gastric emptying studies. McCallum's patients were not studied with abdominal binders.

In a relatively small series, we have also found low sensitivity in detecting GE reflux using the standard technique of Malmud et al with a cutoff of 4% GER index. Only 4 (27%) of 15 adult patients with severe esophagitis had abnormal results by this criteria. Standard acid reflux tests were not performed on our patients, and scintigraphic imaging was obtained for only 7 minutes. Whether the variation in results reflects unrecognized differences in technique, the intermittent nature of esophageal reflux, different patient populations (some series included only those with positive acid reflux) or other unknown variables will require further investigation.

Following the initial description of radionuclide imaging for gastroesophageal reflux, Reich et al[9] modified the technique to allow evaluation of pulmonary aspiration of gastric contents. A bedtime feeding of 3 to 5 mCi ^{99m}Tc-sulfur colloid was given along with 30 to 50 ml of water. Images over the chest the following morning were positive for pulmonary activity in 2/7 adults with severe fibrotic lung disease. Chernow et al[10] using a similar procedure in adults reported abnormal studies in 3/6 patients with suspected pulmonary aspiration.

Ghaed et al,[11] however, had 20 negative studies in 10 patients with clinical asthma and other evidence of reflux. They were uncertain whether this represented lack of sensitivity of the technique, only intermittent occurrence of aspiration, or actual lack of significant aspiration in their group of asthmatics with esophageal reflux. It has been suggested that results might be improved if a more complex radiolabeled meal such as an egg salad sandwich was given at bedtime to retard gastric emptying and provide a longer opportunity for reflux and aspiration.[12]

Results in Children

Because of the difficulty of evaluating abnormal GE reflux in infants and children and the need for a definitive test for pulmonary aspiration of refluxate, the radionuclide technique was quickly applied to pediatric patients with modifications of feeding volume and dose administered according to the patient's age and size. Technetium sulfur colloid was usually mixed with the infant's regular feeding. Other technical modifications included immobilization of the patient, sedation if required, and employment of smaller field of view gamma cameras. Rudd and Christie[13] studied 25 infants and children with positive acid reflux tests and found radionuclide evidence of reflux in 80%. Computer quantitation was not employed, and no attempt was made to search for pulmonary aspiration. Although abdominal pressure was used, most of their abnormal studies occurred without pressure or at relatively low levels ($\leqq$5 mmHg).

Heyman et al[14] found abnormal studies in 59% of children referred because of possible reflux compared with only 26% detection with barium techniques. Other reports comparing barium to radionuclide techniques in children have noted similar improved sensitivity with scintigraphy (Table 2). Seibert et al,[18] however, using 24-hour pH probe monitoring as their standard, found slightly lower sensitivity for the radionuclide technique compared with barium. They emphasized the greatly improved specificity of the radionuclide study (93% versus 21%). Of those series using the acid reflux test as the standard, Arasu et al[16,19] found the lowest sensitivity for scintigraphy (56%) compared with barium (50%) and were disappointed at the relatively low detection rate of the radionuclide technique.

Blumhagen et al[20] reported on an expanded series of patients with 75% sensitivity for scintigraphy when the acid reflux test was used as the "gold standard." They discounted the significance of radioactive reflux occurring only during the first few minutes of the study since this was noted in several patients in whom all other tests for reflux were negative. Others, however, have disagreed, feeling reflux at any time was significant.[18]

Some investigators have felt that the abdominal binder was excessively non-physiologic, especially in children, and other tech-

Table 2.
Sensitivity of Detection of Gastroesophageal Reflux in Children

Author/Ref.	Radionuclide	Barium	Acid Reflux
Rudd[13]	80%	60%	100%
Heyman[14]	59%	26%	—
Conway[15]	90%	33%	—
Arasu[16]	56%	50%	96%
Jona[17]	77%	41%	—
Seibert[18]	79%	76%	100%
Averages	74%	48%	99%

niques such as the left lateral decubitus position have been utilized when reflux was not seen in the resting supine position.[17] In a comparison of various patient positions including prone, supine, right posterior oblique, and left lateral decubitus, the supine view was shown to be preferable.[21] Swanson et al[22] also recommended avoiding abdominal pressure. They compared incremental abdominal pressure images without computer processing to non-compression computer-enhanced images. The latter were found to give better results. Unfortunately, comparison was not also made to computer-processed images obtained with abdominal pressure. Most reports have also supported the need for computer manipulation of the images[14,17,18,20,23,24] (Figure 3).

Computer techniques have also been frequently utilized for generation of curves of esophageal activity to allow detection of episodic "peaks" (Figure 4) and to quantitate the severity of reflux by calculation of a reflux index.[14,17,18,20-22] The degree of reflux required to be considered abnormal has varied from the lower limit of 4% suggested by Fisher in adults[1] to a mean value of 3.66 ± 0.81 by Duvos[25] to any value above 0.5% by Piepsz.[24]

Since reflux may occur intermittently, the importance of continuous monitoring over a prolonged period has been stressed in some

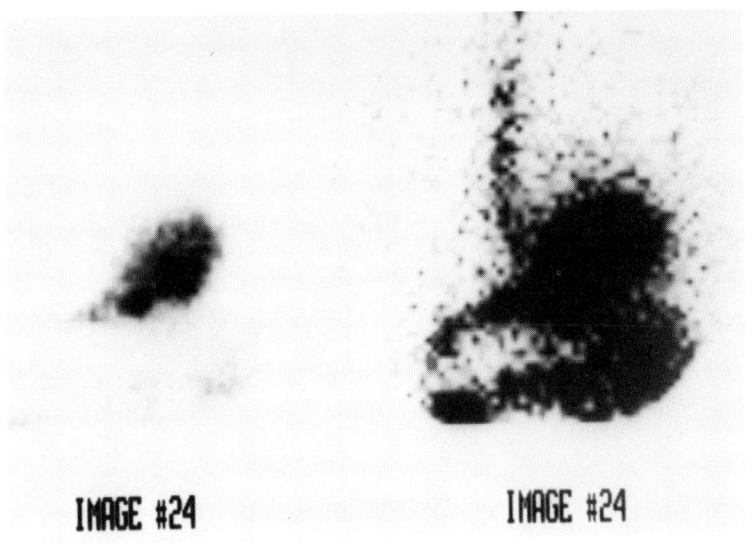

IMAGE #24   IMAGE #24

Figure 3: *Esophageal activity is not evident on the unprocessed image on the left. After computer enhancement (right), esophageal activity is clearly visible.*

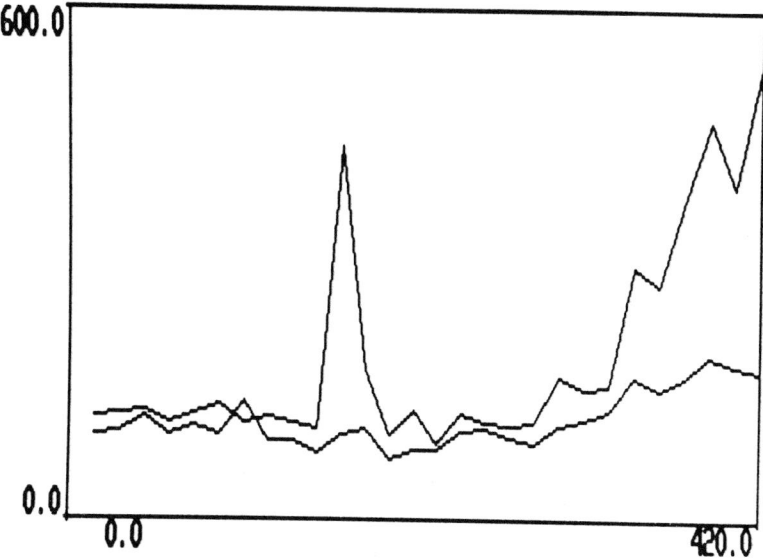

Figure 4: *Time activity curve from the esophageal region of interest demonstrating peak of esophageal activity during episode of reflux. The lower curve represents background activity over the chest. The X axis represents time in seconds, and the Y axis reflects counts.*

reports. Piepsz et al[21] found 25% of their abnormal studies did not demonstrate reflux until the second half-hour of the study.

Most studies have also employed delayed images over the lungs to search for evidence of pulmonary aspiration. The results have been variable (Table 3), but no suitable "gold standard" has been available for comparison. Since aspirated material can be cleared from the lung with time, relatively early images at 2 to 4 hours have been recommended in addition to overnight views.[26,27] Howman–Giles and Trochei[27] found that 78% of their scans that were positive for pulmonary aspiration were abnormal by 2 hours with only minimal gain in sensitivity by the addition of 24-hour images. Provided no aspiration occurs during the initial swallowing and the upper passages are shown to be clear, subsequent appearance of activity within the lung should be considered as evidence of aspiration of gastric contents. As with detection of esophageal activity, image enhancement should be employed.

Table 3. Detection of Pulmonary Aspiration in Children by Radionuclide Imaging		
Author/Ref.	Sensitivity (%)	
Heyman[14]	2/29	(6.9)
Arasu[16]	0/30	(0.0)
Blumhagen[20]	0/10	(0.0)
Boonyaprapa[26]	5/20	(25.0)
Jona[17]	18/125	(14.4)
Piepsz[24]	0/35	(0.0)
Howman–Giles[27]	9/19	(47.4)
MacFadyen[28]	4/9	(44.4)
Totals	38/277	(13.7)

Conclusion

Radionuclide techniques offer an attractive alternative to other more cumbersome (acid reflux) or less sensitive (barium) tests for detection of gastroesophageal reflux. Although the technique was initially described in adults, it appears to have been more widely utilized in the pediatric group. Advantages include lack of patient discomfort, ability to employ physiological substances (milk, juice, semi-solid food), capability for prolonged continuous monitoring, and ability to semi-quantitate the "esophageal exposure to gastric refluxate." Patient radiation is low (< 200 millirads to the GI tract and < 10 millirads total body) and is not increased by additional images. In comparison, fluoroscopy results in approximately 5,000 millirads per minute of exposure.[29] Careful technique must be employed including use of computer enhancement of the images, and reasonably long data collection periods may be important. Additional questions remain to be answered regarding its practical clinical usefulness as a screening procedure since intermittent reflux may go undetected.

Radionuclide techniques are not as sensitive as the acid reflux test but in almost all series have been superior to barium studies. It will not, however, replace barium since the low anatomic detail may allow important structural abnormalities to be missed. Although the reported sensitivity is variable, it offers the simplest test to detect pulmonary aspiration.

Gastric Emptying

Radionuclide techniques have also been extensively investigated for the measurement of gastric emptying rates. Since the initial description by Griffith[30] in which passage of chromium-51 labeled porridge was monitored by a dual-headed scanner, a wide assortment of radiolabeled meals have been evaluated.[31-35] It was recognized early that test meal composition, particularly liquid versus solid components, was an important variable influencing measured emptying rates[36] (Figure 5). Emptying rates for liquids approximated an

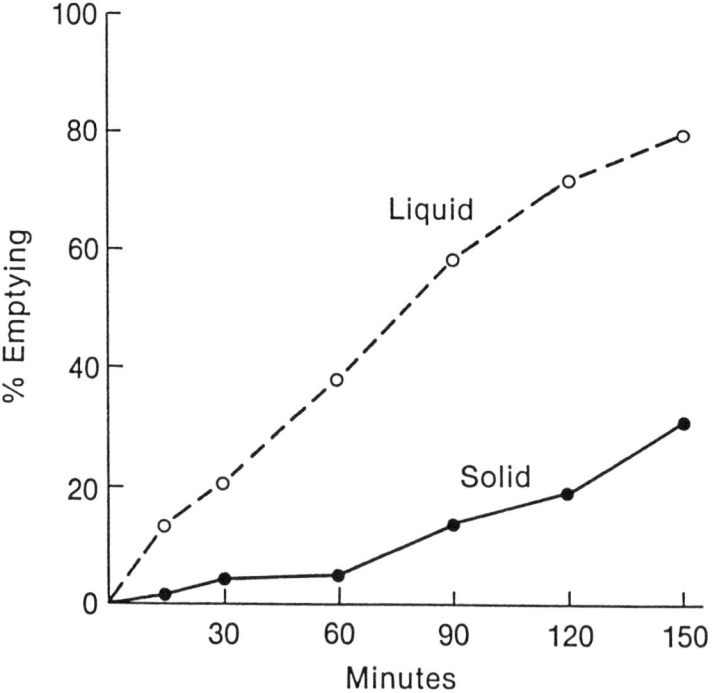

Figure 5: *Curves of percent gastric emptying for liquid and solid phase material. Although both curves are delayed compared with our normal range, there is considerably more rapid emptying of the liquid phase.*

exponential function while solid emptying was more nearly linear. Because of the limitations of a purely liquid test meal, a variety of solid phase radiolabeled materials have been tested. Meyer et al[37] utilized the hepatic uptake of intravenous radiocolloid ([99mTc-sulfur colloid) to label chicken liver *in vivo*. Testing of the radiolabeled liver revealed minimal dissociation of the technetium-99m from the solid phase on comparison with test meals of chromium-51 labeled eggs, which showed up to 90% dissociation. Others[38-41] have confirmed the excellence of the *in vivo* chicken liver tag; however, the inconvenience of this method in a hospital setting has prompted the search for suitable alternatives. *In vitro* labeling of raw harvested chicken liver with subsequent cooking of the radiolabeled preparation has been shown to have minimal dissociation in both hydrochloric acid and human gastric juice and to be suitable for most clinical applications.[35,39,41,42] *In vivo* and *in vitro* labeled chicken liver is usually administered mixed with other solids such as stew or hamburger to increase patient acceptance. Technetium-99m labeled purified ovalbumin and ^{99m}Tc-sulfur colloid labeled scrambled eggs have also been endorsed as satisfactory agents,[40,43] although ^{99m}Tc labeled eggs may exhibit some dissociation in the presence of gastric juice.[39] Other potentially useful solid phase markers include labeled polystyrene resins and radiolabeled fibers.[44-46] Patient radiation from technetium-99m is low because of the short physical half-life of 6 hours. A typical dose of 500 uCi of ^{99m}Tc chicken liver is estimated to deliver 230 millirads to the colon and < 10 millirads to the total body.[29]

Solid phase studies are more sensitive for subtle abnormalities of gastric emptying than pure liquid techniques.[47-49] and if a single agent is to be employed, a solid phase marker is usually preferable. At times, for a more complete description of gastric emptying, knowledge of both liquid and solid rates may be important. If the liquid phase study is being performed alone, technetium labeled agents such as ^{99m}Tc-DTPA or ^{99m}Tc-sulfur colloid in a suitable volume of liquid are satisfactory. However, if the liquid phase agent is intended for simultaneous use with a solid phase marker, the liquid marker must not become associated with the solid component and must differ sufficiently in gamma emissions to permit detection in the presence of the ^{99m}Tc solid label. Indium-111 or indium-113m-DTPA meet these criteria and have become accepted radiopharmaceuticals for dual liquid–solid studies.[35,38,42,47] The longer half-life of indium-111 results in a slightly higher patient radiation exposure with 250 uCi delivering approximately 2,000 millirads to the large intestine.[29]

When dual isotopic studies are performed, appropriate corrections must be made for downscatter from the higher energy label into the energy range of the second isotope. Downscatter interference can be minimized by using enough low energy isotope to result in a count rate at least six times greater than that from the higher energy label.[50] When higher energy isotopes, such as indium-111 or indium-113m, are employed, correction for septal penetration has also been suggested.[51]

Emptying rates of radiolabeled liquids may be slightly altered by the simultaneous feeding of solids, and it is imperative to establish normal limits for the particular combination of agents employed.[52,53]

Volume of the test meal will also influence observed emptying rates. In general, the larger the amount administered, the more prolonged will be the measured emptying half-time.[38] Typically, meals of 250 to 300 ml are used for adults although some investigators have utilized more generous portions. Again, standardization of technique is imperative if reproducible and comparative results are to be realized.

Initial radiation detecting equipment consisted of stationary probes or rectilinear scanners,[30,33] but the superiority of the gamma camera with its associated image and rapid acquisition time was recognized early[31,34,54] (Figure 6). Current state-of-the-art gamma cameras have sufficiently large fields of view to monitor the entire stomach plus portions of the esophagus and bowel. This permits more precise placement of appropriate regions of interest for generation of quantitative information (Figure 7). A computer interface allows for correction for background activity, isotope decay, and attenuation. Appropriate indices can then be generated.

Considerable controversy has existed over the question of need for collection of data from more than one projection. Initial investigators used primarily the anterior view, but concern arose over potential variation in overlying attenuation between different portions of the stomach and of possible changes in shape and position of the stomach during emptying. The anterior view alone may overestimate emptying measurements and may even produce a paradoxical initial increase in gastric counts during the early phase of the study.[38] Use of the geometric mean of both anterior and posterior views was suggested as a preferable technique.[47,55,56] This is of greater importance with relatively low energy isotopes such as technetium-99m and with relatively large volume test meals, especially in obese patients; however, some effect of varying attenuation may be seen with higher energy labels such as indium-111 or indium-113m and with smaller meal size.[38] Some investigators have felt attenuation correction with the geometric mean technique to be unnecessary.[57,58]

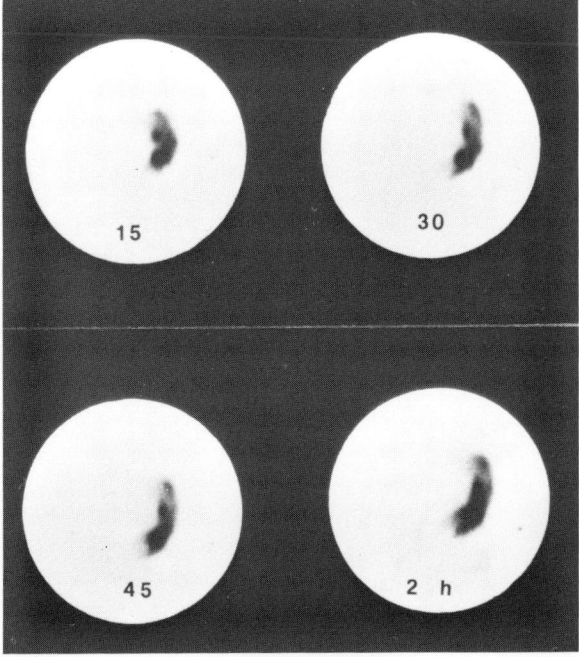

Figure 6: *Sequential anterior images of the stomach revealing minimal visual evidence of gastric emptying by 2 hours.*

Others have attempted to compensate by waiting until counts within the stomach reach maximum before beginning measurement[59] or through the use of peak-to-scatter ratio corrections from the anterior image alone.[60] Although attenuation correction may be unnecessary in thin individuals, it is recommended for the greatest accuracy,[50] and the geometric mean technique is probably the most straightforward approach.

Typically, results of gastric emptying studies have been expressed as the time for gastric activity to decline to one-half of the initial (or maximal counts) or as a given percentage of emptying at a specific time (60 minutes, 90 minutes, etc.). Other more intricate "indices" have been suggested but have not gained widespread acceptance.[59] Inspection of the entire curve rather than selected "arbitrary" points may provide additional information, and superimposition of the patient's results onto established normal curves provide a convenient expression of the data.[35]

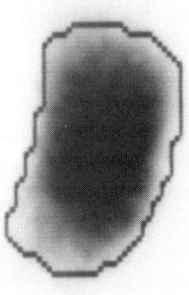

IMAGE #3

Figure 7: *Typical region of interest placement for quantitation of gastric emptying.*

Application to Gastroesophageal Reflux

Radionuclide techniques have been employed to investigate the possible role of abnormalities in gastric emptying in esophageal reflux disease.[48,61–66] Abnormal retention of liquid and/or solid food within the stomach has been suggested as an aggravating factor in gastroesophageal reflux by increasing the volume of material available for reflux. Although some investigators have found no abnormalities in gastric emptying,[62] McCallum et al[63] demonstrated slower gastric emptying rates with a mixed liquid–solid meal in 20 patients with reflux disease compared with age matched controls. In a larger group of 100 patients with gastroesophageal reflux, 41% were shown to have delayed gastric emptying. Others have also used radionuclide techniques to demonstrate gastric emptying disturbances in patients with reflux esophagitis[61,65,66] and to evaluate the effect of pharmacological therapy.[62,66] The Yale group also investigated liquid meal emptying rates in infants with symptomatic gastroesophageal reflux.[64] They found a significant delay in gastric emptying at one hour in the severe reflux group and postulated that abnormal motor function of the gastric fundus might be a significant factor in infants with reflux.

Conclusion

Radionuclide techniques for evaluation of gastric emptying offer the advantages of being physiologic and non-invasive with minimal patient discomfort. Various radionuclide labels can be incorporated into liquid or solid meal components permitting evaluation of either or both of these types of materials. Radiation exposure to the patient is low, considerably less than with techniques requiring prolonged fluoroscopy or repeated radiographs, and quantitation of the data is readily achieved.

Because of the wide variety of techniques currently in vogue for gastric emptying and the effect of alterations in test meal composition, volume, method of detection, and data calculation on the final results, each laboratory is encouraged to verify its specific normal range and to standardize its procedure.

Abnormalities in gastric emptying have been identified in many patients with severe gastroesophageal reflux. Radionuclide techniques are providing further information to assess the significance of this in reflux disease and to aid in monitoring the response to therapy.

Esophageal Function

Esophageal emptying and/or transit times may be readily studied with radionuclide techniques. Kazem[67] initially reported a scintigraphic technique for following transit through the esophagus of a ^{99m}Tc-pertechnetate liquid bolus and studied both normals and patients with obstructive lesions. Other, after modifying the technique by using a smaller semi-solid (gelatin) bolus and dividing the esophagus into two segments for histogram generation, evaluated a larger number of normals and a few patients with obstruction.[68] Tolin et al[69] used non-absorbable ^{99m}Tc-sulfur colloid in a liquid bolus with the patient supine to minimize gravitational effect. They introduced a quantitative index of percent esophageal transit through a single esophageal region of interest to permit more objective evaluation of the study and investigated a variety of esophageal motility disorders including achalasia and diffuse esophageal spasm. Several centers employed variations of this technique to quantitate esophageal emptying in patients with achalasia and to evaluate the results of various forms of treatment including dilatation, surgery, and medication.[70-72] Relatively long individual data collection periods were used ($\geq$ 10 seconds), and primary emphasis was on the percent retention several minutes after swallowing. Review of the cine display of the images was also recommended.[73]

Both liquid (^{99m}Tc-s-colloid or ^{99m}Tc-DTPA in water) and solid (^{99m}Tc-chicken liver or eggs) materials have been employed. As with the other GI scintigraphic techniques using technetium-99m, the radiation to the patient is low.[29]

Russell et al[74] employed considerably shorter acquisition times (0.4 seconds per frame) to monitor the early dynamics of esophageal transit. Three esophageal regions of interest were used, and an esophageal transit time (time for 90% clearance of activity) was determined (Figure 8). They were able to detect abnormal transit times in a

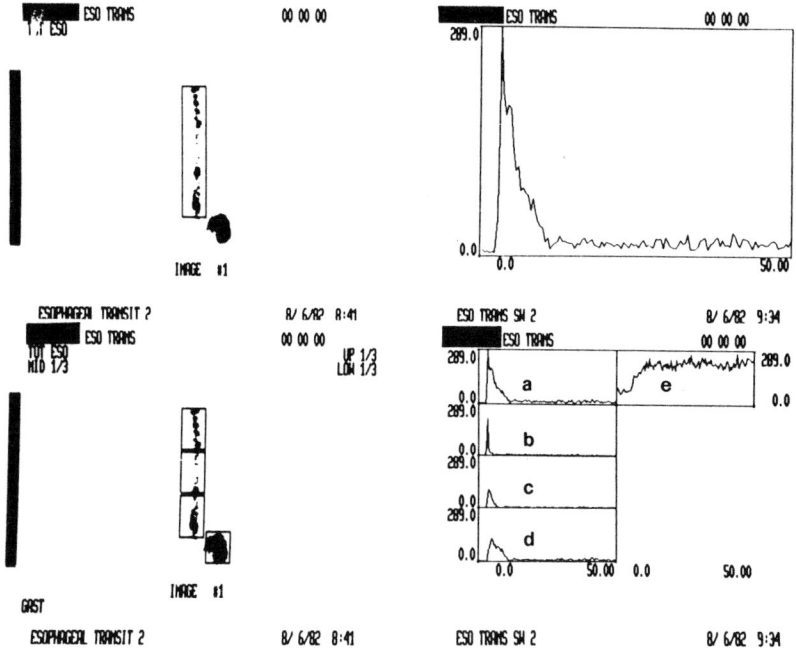

Figure 8: *Normal rapid sequence liquid bolus esophageal transit study. Upper right-hand curve reflects total esophageal activity obtained from region of interest seen at upper left. Curves at lower right consist of: (a) total esophageal activity, (b–d) segmental esophageal activity, and (e) gastric activity from regions of interest at lower left. The X axis indicates time from 0 to 50 seconds, and the Y axis represents counts.*

variety of motility disorders and, by inspection of the various segmental histograms, to characterize the abnormalities into adynamic or incoordination patterns. Nine of fourteen patients with dysphagia but normal manometry and without radiographic evidence of obstruction had abnormal radionuclide studies. Other reports have supported the utility of rapid sequence imaging in detecting and clarifying esophageal motility disorders[75-77] (Figure 9). Liquid bolus techniques (labeled water or milk) have been adapted for investigation of pediatric patients.[78,79] In infants and young children, repetitive swallows rather than a single swallow on command may have to be accepted.

Potential technical pitfalls have been recently reviewed and include double swallowing by the patient, unrecognized gastroesophageal reflux, residual activity in hiatal hernias, and employment of an esophageal region of interest which impinges on the gastric fundus.[80] Practice swallows by the patient, meticulous attention to detail, and

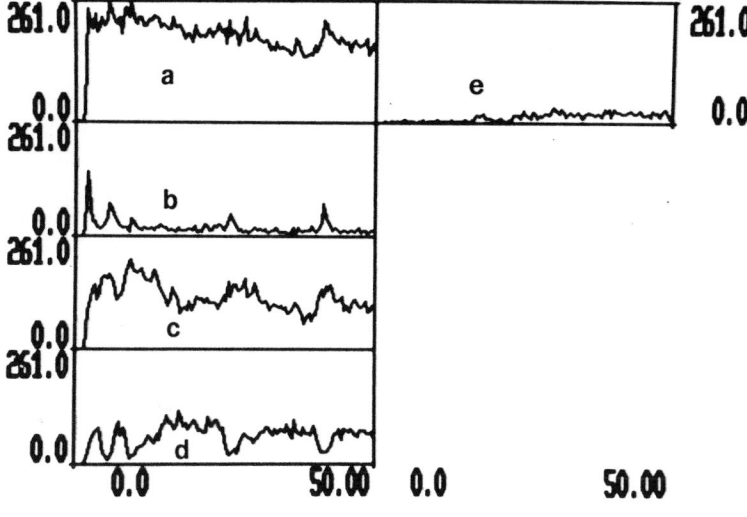

ESO TRANS CUR SM1 JH   **9/10/82 17:41**

Figure 9: *Curves from abnormal liquid bolus esophageal transit study in a patient with achalasia. (a) total esophageal curve, (b–d) segmental esophageal curves, and (e) gastric activity. The curves reflect a relative adynamic pattern, and minimal activity is seen to reach the stomach by the end of 50 seconds.*

visual inspection of the radionuclide images will help to minimize technical problems.

Simultaneous manometric measurements and liquid bolus transit times in the supine position have shown that esophageal transit time is primarily dependent upon peristaltic esophageal contractions and is not altered by the amplitude or duration of the peristaltic wave. Simultaneous contractions were shown to result in prolonged esophageal transit associated with to and fro movement of the liquid bolus.[81] The effect of position (erect and supine) and bolus composition has also been evaluated. Esophageal transit time is generally longer in the supine position, especially with solid or semi-solid material.[82-84]

Application to Reflux

Since the period of exposure of esophageal mucosa to gastric refluxate has been suggested as an important factor influencing development of esophageal mucosal injury, radionuclide transit and emptying studies have been used to evaluate patients with reflux esophagitis. Tolin et al[69] found abnormal transit in patients with symptomatic reflux, especially those with manometric evidence of motor dysfunction. They questioned whether reflux-induced mucosal injury resulted in subsequent motor dysfunction or whether underlying motility problems contributed to increased refluxate contact time causing mucosal injury. Thirty-one pediatric patients referred for possible reflux were studied by Heyman.[78] Eleven of these had abnormal esophageal liquid bolus transit as evaluated by visual inspection of the images. Quantitation was not attempted.

Radionuclide emptying techniques together with acid clearance studies have been used to evaluate mechanisms involved in raising the distal esophageal pH following an episode of acid refluxate.[85] Following instillation of acid into the distal esophagus of normal volunteers, peristaltic activity was shown to rapidly clear the majority of the acid volume but esophageal pH remained low, presumably due to mucosal coating. Restoration of intraluminal pH to normal was shown to be strongly influenced by neutralization of residual acid by swallowed saliva.

Conclusion

Radionuclide techniques can be used to evaluate the passage of a bolus through the esophagus by visual inspection of serial images and analysis of activity curves produced from various esophageal segments. Characteristic patterns may be seen in different motility disorders. Indices quantitating the degree of esophageal retention may be used to follow patients with disorders such as achalasia. These techniques are now being applied to patients with gastroesophageal reflux to further evaluate the incidence and type of esophageal dysfunction in this group and to investigate the pathophysiology of reflux esophagitis.

Summary

A variety of procedures which employ radiolabeled feedings to evaluate functional disturbances of the esophagus and stomach have been described. Such techniques are more physiologic and quantitative than other radiographic procedures and result in minimal patient radiation exposure. The methodology is still evolving as evidenced by considerable variation between laboratories. Standardization of technique is imperative for consistent results. Radionuclide techniques have provided a better understanding of the interrelationship of esophageal and gastric functional disorders in patients with reflux disease and in assessing response to therapy.

References

1. Fisher RS, Malmud LS, Roberts GS, Lobis IF: Gastroesophageal (GE) scintiscanning to detect and quantitate GE reflux. *Gastroenterology* 1976; 70:301–308.
2. Malmud LS, Fisher RS: Gastroesophageal scintigraphy. *Gastrointest Radiol* 1980; 5:195–204.
3. Menin RA, Malmud LS, Peterson RP, et al: Gastrointestinal scintigraphy to assess the severity of gastroesophageal reflux disease. *Ann Surg* 1980; 191:66–71.
4. Malmud LS, Fisher RS: The evaluation of gastroesophageal reflux before and after medical therapies. *Semin Nucl Med* 1981; 11:205–215.
5. Dodds WJ, Hogan WJ, Palmer DW: Scintiscanning for GE reflux. *Gastroenterology* 1977; 73:418–419.
6. Hoffman GC, Vansant JH: The gastroesophageal scintiscan: Comparison of methods to demonstrate gastroesophageal reflux. *Arch Surg* 1979; 114:727–728.
7. Velasco N, Pope CE, Gannan RM, Hill LD: Gastroesophageal scintigraphy for evaluation of gastroesophageal reflux and esophageal clearance. *Gastroenterology* 1982; 82:1204 (abstract).

8. McCallum RW: Radionuclide scanning in esophageal disease. Editorial comments. *J Clin Gastroenterol* 1982; 4:67–70.

9. Reich SB, Earley WC, Ravin TH, et al: Evaluation of gastro-pulmonary aspiration by a radioactive technique: Concise communication. *J Nucl Med* 1977; 18:1079–1081.

10. Chernow B, Johnson LF, Janowitz WR, Castell DO: Pulmonary aspiration as a consequence of gastroesophageal reflux. A diagnostic approach. *Dig Dis Sci* 1979; 24:839–844.

11. Ghaed N, Stein MR: Assessment of a technique for scintigraphic monitoring of pulmonary aspiration of gastric contents in asthmatics with gastroesophageal reflux. *Ann Allergy* 1979; 72:306–308.

12. Greyson ND, Reid RH, Liu YC, Thomas P: Radionuclide assessment in nocturnal asthma. *Clin Nucl Med* 1982; 7:318–319.

13. Rudd TG, Christie DL: Demonstration of gastroesophageal reflux in children by radionuclide gastroesophagography. *Radiology* 1979; 131: 483–486.

14. Heyman S, Kirkpatrick JA, Winter HS, Treves S: An improved radionuclide method for the diagnosis of gastroesophageal reflux and aspiration in children (milk scan). *Radiology* 1979; 131:479–482.

15. Conway JJ, Weiss SC, Luck SR, Goldstein RI: Radionuclide evaluation of gastroesophageal reflux in children. *J Nucl Med* 1979; 20:680 (abstract).

16. Arasu TS, Franken EA, Wyllie R, et al: The gastroesophageal (GE) scintiscan in detection of GE reflux and pulmonary aspiration in children. *Ann Radiol* 1980; 23:187–192.

17. Jona JZ, Sty JR, Glicklich M: Simplified radioisotope technique for assessing gastroesophageal reflux in children. *J Pediatr Surg* 1981; 16:114–117.

18. Seibert JJ, Byrne WR, Euler AR, et al: Gastroesophageal reflux—the acid test: Scintigraphy or the pH probe? *AJR* 1983; 140:1087–1090.

19. Arasu TS, Wyllie R, Fitzgerald JF, et al: Gastroesophageal reflux in infants and children—comparative accuracy of diagnostic methods. *J Pediatr* 1980; 96:798–803.

20. Blumhagen JD, Rudd TG, Christie DL: Gastroesophageal reflux in children: Radionuclide gastroesophagography. *AJR* 1980; 135:1001–1004.

21. Piepsz A, Georges B, Rodesch P, Cadranel S: Gastroesophageal scintiscanning in children. *J Nucl Med* 1982; 23:631–632.

22. Swanson MA, Cox KL, Kannon RA: Gastroesophageal scintigraphy with and without compression. *Clin Nucl Med* 1981; 6:62–67.

23. Gelfand MJ, Thomas SR: Scintigraphy for detection of gastroesophageal reflux. *J Pediatr* 1981; 98:172.

24. Piepsz A, Georges B, Perlmutter N, et al: Gastro-oesophageal scintiscanning in children. *Pediatr Radiol* 1981; 11:71–74.

25. Devos PG, Forget P, De Roo M, Eggermont E: Scintigraphic evaluation of gastroesophageal reflux (GER) in children. *J Nucl Med* 1979; 20:636 (abstract).

26. Boonyaprapa S, Alderson PO, Garfinkel DJ, et al: Detection of pulmonary aspiration in infants and children with respiratory disease: Concise communication. *J Nucl Med* 1980; 21:314–318.

27. Howman–Giles R, Trochei M: Radionuclide "milk" scan for detection of pulmonary aspiration in infants and children. *J Nucl Med* 1980; 21:P9.

28. MacFadyen UM, Hendry GMA, Simpson H: Gastro-oesophageal reflux in near-miss sudden infant death syndrome or suspected recurrent aspiration. *Arch Dis Child* 1983; 58:87–91.

29. Seigel JA, Wu RK, Knight LC, et al: Radiation dose estimates for oral agents used in upper gastrointestinal disease. *J Nucl Med* 1983; 24: 835–837.
30. Griffith GH, Owen GM, Kirkman S, Shields R: Measurement of rate of gastric emptying using chromium-51. *Lancet* 1966; 1:1244–1245.
31. Harvey RF, Mackie DB, Brown NJG, Keeling DH: Measurement of gastric emptying time with a gamma camera. *Lancet* 1970; 1:16–17.
32. Chaudhuri TK, Greenwald AJ, Heading RC, Chaudhuri TK: A new radioisotopic technique for the measurement of gastric emptying time of solid meal. *Am J Gastroenterol* 1976; 65:46–51.
33. Coates G, Gilday DL, Cradduck TD, Wood DE: Measurement of the rate of stomach emptying using Indium-1113m and a 10 crystal recilinear scanner. *Can Med Assoc J* 1977; 108:180–182.
34. vanDam APM: The gamma camera in clinical evaluation of gastric emptying. *Radiology* 1974; 110:155–157.
35. Malmud LS, Fisher RS, Knight LC, Rock E: Scintigraphic evaluation of gastric emptying. *Semin Nucl Med* 1982; 12:116–125.
36. Sheiner HJ: Progress report. Gastric emptying tests in man. *Gut* 1975; 16:235–247.
37. Meyer JH, MacGregor IL, Gueller R, et al: ^{99m}Tc-tagged chicken liver as a marker of solid food in the human stomach. *Am J Dig Dis* 1976; 21:296–304.
38. Christian PE, Moore JG, Sorenson JA, et al: Effects of meal size and correction technique on gastric emptying time: Studies with two tracers and opposed detectors. *J Nucl Med* 1980; 21:883–885.
39. Christian PE, Moore JG, Datz FL: In vitro comparison of solid food radiotacers for gastric emptying studies. *J Nucl Med Technol* 1981; 9:116–117.
40. Knight LC, Malmud LS: Tc-99m-ovalbumin labeled eggs: Comparison with other solid food markers in vitro. *J Nucl Med* 1981; 22:P28.
41. McCallum RW, Saladino T, Lange R: Comparison of gastric emptying rates of intracellular and surface-labeled chicken liver in normal subjects. *J Nucl Med* 1980; 21:P67.
42. Wright RA, Thompson D, Syed I: Simultaneous markers for fluid and solid gastric emptying: New variations on an old theme: Concise communication. *J Nucl Med* 1981; 22:772–726.
43. Drane WE, Marks DS, Simms SM, et al: Work in progress: Radioisotopic evaluation of gastroplasty patients. *Radiology* 1983; 147:215–220.
44. Theodorakis MC, Digenis GA, Beihn RM, et al: Rate and pattern of gastric emptying in humans using ^{99m}Tc-labeled triethylenetetraamine-polystyrene resin. *J Pharm Sci* 1980; 69:568–571.
45. Carlson GL: Radiolabel fiber: A physiologic marker for gastric emptying and intestinal transit of solids. *Dig Dis Sci* 1980; 25:81–87.
46. Theodorakis MC, Groutas WC, Whitlock TW, Tran K: Tc-99m-labeled polystyrene and cellulose macromolecules: Agents for gastrointestinal scintigraphy. *J Nucl Med* 1982; 23:693–697.
47. Heading RC, Tothill P, McLoughlin GP, Shearman DJC: Gastric emptying rate measurement in man. *Gastroenterology* 1976; 71:45–50.
48. Ippoliti AF, McCallum RW, Sturdevant RAL: Impaired gastric emptying in patients with gastroesophageal reflux. *Clin Res* 1976; 24:535A.
49. Goldstein HA, Alavi A, Snape WJ: The increased sensitivity of solid scintigraphic gastric emptying. *J Nucl Med* 1980; 22:P29.

50. Christian PE, Datz FL, Sorenson JA, Taylor A: Technical factors in gastric emptying studies. *J Nucl Med* 1983; 24:262–268.
51. VanDeventer J, Thomson J, Graham LS, et al: Validation of corrections for errors in collimation during measurement of gastric emptying of nuclide-labeled meals. *J Nucl Med* 1983; 24:187–196.
52. Bandini P, Malmud L, Applegate G, et al: Dual radionuclide studies of gastric emptying using a physiologic meal. *J Nucl Med* 1980; 21:P66–7 (abstract).
53. Fisher RS, Malmud LS, Bandini P, Rock E: Gastric emptying of a physiologic mixed solid–liquid meal. *Clin Nucl Med* 1982; 7:215–221.
54. Calderon M, Sonnemaker RE, Hersh T, Burdine JA: ^{99m}Tc-human albumin microspheres (HAM) for measuring the rate of gastric emptying. *Radiology* 1971; 101:371–374.
55. Delin NA, Axelson B, Johansson C, Poppen B: Comparison of gamma camera and withdrawal methods for the measurement of gastric emptying. *Scand J Gastroenterol* 1978; 13:867–872.
56. Tothill P, McLoughlin GP, Holt S, Heading RC: The effect of posture on errors in gastric emptying measurements. *Phys Med Biol* 1980; 25:1071–1077.
57. Rattnur Z, Charkes ND, Malmud LS: Meal size and gastric emptying. *J Nucl Med* 1981; 22:831–832.
58. Wright RA, Krinski S: The use of a single γ camera in radionuclide assessment of gastric emptying. *Am J Gastroenterol* 1982; 77:890–891.
59. Dugas MC, Schade RR, Lhotsky D, Van Thiel D: Comparison of methods for analyzing gastric isotopic emptying. *Am J Physiol* 1982; 243:G237–242.
60. Meyer JH, VanDeventer G, Graham LS, et al: Error and corrections with scintigraphic measurements of gastric emptying of solid foods. *J Nucl Med* 1983; 24:197–203.
61. Donovan IA, Harding LK, Keighley MRB, et al: Abnormalities of gastric emptying and pyloric reflux in uncomplicated hiatus hernia. *Br J Surg* 1977; 64:847–848.
62. Behar J, Ramsby G: Gastric emptying and antral motility in reflux esophagitis. *Gastroenterology* 1978; 74:253–256.
63. McCallum RW, Berkowitz DM, Lerner E: Gastric emptying in patients with gastroesophageal reflux. *Gastroenterology* 1981; 80:285–291.
64. Hillemeier AC, Lange R, McCallum R, et al: Delayed gastric emptying in infants with gastroesophageal reflux. *J Pediatr* 1981; 98:190–193.
65. Baldi F, Corinaldesi R, Ferrarini F, et al: Gastric secretion and emptying of liquids in reflux esophagitis. *Dig Dis Sci* 1981; 26:886–889.
66. Valenzuela JE, Miranda M, Ansari AN, Lim BR: Delayed gastric emptying in patients with reflux esophagitis. *Gastroenterology* 1981; 80:1307 (abstract).
67. Kazem I: A new scintigraphic technique for the study of the esophagus. *AJR* 1972; 115:681–688.
68. Bosch A, Dietrich R, Lanaro AE, Frias Z: Modified scintigraphic technique for dynamic study of the esophagus. *Int J Nucl Med Biol* 1977; 4:195–199.
69. Tolin RD, Malmud LS, Reilley J, Fisher RS: Esophageal scintigraphy to quantitate esophageal transit. *Gastroenterology* 1979; 76:1402–1408.
70. Gross R, Johnson LF, Kaminski RJ: Esophageal emptying in achalasia quantitated by a radioisotope technique. *Dig Dis Sci* 1979; 24:945–949.

71. Holloway RH, Krosin G, Lange R, et al: Radionuclide esophageal emptying of a solid meal to quantitate results of therpy in achalasia. *Gastroenterology* 1983; 84:771−776.
72. Rozen P, Gelfond M, Zaltzman S, et al: Radionuclide confirmation of the therapeutic value of isosorbide dinitrate in relieving the dysphagia in achalasia. *J Clin Gastroenterol* 1982; 4:17−22.
73. Rozen P, Gelfond M, Zaltzman S, et al: Dynamic, diagnostic, and pharmacologic radionuclide studies of the esophagus in achalasia. *Radiology* 1982; 144:587−590.
74. Russell COH, Hill LD, Holmes ER, et al: Radionuclide transit: A sensitive screening test for esophageal dysfunction. *Gastroenterology* 1981; 80:887−892.
75. Blackwell JN, Hannan WJ, Adam RD, Heading RC: A radionuclide technique for assessing oesophageal function. *Nucl Med Commun* 1982; 3:291−296.
76. Blackwell JN, Hannan WJ, Adam RD, Heading RC: Radionuclide transit studies in the detection of oesophageal dysmotility. *Gut* 1983: 24: 421−426.
77. Kramer CM, Harp GD, Lovgren K, et al: Quantitation of fluid transport by the human esophagus. *Gastroenterology* 1982; 82:1106 (abstract).
78. Heyman S: Esophageal scintigraphy (milk scans) in infants and children with gastroesophageal reflux. *Radiology* 1982; 144:891−893.
79. Guillet J, Wynchank S, Basse−Cathalinat B, et al: Pediatric esophageal scintigraphy. Results of 200 studies. *Clin Nucl Med* 1983; 9:427−433.
80. Blackwell JN, Richter JE, Wu WC, et al: Esophageal radionuclide transit test: Potential false positive results. *Gastroenterology* 1983; 84:1108.
81. Richter JE, Blackwell JN, Wu WC, et al: Assessment of liquid bolus transit (LBT) by simultaneous radionuclide transit and esophageal manometry. *Gastroenterology* 1983; 84:1285 (abstract).
82. Fisher RS, Malmud LS, Applegate G, et al: Effect of bolus composition on esophageal transit: Concise communication. *J Nucl Med* 1982; 23: 878−882.
83. O'Sullivan G, Ryan J, Brunsden B, et al: Quantitation of esophageal transit: A scintigraphic and manometric analysis. *Gastroenterology* 1982; 82:1143 (abstract).
84. Kjellen G, Tibbling L: Esophageal transit of a radionukleide, solid bolus in normals. *Gastroenterology* 1982; 82:1101.
85. Helm JF, Dodds WY, Pelc LR, et al: Effect of esophageal emptying and saliva on clearance of acid from the esophagus. *N Engl J Med* 1984; 310: 284−288.

THERAPY

13

Overview of Treatment of Gastroesophageal Reflux Disease

Donald O. Castell, M.D.

Chapter Contents

During the past decade, there have been numerous studies on potential new forms of therapy of GE reflux that have resulted in remarkable changes in our approach to these patients. In the early 70s the treatment of reflux consisted of the following: elevation of head of the bed, a bland diet, avoidance of irritants (orange juice, coffee), no eating before bedtime, weight loss, avoidance of tight garments, and the use of antacids.

Notably absent from the above are the now well-accepted medical modalities of bethanechol, metoclopramide, and histamine H_2 receptor blockers. Through the combined approach of manometric

From Castell DO, Wu WC, Ott DJ (eds): *Gastroesophageal Reflux Disease: Pathogenesis, Diagnosis, Therapy.* Mount Kisco, NY, Futura Publishing Co., Inc., 1985.

laboratory investigations and subsequent clinical trials, the potential for these agents as new therapies for GE reflux disease has been developed.

Phase I Medical Management

Patients with symptomatic GE reflux disease who are seen by physicians should be approached with the concept that this is usually a long-standing chronic disease. It is important to begin to educate these patients on modifications of their lifestyle that can produce meaningful long-term effects on the presentation of their disease. For all patients with chronic reflux, therapy must begin with a commitment to modification of habits that are potentially detrimental in their ability to produce reflux.[1] Much attention has been given over the years to some of the simpler and mechanical approaches to prevention of reflux, as listed above. Although clear-cut experimental data are not available to support many of these approaches, there is ample reason to build the therapeutic program on these measures. Phase I therapy of chronic reflux disease can be better identified as *lifestyle modification* and includes those modalities listed in Table 1. These simple, but often effective, changes in lifestyle can produce meaningful results in the long-term treatment of GE reflux. Similar to the treatment recommended a decade ago, instructing the patient to eat three meals daily and to take his evening meal several hours before retiring, and to avoid lying down after meals is a good recommendation. Modifying the diet to include a lower fat content, usually with higher protein, and to result in significant weight loss in the overweight patient is also recommended. The simple maneuver of elevation of the head of the bed by at least 6 inches has been recommended for many years because of its apparent effect. Recent studies with overnight pH monitoring have shown a significant decrease in esophageal acid exposure with this maneuver.[2] Drugs that have a potential for decreasing lower esophageal sphincter (LES) pressure or interfering with esophageal peristalsis are to be avoided. These may include progesterone, theophylline, prostaglandins, anti-cholinergics, beta adrenergic agonists, alpha adrenergic antagonists, dopamine, diazapam, narcotics, and even the new calcium channel blocking agents. Cigarette smoking has been shown to produce a marked reduction in LES pressure and therefore should be avoided. Finally, regular use of antacids and/or alginic acid completes the basic Phase I program to be followed by all patients with chronic reflux. It can be

Table 1. **Medical Therapy of GE Reflux**	
Phase I Therapy (Lifestyle modifications)	**Phase II Therapy**
Elevation of head of the bed (6 inches)	Increase lower esophageal sphincter pressure
Dietary modifications	
1. Lower fat, higher protein	Bethanechol (also improves esophageal clearance)
2. Avoid specific irritants	Metoclopramide (also improves gastric emptying)
a. Citrus juices	
b. Tomato products	Inhibit gastric acid output
c. Coffee	Cimetidine
d. Alcohol ?	Ranitidine
3. Weight loss if overweight	
4. Do not eat prior to sleep	
Decrease or stop smoking	
Avoid potentially harmful medications	
1. Anticholinergics	
2. Sedatives/tranquilizers	
3. Theophylline	
4. Prostaglandins	
5. Calcium channel blockers	
Antacids or alginic acid	

expected that many patients with uncomplicated chronic reflux disease will find that Phase I modifications will effectively control their symptoms most of the time.

Phase II Medical Management

In those patients in whom the lifestyle modifications suggested above do not result in a satisfactory level of symptom control, more aggressive medical therapy is recommended. The Phase II medications include either those drugs that will potentially increase the level of pressure in the LES or drugs that will produce a significant degree of inhibition of gastric acid secretion. (Table 1). It has been my approach to attempt to use Phase II therapy in an intermittent fashion to suppress active manifestations of GE reflux disease as additives to chronic Phase I therapy.

The possibility of decreasing reflux by increasing LES pressures via a cholinergic agent was first studied as early as 1960 by investigators in the laboratory of the late Morton Grossman.[3] Injections of bethanechol were shown to significantly decrease acid reflux and produce concurrent increases in LES pressure. The pressure changes were minimal, however, since they were measured with infusion systems now known to be inadequate. Subsequent laboratory studies confirmed the ability of bethanechol to produce major increases in LES pressure both in normal individuals and in patients with GE reflux.[4] As discussed by Dr. Richter in Chapter 14, numerous clinical trials have now shown the effectiveness of bethanechol as an adjunct to the treatment of chronic reflux symptoms in both adult patients and children. Thus, the concept of increasing the anti-reflux pressure barrier through medical modalities has received good support and is currently an accepted therapeutic practice. One note of warning seems appropriate. It has been my observation that patients with severe long-standing reflux disease who have very low resting LES pressure are not likely to respond to bethanechol therapy. This is based on the observation that their sphincter contraction pressures are so low that this circular muscle has lost its ability to respond to any meaningful degree. Therefore, bethanechol is least likely to be effective in patients with the more severe forms of reflux disease who might benefit the most from adjunctive therapy.

The early laboratory studies with metoclopramide indicated that it, like bethanechol, would increase LES pressures considerably.[5] The more exciting potential use of this drug, however, resulted from studies showing that it would also improve gastric emptying. This observation, combined with studies showing that patients with chronic GE reflux often have delayed gastric emptying, has led to the recommendation that metoclopramide also be used as an adjunctive form of therapy in patients with chronic reflux.[6] This drug would particularly be useful, of course, in those patients in whom abnormalities of gastric emptying have been demonstrated. As Dr. Richter tells us in Chapter 14, there are ample supporting clinical trials to indicate the effectiveness of this drug in patients with chronic reflux symptoms. One has to be somewhat wary of the potential side effects of metoclopramide. We do note that the neurologic and/or psychiatric side effects tend to limit the use of this drug in a certain percentage of patients.

It has been the histamine H_2 receptor blockers that have brought the greatest excitement in their potential as effective therapeutic agents in treating acid reflux disease. These drugs have been shown to dramatically decrease gastric acid output and to have no adverse effect on resting or stimulated LES pressure measurements. Numerous clinical trials have demonstrated a definite effect of cimetidine in short-term (4–8 weeks) studies of patients with chronic heartburn. These studies are described in detail by Dr. Richter in Chapter 14. More recent studies with ranitidine have indicated similar effectiveness in the short-term therapy of reflux patients.[7] Yet to be determined is the long-term role or proper usage of these drugs in the treatment of these patients with this chronic, often unrelenting, problem.

A word about the future: It seems likely that we can anticipate that a great number of potential new medical therapies for patients with reflux will be seen over the new few years.

- Newer drugs in the family of histamine receptor blockers, potentially having greater potency and longer duration of action, are surely to be available to us in the future.
- Other forms of acid-suppressing drugs are likely to be developed. Drugs of the pharmacologic class that inhibit H^+/K^+ ATPase such as omeprazole offer a real potential in treatment of reflux disease. This drug has been shown to inhibit acid secretion for greater than 24 hours after a single dose, promising the one-a-day dose regimen that may provide greater patient compliance.
- An exciting class of drugs are the so-called antimuscarinic M_1 receptor antagonists. The prototype of this kind is pirenzepine, which has been proposed to selectively inhibit gastric acid production from the parietal cell with minimal effects on GI tract smooth muscle. This effect relates to the potential site of action as an inhibitor of the ganglionic M_1 receptor (Figure 1). Studies from our laboratory indicate that pirenzepine is quite different than typical anticholingeric drugs. It does not decrease LES pressure or peristaltic contraction pressures as produced by a classical anticholinergic such as propantheline (Figure 2). Because of its ability to inhibit acid secretion without adverse effects on smooth muscle contractions, pirenzepine may have a role in the treatment of chronic reflux disease.
- There are continuing attempts to develop newer drugs with

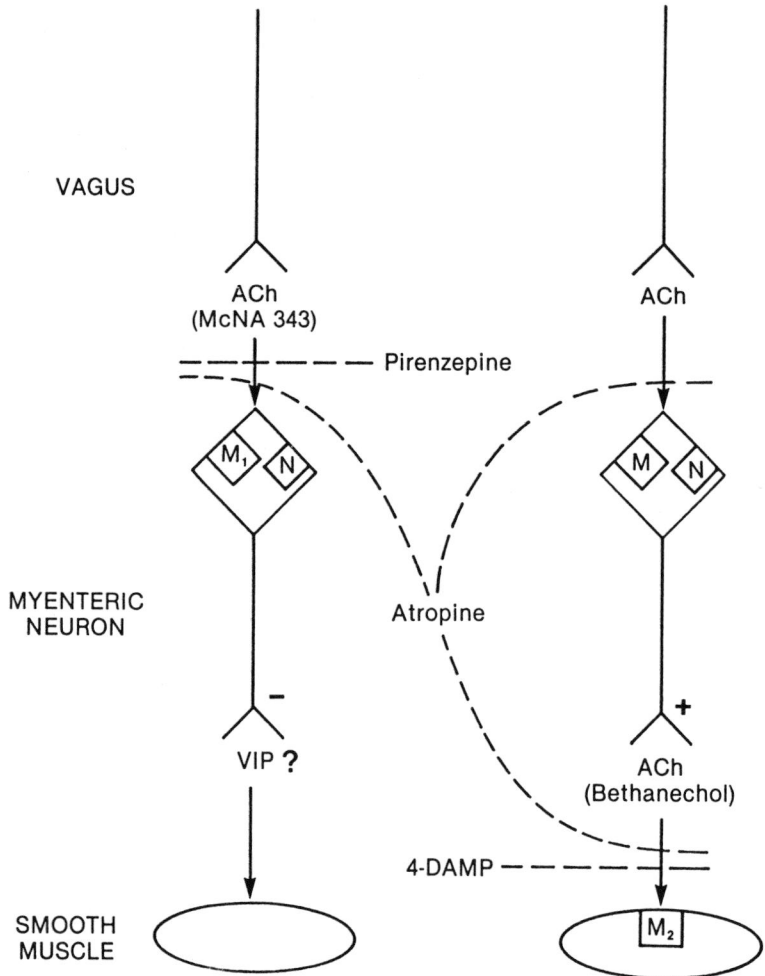

Figure 1: *Schematic representation of the site of action of various neurotransmitters and pharmacologic agents on the stimulatory (right) and inhibitory (left) pathways to esophageal smooth muscle. ACh = acetyl choline; McNA-343 = McNeil compound 343, a specific stimulant to the M_1, muscarinic inhibitory receptor; VIP = vasoactive intestinal peptide; 4-DAMP = 4-diphenylacetoxy-N-methylpiperodine-methiodide, a specific inhibitor of the postganglionic neurotransmitter on the smooth muscle muscarinic receptor; M = muscarinic receptors; N = nicotinic receptors. As illustrated, pirenzepine is believed to selectively inhibit preganglionic transmission in the inhibitory pathway (the M_1 receptor). In contrast, classical anticholinergics like atropine have a more non-specific inhibitory action at all muscarinic receptors. M_2 indicates the stimulatory muscarinic receptor on the smooth muscle.*

either cholinergic stimulatory effects on GI tract smooth muscle or dopamine antagonists with selective peripheral actions, such as domperidone. Preliminary studies with this drug suggest that it may well promote increased gastric emptying without the central side effects noted by metoclopramide.

• Sucralfate is a new agent being advocated in the treatment of acid-peptic mucosal injury. This compound has been shown to selectively bind to areas of injured GI tract mucosa and to form a local protective layer with additional antipeptic activity. It has been shown to be effective in the treatment of acute duodenal ulcers and has been proposed as possible therapy for other mucosal lesions, including peptic esophagitis. At present, there are no clinical studies to support this latter hypothesis, although occasional clinical antedotes indicate that patients experience considerable symptomatic relief of heartburn after

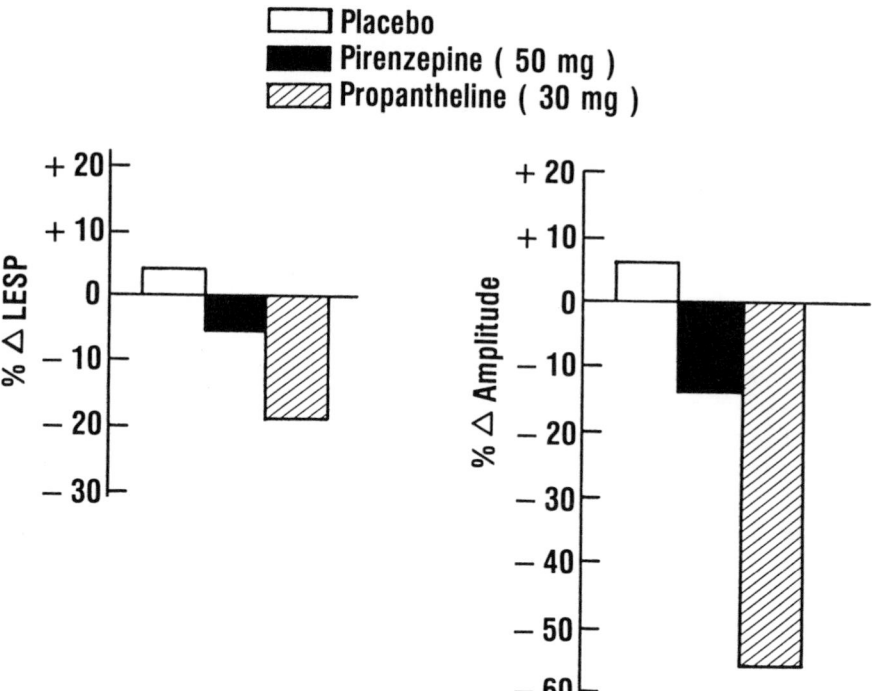

Figure 2: *Comparison of the effects of pirenzepine (50 mg), propantheline (30 mg), and placebo on lower esophageal sphincter pressure (LESP) and amplitude of esophageal contraction in a group of normal volunteers. Only propantheline produced significant decreases in pressures.*

ingestion of a suspension of crushed sucralfate tablets. Further studies with this compound are needed before any conclusion relative to its use in patients with GE reflux can be made.

Surgical Therapy

In Chapter 15, Dr. DeMeester provides a thorough review of the surgical approach to the treatment of the patient with chronic reflux disease. Based on his years of experience, he has suggested that the Nissen fundoplication is the preferred approach to these patients. The silicone prosthetic device proposed by Dr. Angelchik has been the newest potential addition to the surgical therapy of chronic reflux disease.[8] Although it has been used in a number of patients on this continent, the studies to date are still quite preliminary and do not allow any definite conclusion about the appropriate use of this device or whether it should be used at all.

Conclusions

In those patients with chronic GE reflux disease who are seen by the physician, an outline of my proposed therapeutic approach is shown in Figure 3. All patients should be advised of the lifestyle modifications that are included in Phase I therapy. For those patients who do not respond satisfactorily to this approach, the addition of Phase II medications should be considered. Whenever possible, one should attempt to back down to only the continuing Phase I therapy. It is often more difficult to determine when Phase III treatment, or anti-reflux surgery, is indicated. This is a very controversial question that is dealt with by Dr. DeMeester in Chapter 15. Some of those patients with severe persistent symptoms and without complications may be candidates for surgery. Many patients with complications of chronic GE reflux are candidates for anti-reflux therapy. The management of these problems is discussed by Drs. Barish and Wu in Chapter 16. The special problems associated with Barrett's esophagus are reviewed by Drs. Eastwood and Bonnice in Chapter 17.

GERD ICEBERG

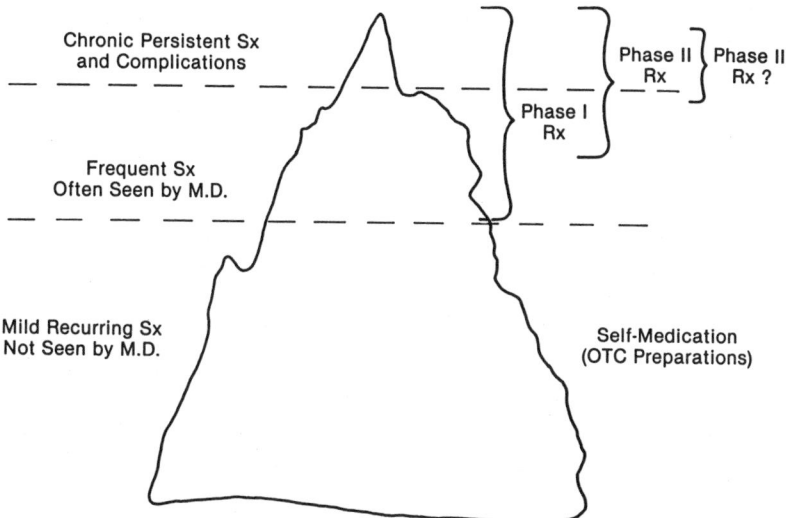

Figure 3: *The gastroesophageal reflux disease (GERD) iceberg is again shown as in Chapter 1. In this figure, usual therapy for the different presentations of reflux is indicated on the right. The great majority of reflux patients with mild intermittent symptoms, usually not seen by a physician, treat themselves for symptoms with a variety of over-the-counter (OTC) antacid-type medications. All patients seen by the physician should initially be treated with Phase I therapy, and these measures should be continued chronically. For persistence of symptoms, Phase II therapy should be invoked. Exactly when to recommend surgery (Phase III) in those patients with chronic symptoms or with complications of reflux remains controversial.*

References

1. Richter JE, Castell DO: Gastroesophageal reflux. Pathogenesis, diagnosis, and therapy. *Ann Intern Med* 1982; 97:93–103.
2. Johnson LF, DeMeester TR: Evaluation of elevation of the head of the bed, bethanechol, and antacid foam tablets on gastroesophageal reflux. *Dig Dis Sci* 1981; 26:673–680.

3. Bettarello A, Tuttle G, Grossman MI: Effect of autonomic drugs on gastro-esophageal reflux. *Gastroenterology* 1960; 39:340–346.
4. Farrell RL, Roling GT, Castell DO: Stimulation of the incompetent lower esophageal sphincter: A possible advance in therapy of heartburn. *Am J Dig Dis* 1978; 18:646–650.
5. Behar J, Biancani P: Effect of oral metoclopramide on gastroesophageal reflux in the post-cibal state. *Gastroenterology* 1976; 70:331–335.
6. McCallum RW, Ippoliti AF, Cooney C, Sturdevant R: A controlled trial of metoclopramide in symptomatic gastroesophageal reflux. *N Engl J Med* 1977; 296:354–357.
7. Wesdorp IC, Dekker W, Klinkenberg–Knol EC: Treatment of reflux oesophagitis with ranitidine. *Gut* 1983; 24:921–924.
8. Angelchik JP, Cohen R: A new surgical procedure for the treatment of gastroesophageal reflux and hiatal hernia. *Surg Gynecol Obstet* 1979; 148:246–248.

14

Gastroesophageal Reflux Disease: A Review of Medical Therapy

Joel E. Richter, M.D.

Chapter Contents

Symptomatic gastroesophageal (GE) reflux is one of the most common problems encountered by physicians of all specialties. The incidence of reflux and its primary symptom, heartburn, in the general population is extremely difficult to obtain, because many patients consider the sensation normal and do not seek medical attention. A study that surveyed presumably healthy hospital staff and employees found that 7% of the individuals experienced daily heart-

From Castell DO, Wu WC, Ott DJ (eds): *Gastroesophageal Reflux Disease: Pathogenesis, Diagnosis, Therapy.* Mount Kisco, NY, Futura Publishing Co., Inc., 1985.

burn, although 36% of the "normals" had this symptom at least once a month.[1] Heartburn reaches its maximal frequency during pregnancy, when 25% of patients may be found to have daily symptoms.[1] The magnitude of the problem is further increased by the observation that gastroesophageal reflux can masquerade as atypical chest pain[2] or present with pulmonary symptoms, particularly in the pediatric age group.[3]

The major anti-reflux mechanism is generally considered to be the level of pressure, and therefore competence, of the lower esophageal sphincter (LES). There is, as reviewed in previous chapters, good evidence to support the concept that at least four potential components may be important in the pathogenesis of gastroesophageal reflux disease (Figure 1): (a) an incompetent anti-reflux barrier; (b) the irri-

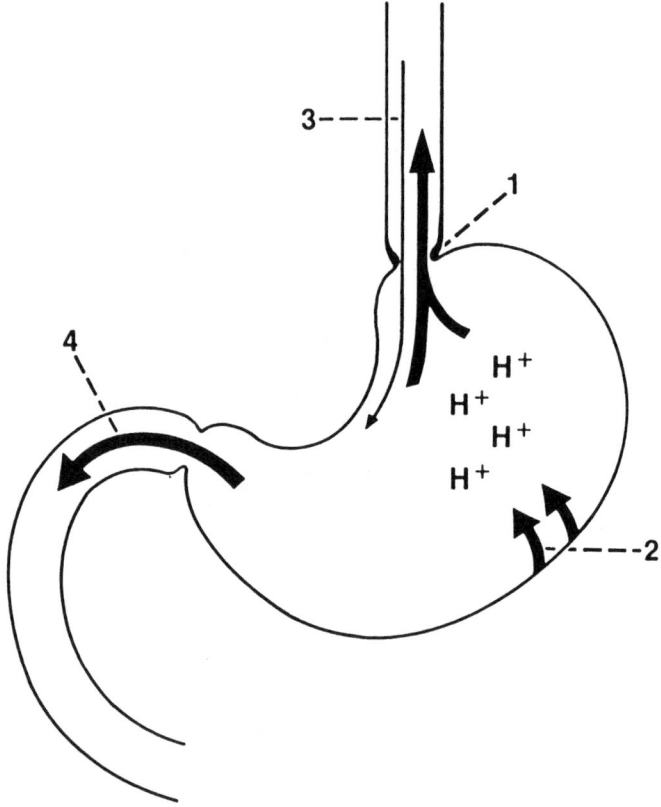

Figure 1: *Schematic representation of classical concept of the pathogenesis of gastroesophageal (GE) reflux disease and various cyclic mechanisms of potential importance. Details in text.*

tant effect of refluxed material on the esophageal mucosa: primarily gastric acid, but also pepsin and bile; (c) abnormal esophageal clearing; (d) abnormal gastric emptying. Many common drugs and foods may aggravate GERD by potentiating these factors. A rational treatment program including traditional approaches and newer forms of therapy can be developed based on attempts to improve each of the four possible defects listed above.[4,5]

Improving the Anti-reflux Barrier

A variety of modalities may improve LES pressure or otherwise decrease reflux: modification of diet, cessation of smoking, antacids, alginic acid, bethanechol, metoclopramide, domperidone (?), weight loss (?). Specifics of most of these therapies will be discussed below.

Smoking causes a marked reduction in lower esophageal sphincter pressure. The smoking of two cigarettes over a 20-minute period has been shown to result in a 50% decrease in LES pressure. Pressure fell within 2 to 3 minutes after smoking began, and remained low until smoking was stopped.[6] Another study utilizing overnight esophageal pH measurements found that one-third of all reflux episodes occurred while the patients were smoking, and reflux was seen during the smoking of two-thirds of all the cigarettes consumed.[7] The exact mechanism by which cigarette smoking lowers sphincter pressure is not clear, but recent studies indicate that nicotine, by blocking the cholinergic control mechanism, may decrease LES pressure.[8] Although not tested in a clinical trial, stopping or decreasing smoking, therefore, is an important part of the treatment program. Weight loss is a traditional component of reflux treatment. Empirical observations with patients seem to indicate that loss of a few critical pounds may improve symptoms. A recent report, however, has failed to confirm the suggestion that obese patients have low LES pressure, which might predispose to reflux.[9] There have been no clinical trials of weight loss in the therapy of GE reflux.

Decreasing Gastric Acidity

Antacids and the histamine H_2 receptor blocking drugs are used to decrease esophageal irritation from gastric acid and pepsin. Details of specific therapies are discussed subsequently. Classical anti-cholinergic agents should not be used to decrease gastric acidity in patients with GERD. These drugs have also been found to decrease both the resting tone and responsiveness of the LES and also result in increased reflux.[10] Pirenzepine, a new anti-cholinergic that specifically antagonizes M_1 muscarinic receptors, potentially may be useful in the treatment of GERD. While selectively inhibiting acid secretion, pirenzepine has been shown in preliminary reports to have minimal effect on LES pressure or esophageal contractions.[11]

Improving Esophageal Clearing

Specific measures directed at improving esophageal clearing are elevation of the head of the bed, avoidance or use of alcohol in moderation, bethanechol, and possibly metoclopramide or domperidone. The effects of specific agents will be discussed below.

Elevation of the head of the bed has been a standard component of therapy of GE reflux for many years. Recent studies with overnight intra-esophageal pH recordings have documented a significant increase in esophageal acid clearance time at night, lending strong support for the value of this mode of therapy.[12] No clinical trial of elevation of the head has been performed. Intoxicating doses of alcohol given orally or intravenously to normal volunteers have been shown to decrease LES pressure, amplitude of primary peristalsis in the distal esophagus, and upper esophageal sphincter pressure.[13] These effects are reversible, but chronic alcoholics with peripheral neuropathy may have similar permanent esophageal motor dysfunction.

Improving Gastric Emptying

Metoclopramide and possibly bethanechol and domperidone might improve abnormal gastric emptying in patients with reflux.

Specific Therapy

Drugs to Avoid

Recent investigations have indicated that a variety of drugs will decrease LES pressure and thereby produce a greater tendency toward incompetence of the anti-reflux barrier. These drugs include progesterone, theophylline, prostaglandins E_1, E_2, A_2, classical anticholinergic agents, beta-adrenergic agonists (isoproterenol), alpha-adrenergic antagonists (phentolamine), dopamine, valium, meperidine, morphine, and the new calcium-channel blocking agents.[14] Many of these drugs have been studied only in animals with little clinical data in patients with GE reflux. The progesterones, however, may have the most clinically important drug action on LES pressure. Sphincter pressures are progressively decreased during pregnancy,[15] and in women taking birth control pills containing progesterone.[16] These effects correlate well with increased levels of serum progesterone and increased demonstration of gastroesophageal reflux.

Dietary Therapy

There are at least two potential beneficial effects of diet modification in the treatment of reflux disease. The first relates to the effect of foods on LES pressure. Primary foods to avoid include fats, chocolate, alcohol, and carminatives as these have been shown to impair sphincter function. Volunteer studies with equal caloric test meals have shown significant decreases of pressures after fat ingestion and augmentation of sphincter pressures particularly after protein meals.[17] This has suggested to some the efficacy of a protein-rich "anti-reflux" diet. Although the lowering of LES pressure by chocolate was originally considered to be due to the high fat content of most chocolate preparations, the use of defatted chocolate syrup has indicated that chocolate itself decreases sphincter pressure. The mechanism of action is most likely explained by the high content of methyl xanthines, and their inhibition of phosphodiesterase, resulting in accumulation of cyclic AMP. Increased levels of cyclic AMP have a relaxant effect on the smooth muscle of the stomach and small intestine, and thus it is reasonable to anticipate a similar effect on the smooth muscle of the LES.[18] Carminatives, including peppermint and spearmint, which are often included in foods and after-dinner liqueurs, have been shown to result in decreased LES pressure and may provide another explanation for postprandial heartburn.[19]

The second effect of dietotherapy derives from avoiding those foods that may have a direct irritating effect on the esophagus. Citrus juices, tomato products (base in many spicy products), and coffee are frequently associated with exacerbations of heartburn. While generally not affecting LES pressure, these food substances have a direct pH-independent irritating effect of the inflamed esophageal mucosa.[20] Recent studies suggest that this effect may be related to high osmolarity.[21]

Coffee may have more than an irritating effect on the esophagus.

Studies of the response of LES pressure to coffee and caffeine ingestion have been conflicting. Initial studies with caffeine alone suggested minimal lowering of LES pressure.[22] Cohen and Booth demonstrated that brewed regular and decaffeinated coffee both increased
LES pressure and augmented acid production, while caffeine alone
had no effect on sphincter pressure.[23] In patients with gastroesophageal reflux, ingestion of coffee augmented acid production but only
minimally increased LES pressure, resulting in worsening of acid
reflux.[24] Thomas et al subsequently reached opposite conclusions.[25]
They found one cup of instant caffeinated coffee decreased LES pressure over 60 minutes in healthy volunteers and patients with reflux.
More recently, a British group has noted that caffeinated coffee had
no significant effect on LES pressure in the fasting or the postprandial
state.[26] Although it is difficult to reconcile these conflicting data,
coffee most likely aggravates heartburn not by a primary effect on
LES pressure but by increasing acid production in addition to its
direct irritant effect on the inflamed esophagus. The effect on acid
secretion is supported by the findings that coffee itself, even in high
doses, fails to elicit heartburn when acid secretion is inhibited.[24]

Antacids

Antacid therapy has been the backbone of effective medical
therapy of reflux disease for many years. Although these drugs were
originally proposed for their acid neutralizing effect, they have also
been shown to increase LES pressure and decrease gastroesophageal
reflux.[27,28] Antacids would appear to represent the most widely
used drugs for the treatment of heartburn, although there is only
meager evidence to support this widespread popularity. Two published trials have shown that either antacids or Gaviscon produced
significant decreases in reflux symptoms and healing of esophagitis
compared with pre-treatment levels. There was no true placebo group
in these studies.[29,30] A recent study has suggested that antacids are
no better than placebo in the treatment of GERD.[31] Drug treatment
consisted of 15 ml (80 mEq) doses of antacids (Maalox Therapeutic
Concentration, William H. Rorer) or placebo taken one and three
hours after meals and at bedtime. Both groups showed significant
improvement in both frequency and severity of heartburn. The time
to reproduce heartburn with a timed Bernstein test was increased by
both active drug and placebo. Both the antacid and placebo groups
showed improvements in the endoscopic degrees of esophagitis. In
clinical practice, antacids appear to be effective in the control of mild

to moderate symptoms of reflux disease. Whether this represents true pharmacologic efficacy or a placebo effect remains to be ascertained.

Alginic Acid

Gaviscon, containing alginic acid and antacids, is a popular agent proposed for the treatment of heartburn. The active component of this medication is alginic acid, which has been proposed to react with saliva to form a highly viscous solution that floats on the surface of the gastric pool, acting as a mechanical barrier. This compound is not an antacid, and it has been clearly shown to result in little, if any, change in the pH of the gastric contents below the foam barrier. In addition, alginic acid has not been shown to have any effect on LES pressure. Initial studies with both intra-esophageal pH monitoring and radioisotopes have demonstrated a significant decrease in episodes or quantity of reflux after the administration of alginic acid.[28,32] A more recent study utilizing prolonged intra-esophageal pH monitoring, however, found that Gaviscon failed to significantly diminish acid exposure despite doses as high as four tablets every two hours while awake and at bedtime.[12]

There have been five reported clinical trials with Gaviscon (Table 1). Bernardo et al showed that one tablet four times daily produced a significant decrease in reflux symptoms compared with administration of placebo in the same patients.[33] Antacid use and healing of esophagitis were not evaluated. Graham et al compared the effect of Gaviscon to antacids. Although both treatment regimens produced a significant decrease in symptoms and significant healing in four weeks compared with the pretreatment evaluation, there was no significant difference between the effect of the two programs.[29] A similar result was obtained by McHardy et al in a four-week, multi-center trial of 133 patients.[30] Again, Gaviscon was compared with antacids, with both regimens producing significant improvement in reflux symptoms and degree of esophagitis. Chevrel found liquid Gaviscon superior to liquid antacids in the relief of reflux symptoms in 44 patients studied in a two-week crossover trial.[34] Good relief of symptoms was reported by 85% of patients during therapy with Gaviscon compared with only 23% during antacid therapy. Prolonged symptomatic relief may also be maintained with Gaviscon. In an uncontrolled study, Hasan showed that 23/38 patients (62%) had complete relief of their chronic reflux symptoms at six months while taking an alginic acid/antacid combination (Gastrocote, MCP Pharmaceutical Ltd.) and an additional 7 patients experienced only occa-

Table 1.
Clinical Trials of Alginic Acid Therapy of GE Reflux Disease

Author	Year	No. Patients	Dose	Duration	↓ Sx	↓ Antacid Use	Healing
					____Effect____		
Bernardo	1975	26 (c/o)	1 tab qid	6 wks	+	—	—
Graham	1977	41 (20 Alg) (21 Ant)	2 tab qid	4 wks	*	–(Pl)	*
McHardy	1978	133 (65 Alg) (68 Ant)	2 tab	4 wks	*	–(Pl)	*
Chevrel	1980	44 (c/o) (Alg vs Ant)	10 ml qid	15 days	+	—	—
Hasan	1980	37 (No Pl)	2 tab qid	6 mos	+	—	—

*Significant improvement in both groups (alginic acid and antacid), but no difference between groups.

c/o = cross-over study　　　+ = significant effect
Alg = Alginic Acid　　　　　NS = not significant
Ant = Antacid　　　　　　　— = not studied
Pl = Placebo

sional symptoms.[35] Overall, these clinical studies suggest that alginic acid is effective in the treatment of GERD, but probably no better than antacid therapy.

Bethanechol

This cholinergic agent has great potential in the therapy of GE reflux disease, since it has been shown to increase resting LES pressure, to decrease reflux, and to also improve esophageal acid clearing in patients with reflux.[10,36,37] Recent prolonged pH studies suggest bethanechol is most effective in improving recumbent acid exposure; upright acid exposure is unchanged.[12] Although bethanechol has also been proposed as a drug that might improve gastric emptying, good support for this effect is not available.

There have been five published clinical trials of bethanechol in the treatment of gastroesophageal reflux disease (Table 2). Farrell et al showed that 25 mg four times a day produced significant decrease in reflux symptoms and decreased antacid use in 8 weeks as compared with placebo in a cross-over study of 20 patients with chronic reflux.[38] The extent of esophagitis was not assessed. Thanik et al have shown that the same dose of bethanechol produced significant healing of esophagitis (evaluated during endoscopy) when compared to placebo in a 4-week trial. Although there was greater improvement in symptoms with bethanechol, the level was not significant.[39] The amount of antacid usage was not evaluated in these patients. More recently, the same group has compared bethanechol and cimetidine in a six-week double-blind control trial.[40] To a similar degree, both drugs significantly decreased symptoms and improved the endoscopic healing of esophagitis. The 52% complete endoscopic healing rate in the bethanechol group was comparable to the healing rate seen with cimetidine in this and other studies.[41] In contrast, Saco et al found that bethanechol and intensive antacids were not better than placebo and antacids in the improvement of symptoms and healing of esophagitis in 28 patients with erosive esophagitis.[42] The clinical trial by Euler was performed in 45 pediatric patients. In these infants and

Table 2.
Clinical Trials of Bethanechol Therapy of GE Reflux Disease

Author	Year	No. Patients	Dose	Duration	↓ Sx	↓ Antacid Use	Healing
Farrell	1974	20 (c/o)	25 mg qid	8 wks	+	+	—
Thanik	1980	44 (22 Beth) (22 Pl)	25 mg qid	4 wks	NS	—	+
Euler	1980	45 (Peds) (c/o)	3 mg/m^2 tid	6 wks	+	—	—
Saco	1982	28 (14 Beth) (14 Pl)	25 mg qid	8 wks	NS	—	NS
Thanik	1982	43 (21 Beth) (21 Cim)	25 mg qid	6 wks	*	—	*

*Significant improvement in both groups (bethanechol and cimetidine), but no difference between groups.

c/o	= cross-over study	+	= significant effect
Beth	= Bethanechol	NS	= not significant
Cim	= Cimetidine	—	= not studied
Pl	= Placebo	Peds	= Pediatric patients

children, a significant improvement in reflux symptoms was noted compared with placebo therapy in the same patients over six weeks.[43] Antacid use and the healing of esophagitis were not evaluated. At a dose of 25 mg four times a day, bethanechol is well tolerated with few side effects. Abdominal cramps, diarrhea, urinary frequency, and blurred vision may occur, but the symptoms are usually mild and transient.

Metoclopramide

This dopamine antagonist offers promise as an effective agent in the treatment of reflux. It has been shown to increase LES pressure[44] and, more recently, to increase gastric emptying in reflux patients with normal as well as delayed gastric emptying.[45] The proposed ability of metoclopramide to increase esophageal clearing awaits documentation.

There have been six published clinical trials with metoclopramide in the treatment of reflux disease (Table 3). Venables et al were unable to show any significant effect on symptoms in a short (4-week) study, which included only 15 patients in a cross-over design.[46] Antacid use and healing of esophagitis were not studied. Similarly, Paull and Kerr failed to show a significant improvement in reflux symptoms compared with placebo treatment for 6 weeks. Again, antacid use and healing were not evaluated.[47] In the most positive published study of 31 patients, metoclopramide (10 mg four times daily) resulted in significant improvement in symptoms and antacid use compared with placebo in patients with reflux.[48] A more recent study supported the effectiveness of this dose regimen in producing significant decreases in symptoms and antacid use compared with placebo, but failed to document healing of esophagitis.[49] A disconcerting element in this report was the observation that one-third of the patients experienced important side-effects of a neurologic or psychotropic nature while taking metoclopramide. These side effects included restlessness, anxiety, insomnia, and acute extrapyramidal reactions necessitating discontinuation of metoclopramide. In a rare combination study, Temple et al found cimetidine plus metoclopramide (10 mg three times daily) to be no better than cimetidine alone in decreasing symptoms and healing esophagitis.[50] Adverse effects were more common in patients receiving combination therapy and severe enough to necessitate withdrawal in one-third of patients. A recent six-week trial by Guslandi et al has compared metoclopramide and ranitidine in 42 reflux patients.[51] Both drugs were equally effica-

Table 3.
Clinical Trials Metoclopramide Therapy of GE Reflux Disease

Author	Year	No. Patients	Dose	Duration	↓ Sx	↓ Antacid Use	Healing
Venables	1973	15 (c/o)	10 mg tid	4 wks	NS	—	—
Paull	1974	31 (15 Met) (16 Pl)	10 mg qid	6 wks	NS	—	—
McCallum	1977	31 (c/o)	10 mg qid	8 wks	+	+	—
Bright– Asare	1980	30 (20 Met) (10 Pl)	10 mg qid	8 wks	+	+	NS
Temple	1983	73 (40 Cim) (33 Cim & Met)	10 mg tid	12 wks	*	—	*
Guslandi	1983	42 (21 Met) (21 Ran)	10 mg tid	6 wks	*	—	*

*Significant improvement in both groups, but no difference between groups

c/o = cross-over study	+ = significant effect
Met = Metoclopramide	NS = not significant
PL = Placebo	— = not studied
Cim = Cimetidine	
Ran = Ranitidine	

cious in symptoms relief and endoscopic healing of esophagitis. Metoclopramide was significantly inferior to ranitidine in reducing the histologic changes of esophagitis.

Histamine H₂ Receptor Blockers

Histamine H_2 receptor blocking agents such as cimetidine and ranitidine have only one known mechanism of action in the treatment of reflux disease, decrease in gastric acid production. These drugs have not been shown to have any effect on LES pressure or esophageal or gastric emptying. Because of the great excitement over the therapeutic potential of an effective acid-suppressing agent in the treatment of gastroesophageal reflux disease, many clinical studies have been performed in a relatively short period, as summarized in Table 4. The large multicenter study by Behar et al showed that 8 weeks of therapy with cimetidine (300 mg four times daily) produced significant decrease in symptoms of reflux and use of antacids compared with placebo, but showed no greater effect on healing of esophagitis.[52] An identical result was obtained by Powell–Jackson in a smaller series of patients.[53] The possibility that cimetidine might

Table 4.
Clinical Trials of Cimetidine and Ranitidine Therapy of GE Reflux Disease

Author	Year	No. Patients	Dose	Duration	↓ Sx	↓ Antacid Use	Healing
Behar	1978	94 (49 Cim) (45 Pl)	300 qid	8 wks	+	+	NS
Powell– Jackson	1978	27 (c/o)	400 qid	6 wks	+	+	NS
Wesdorp	1978	24 (12 Cim) (12 Pl)	300 qid	8 wks	NS	NS	+
Petrokubi	1979	15 (PSS) (c/o)	300 qid	8 wks	+	–(Pl)	+*
Ferguson	1979	14 (St) (c/o)	400 qid	6 mos	NS	—	+*
Fiasse	1980	34 (19 Cim) (15 Pl)	400 qid	8 wks	+	+(G)	NS
Bright– Asare	1980	30 (20 Cim) (10 Pl)	300 qid	8 wks	+	+	NS
Bennett	1983	84 (51 Cim) (33 Pl)	1–2 gm daily	12 wks	+	+	—
Wesdorp	1983	36 (18 Ran) (18 Pl)	150 bid	6 wks	+	—	+

c/o = cross-over study   + = significant effect
Cim = Cimetidine   NS = not significant
Ran = Ranitidine   — = not studied
Pl = Placebo   G = Gaviscon
PSS = scleroderma   * = No improvement in stricture
St = peptic stricture

result in significant healing of esophagitis was shown by Wesdorp et al in an 8-week controlled trial of 24 patients receiving 300 mg four times daily compared with placebo.[41] These authors failed to find a significant decrease in reflux symptoms and antacid use, although a trend toward greater improvement was seen in the cimetidine-treated patients. The small number of patients in this series may have accounted for the lack of significance in this effect. The study by Petrokubi and Jeffries of 15 patients with chronic reflux symptoms secondary to esophageal scleroderma is of particular interest.[54] In these patients, having potentially the most severe form of esophageal disease, cimetidine, 300 mg four times daily, produced a significantly greater decrease in reflux symptoms and greater healing of esophagitis in 8 weeks than did an antacid placebo given in a cross-over design. The authors, however, noted no improvement of distal esophageal peptic strictures in 9 of these patients. Fiasse et al also reported a significant decrease in reflux symptoms and the use of Gaviscon compared with placebo treatment in a small group of patients.[55] They were not able to show a significant effect on healing of esophagitis in 8 weeks. The same observation was made by Bright–Asare and El-Bassoussi. Cimetidine produced significantly decreased symptoms and decreased antacid use but no improved healing in an 8-week trial when compared with placebo therapy.[49] In this study, a similar group of patients were treated with metoclopramide, and showed a similar therapeutic response. Thanik et al[40] found cimetidine as effective as bethanechol in the reduction of symptoms and healing of esophagitis while Temple et al[50] reported the combination of cimetidine and metoclopramide was no better than cimetidine alone in treating reflux patients. Neither study employed placebo controls. Most recently, Bennett et al compared the effect of cimetidine, 1 or 2 gm daily with placebo during a twelve-week trial in patients with GE reflux.[56] Nocturnal pain and antacid consumption were significantly reduced by cimetidine. No difference between the groups was detected on analysis of global assessment, daytime pain, dysphagia, or odynophagia. Of all the prolonged esophageal pH variables analyzed, only the number of reflux episodes during the 15-hour recording period showed a significant decrease in the cimetidine-treated group. These authors concluded the place of cimetidine in the treatment of GERD should be as an adjunct to the physical prevention of reflux rather than as a first-line agent.

One study of the effect of cimetidine (400 mg four times daily) to promote healing of peptic strictures over a longer term (6 months) has been reported. Although there was significant endoscopic improvement in esophagitis, the need for dilation was not reduced compared with placebo therapy.[57]

Initial studies with ranitidine, a new, more potent, long-acting histamine H_2 antagonist, suggest it is also effective in alleviating symptoms and healing esophagitis. In the only placebo-controlled trial reported to date, Wesdorp et al studied the efficacy of ranitidine (150 mg twice daily) in 36 reflux patients.[58] There was significant improvement in symptoms in the ranitidine-treated patients, although antacid consumption was not different from control patients. Endoscopic healing of esophagitis improved significantly in 15 of 19 ranitidine-treated patients compared with 4 of 19 patients in the placebo treated group. Guslandi et al randomly treated 45 reflux patients with either ranitidine (150 mg twice daily) or metoclopramide for six weeks.[51] Both drugs proved significantly effective in inducing symptomatic and endoscopic improvement, but ranitidine appeared significantly superior in promoting disappearance or improvement of endoscopic esophagitis.

An overall analysis of the clinical trials of chronic reflux patients with medical therapy is summarized in Table 5. These studies would suggest that the histamine H_2 antagonists and bethanechol are the most effective therapeutic agents. Both treatment modalities appear to show a significant improvement in symptoms with a trend toward healing of esophagitis. The short trials (usually 8 weeks or less) may account for the inconsistent evidence of healing in these patients having long-standing disease.

Table 5.
Summary of Clinical Trials in the Medical Therapy of GE Reflux Disease

Drug	↓ Sx	↓ Esophagitis	Healing of Strictures
Antacids	?	?	—
Alginic Acid	Yes	?	—
Bethanechol	Yes	Yes	—
Metoclopramide	Yes	?	—
Histamine H_2 Antagonists	Yes	Yes	No

? = uncertain or no placebo controlled trials

— = not studied

A Proposed Therapeutic Approach

It is clear that a variety of therapeutic modalities either have good laboratory support or have been shown to be effective in clinical trials in the treatment of patients with chronic reflux disease. Based on the concept that the pathogenesis of reflux has many components, therapy directed at different aspects seems rational. An overall approach to the patient presenting with gastroesophageal reflux may be structured, dividing the current therapies into three phases (Table 6). With the initial approach to the patient, it is reasonable to use the simpler forms of therapy with long-term established safety records. These would include: elevation of the head of the bed, dietary modification, decreasing or stopping smoking, avoiding potentially harmful medications, and use of antacids or alginic acid.

It should be anticipated that a therapeutic regimen of this kind will be effective in the majority of patients who have uncomplicated reflux. In those patients who fail to respond, more vigorous therapy should be entertained, to include the use of either drugs that increase LES pressure (bethanechol or metoclopramide) or decrease gastric acid output (histamine H_2 antagonist). It should be noted that an additional action of bethanechol is the improved esophageal acid clearing. Similarly, with metoclopramide, improvement in abnormal gastric emptying may be an additional effect. Some patients may respond well to a combination of histamine H_2 antagonist and bethanechol, particularly at bedtime, although no clinical trial of this combination therapy has been performed.

Table 6. Therapeutic Approach to GE Reflux Disease
Phase I
Elevation of head of the bed
Dietary modification
Decrease or stop smoking
Avoid potentially harmful medications
Antacids or alginic acid
Phase II
Bethanechol or metoclopramide
Histamine H_2 antagonist (cimetidine or ranitidine)
Phase III
Anti-reflux surgery

Though difficult to quantitate, about 5 to 10% of patients with GERD will fail to respond to the best in medical therapy. For these patients with medically intractable symptoms and complications, a surgical anti-reflux procedure is warranted. Phase III of reflux therapy then would include a surgical procedure, either a Belsey or Nissen fundoplication, or a Hill gastropexy.

One must keep in mind that ordinary reflux disease is a chronic problem, tends to have a varying course, and even may remit spontaneously. The multifactorial components of GERD may be both a cause and result of chronic reflux injury thereby perpetuating the process.[5] This complex interaction may account for the failure of many short-term medical trials and uncertainty about the duration of therapy. A recent study has shown that endoscopic healing of esophagitis is not associated with the disappearance of histologic inflammation or abnormal motor function.[59] The persistence of these abnormalities might explain the tendency of esophagitis to recur after endoscopic healing and necessitate the requirement for more prolonged medical treatment. The chronicity of reflux disease therefore probably requires some form of lifelong medical therapy (Figure 2). Simple, but effective, changes in lifestyle should be the cornerstone of treatment regardless of symptomatology. Antacids or alginic acid should be taken for occasional or mild symptoms. Phase II drug therapy may be necessary in the natural history of reflux disease as it waxes and wanes. Surgical intervention will be required infrequently for the most severe forms of reflux disease. In these situations, surgery will be most helpful, however, long-term follow-up studies report recurrence rates as high as 20%.[60]

The Future

Is there any potential for newer modalities with possible greater effectiveness? Several new drugs do appear on the horizon. Domperidone, a dopamine antagonist, which unlike metoclopramide does not cross the blood–brain barrier, offers potential as a new therapeutic agent. Preliminary European studies suggest this drug can increase LES pressure, improve esophageal clearing, and augment gastric emptying.[61] At this time, well designed clinical studies are lacking to support their claims. Prostaglandin $F_{2\alpha}$ has been shown to increase LES pressure after intravenous injection in animals and man.[62] Orally effective analogs have not been studied and may be limited by the diarrhea associated with other oral prostaglandins. Reed and Davies reported an 8-week trial comparing a new product combining

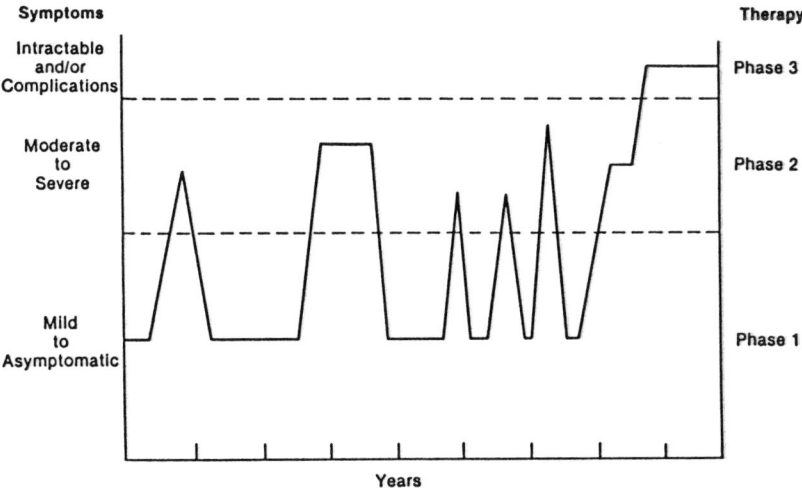

Symptoms   Therapy

Intractable
and/or   Phase 3
Complications

Moderate
to   Phase 2
Severe

Mild
to   Phase 1
Asymptomatic

Years

Figure 2: *Schematic representation of the natural history of GE reflux disease. Note the tendency of symptoms to wax and wane. Phase I medical therapy is the cornerstone of treatment. Worsening disease may require Phase II and eventually Phase III therapy.*

carbenoxolone sodium and alginic acid alone.[63] Significant improvement of symptoms and healing of esophagitis was found with Pyrogastrone as well as 100% healing of esophageal ulcers. The authors suggest this new drug is the most effective agent so far produced for the treatment of reflux esophagitis, but this declaration awaits further placebo-controlled confirmatory studies.

Drugs that have the ability to suppress acid production from the stomach for long periods or "neutralize" stomach contents may, in the final analysis, be most effective in the treatment of GE reflux disease. In the near future, manipulation of the structure of the histamine H_2 receptor antagonists should result in drugs with greater potency and longer duration of action. A new class of drugs that actively inhibits H^+/K^+ ATPase activity in the parietal cell is being developed. The drug that is currently being studied, omeprazole, has been shown to produce marked depression of gastric acid production for at least 24 hours after a single dose.[64] Sucralfate, a nonabsorbable sulfated disaccharide that binds bile salts as well as acid and pepsin, may be particularly useful in the treatment of alkaline reflux esophagitis.[65] Preliminary studies with liquid suspension are now in progress.

A significant amount of work still needs to be done with currently available anti-reflux medications. Further well conducted placebo-controlled trials of the effectiveness of a good antacid regimen are needed. The true effect of alginic acid in the treatment of reflux is difficult to evaluate because of limited studies comparing it with placebo. Long-term studies with cimetidine and bethanechol are needed to better evaluate their potential for healing esophagitis and preventing recurrence. Metoclopramide seems to offer promise, particularly in those patients who might have abnormal gastric emptying, but the potential for side effects is a troubling element. Finally, drug studies comparing and contrasting the available agents alone and in combination are desperately needed in order to better design further therapeutic plans for the treatment of gastroesophageal reflux disease.

References

1. Nebel OT, Fornes MF, Castell DO: Symptomatic gastroesophageal reflux: Incidence and percipitating factor. *Dig Dis Sci* 1976; 21:955–959.
2. Tibbling L, Wranne B: Oesophageal dysfunction in male patients with angina-like pain. *Acta Med Scand* 1976; 200:391–395.
3. Herbst JJ: Gastroesophageal reflux and pulmonary disease. *Pediatrics* 1981; 68:132–134.
4. Richter JE, Castell DO: Drugs, foods and other substances in the cause and treatment of reflux esophagitis. *Med Clin North Am* 1981; 65(6): 1223–1234.
5. Richter JE, Castell DO: Gastroesophageal reflux: Pathogenesis, diagnosis and therapy. *Ann Intern Med* 1982; 97:93–103.
6. Dennish GW, Castell DO: Inhibitory effect of smoking on the lower esophageal sphincter. *N Engl J Med* 1971; 284:1136–1137.
7. Stanciu C, Bennett R: Smoking and gastrooesophageal reflux. *Br Med J* 1972; 3:793–795.
8. Misiewicz JJ, Waller SL, Anthony PP, Gummer JWP: Achalasia of the cardia: Pharmacology and histopathology of isolated cardiac sphincter muscle from patients with and without achalasia. *Q J Med* 1969; 38:17.
9. O'Brien TF, Stroop EM: Lower esophageal sphincter pressure and esophageal function in obese humans. *J Clin Gastroenterol* 1980; 2:145–147.
10. Fisher RS, Malmud LS, Roberts GS, Lobis IF: The lower esophageal sphincter as a barrier to gastroesophageal reflux. *Gastroenterology* 1977; 72:19.
11. Blackwell JN, Dalton CB, Castell DO: Pirenzepine—a unique "anticholinergic" on the esophagus. *Gastroenterology* 1984; 86:1029.
12. Johnson LF, DeMeester TR: Evaluation of evaluation of the head of the bed, bethanechol, and antacid foam tablets on gastroesophageal reflux. *Dig Dis Sci* 1981; 26:673–680.
13. Hogan WJ, Viegas de Andrade SR, Winship DH: Ethanol-induced acute esophageal motor dysfunction. *J Appl Physiol* 1972; 321:775–760.

14. Castell DO: The lower esophageal sphincter. *Ann Intern Med* 1975; 83:390–396.
15. Van Thiel DH, Gravaler JS, Shobha AB, Joshi SN, Sara RK, Stremple J: Heartburn of pregnancy. *Gastroenterology* 1977; 72:666–668.
16. Van Thiel DH, Graveler JS, Stremple J: Lower esophageal sphincter pressure in women using sequential oral contraceptives. *Gastroenterology* 1976; 71:232–234.
17. Nebel OT, Castell DO: Lower esophageal sphincter pressure changes after food ingestion. *Gastroenterology* 1972; 63:778–783.
18. Babka JC, Castell DO: On the genesis of heartburn. *Am J Dig Dis* 1973; 18:391–397.
19. Sigmund CJ, McNallym EF: The action of a carminative on the lower esophageal sphincter. *Gastroenterology* 1969; 56:1318.
20. Price SF, Smithson KW, Castell DO: Food sensitivity in reflux esophagitis. *Gastroenterology* 1978; 75:240–243.
21. Lloyd DA, Borda IT: Food-induced heartburn: Effect of osmolarity. *Gastroenterology* 1981; 80:740–741.
22. Dennish GW, Castell DO: Caffeine and the lower esophageal sphincter. *Dig Dis Sci* 1972; 17:993–996.
23. Cohen S, Booth GH: Gastric acid secretion and lower esophageal sphincter pressure in response to coffee and caffeine. *N Engl J Med* 1975; 293:897–899.
24. Cohen S: Pathogenesis of coffee induced gastrointestinal symptoms. *N Engl J Med* 1980; 303:122–124.
25. Thomas FB, Steinbaugh JT, Fromkes JJ, Mekhjianlts AR, Caldwell JH: Inhibitory effect of coffee on lower esophageal sphincter pressure. *Gastroenterology* 1980; 79:1262–1266.
26. Salmon PR, Fedail SS, Wurzner HP, Harvey RF, Read AE: Effect of coffee on human lower oesophagus function. *Digestion* 1981; 21:69.
27. Higgs RH, Smyth RD, Castell DO: Gastric alkalinization: Effect on lower esophageal sphincter pressure and serum gastrin. *N Engl J Med* 1974; 291:486–488.
28. Malmud LS, Fisher RS: Quantitation of gastroesophageal reflux before and after therapy using the gastroesophageal scintiscan. *South Med J* 1978; 71:10.
29. Graham DY, Lanza F, Dorsch ER: Symptomatic reflux esophagitis: A double-blind controlled comparison of antacids and alginate. *Curr Ther Res* 1977; 22:653.
30. McHardy G: A multicentric, randomized clinical trial of Gaviscon in reflux esophagitis. *South Med J* 1978; 71:16–21.
31. Graham DL, Patterson DJ: Double-blind comparison of liquid antacid and placebo in the treatment of symptomatic reflux esophagitis. *Dig Dis Sci* 1983; 28:559–566.
32. Stanciu C, Bennett JR: Alginate/antacid in the reduction of gastro-oesophageal reflux. *Lancet* 1974; 26:109–111.
33. Bernardo DE, Lancaster–Smith M, Strickland ID, et al: A double-blind controlled trial of "Gavison" in patients with symptomatic gastroesophageal reflux. *Curr Med Res Opin* 1975; 3:388.
34. Chevrel B: A comparison cross-over study on the treatment of heartburn and epigastric pain: Liquid Gaviscon and a magnesium-aluminum antacid gel. *J Int Med Res* 1980; 8:300–302.

35. Hasan SS: Treatment of moderate to severe gastro-oesophageal reflux with an alginate/antacid combination. *Curr Med Res Opin* 1980; 6: 645–648.
36. Farrell RL, Roling GT, Castell DO: Stimulation of the incompetent lower esophageal sphincter: A possible advance in therapy of heartburn. *Am J Dig Dis* 1973; 18:646–650.
37. Miller WN, Ganeshappa KP, Dodds WJ, et al: Effect of bethanechol on gastroesophageal reflux. *Am J Dig Dis* 1977; 22:230–234.
38. Farrell RL, Roling GT, Castell DO: Cholinergic therapy of chronic heartburn. *Ann Intern Med* 1972; 80:573–576.
39. Thanik KD, Chey WY, Shah AN, et al: Reflux esophagitis: Effect of oral bethanechol on symptoms and endoscopic findings. *Ann Intern Med* 1980; 93:805–808.
40. Thanik KD, Chey WY, Shak AN, Hamilton D, Nadelson N: Bethanechol or cimetidine in the treatment of symptomatic reflux esophagitis. *Arch Intern Med* 1982; 142:1479–1481.
41. Wesdorp E, Bartelsman J, Pape K, et al: Oral cimetidine in reflux esophagitis: A double-blind controlled trial. *Gastroenterology* 1978; 74: 821–824.
42. Saco LS, Orlando RC, Levinson SL, Bozymski EM, et al: Double-blind controlled trial of bethanechol and antacid versus placebo and antacid in the treatment of erosive esophagitis. *Gastroenterology* 1982; 82: 1369–1373.
43. Euler AR: Use of bethanechol for the treatment of gastroesophageal reflux. *J Pediatr* 1980; 96:321–324.
44. McCallum RW, Kline MM, Curry N, et al: Comparative effects of metoclopramide and bethanechol on lower esophageal sphincter pressure in reflux patients. *Gastroenterology* 1975; 68:1114–1118.
45. Fink SM, Lange RC, McCallum RW: Effect of metoclopramide on normal and delayed gastric emptying in gastroesophageal reflux patients. *Dig Dis Sci* 1983; 28:1057–1061.
46. Venables CW, Bell D, Eccleston D: A double-blind study of metoclopramide in symptomatic peptic oesophagitis. *Postgrad Med J* 1973: (July Suppl.):73.
47. Paull A, Kerr AK: A controlled trial of metoclopramide in reflux oesophagitis. *Med J Aust* 1974; 2:627.
48. McCallum RW, Ippoliti AF, Conney RN, et al: A controlled trial of metoclopramide in symptomatic gastroesophageal reflux. *N Engl J Med* 1977; 296:354–357.
49. Bright–Asare P, El-Bassoussi M: Cimetidine, metoclopramide, or placebo in the treatment of symptomatic gastroesophageal reflux. *J Clin Gastroenterol* 1980; 2:149–156.
50. Temple JG, Bradley AVH, O'Connor F, et al: Cimetidine and metoclopramide in oesophageal reflux disease. *Br Med J* 1983; 286:1863–1864.
51. Guslandi M, Testoni PA, Passarretti S: Ranitidine vs. metoclopramide in the medical treatment of reflux esophagitis. *Hepato-enterol* 1983; 30:96–98.
52. Behar J, Brand DL, Brown FC, et al: Cimetidine in the treatment of symptomatic gastroesophageal reflux. A double-blind controlled trial. *Gastroenterology* 1978; 74:441–448.
53. Powell–Jackson P, Barkley H, Northfield TC: Effect of cimetidine in symptomatic gastrooesophageal reflux. *Lancet* 2, 1978; 1068.

54. Petrokubi RJ, Jeffries GH: Cimetidine versus antacid in scleroderma with reflux esophagitis. *Gastroenterology* 1979; 77:691–695.
55. Fiasse R, Hanin C, Lepot A, et al: Controlled trial of cimetidine in reflux esophagitis. *Dig Dis Sci* 1980; 25:750–755.
56. Bennett JR, Buckton G, Martin HD: Cimetidine in gastro-esophageal reflux. *Digestion* 1983; 26:166–172.
57. Ferguson R, Dronfield MW, Atkinson M: Cimetidine in treatment of reflux oesophagitis with peptic stricture. *Br Med J* 1979; 2:472–474.
58. Wesdorp IC, Dekker W, Klinkenberg–Knol EC: Treatment of reflux oesophagitis with ranitidine. *Gut* 1983; 24:921–924.
59. Sonnenberg A, Lepsien G, Muller–Liesner SA, et al: When is esophagitis healed? *Dig Dis Sci* 1982; 27:297–302.
60. Negre JB, Markkula HT, Keyrilainen O, Matikainen M: Nissen fundoplication: Results at 10 year follow-up. *Am J Surg* 1983; 146:635–648.
61. Weilhrauch TR, Forstein CF, Krieglstein J: Evaluation of the effect of domperidone on human esophageal and gastroduodenal motility by intraluminal manometry. *Postgrad Med J* 1979; 55 (Suppl 1):7–10.
62. Ratton S, Hersh T, Goyal R: Effect of prostaglandin $F_{2\alpha}$ and gastrin pentapeptide on the lower esophageal sphincter. *Proc Soc Exp Med Biol* 1972; 141:573–575.
63. Reed PI, Davies WA: Controlled trial of a new dosage form of carbenoxolone (pyrogastrone) in the treatment of reflux esophagitis. *Dig Dis* 1978; 23:161–165.
64. Lind T, Cederberg C, Ekenved G, Hoglund U, Oibe L: Effect of omeprazole—a gastric proton pump inhibitor—on pentagastrin stimulated acid secretion in man. *Gut* 1983; 24:270–276.
65. Richardson CT: Sucralfate. *Ann Intern Med* 1982; 97:269–272.

15

Surgical Management of Gastroesophageal Reflux

Tom R. DeMeester, M.D.

Chapter Contents

From Castell DO, Wu WC, Ott DJ (eds): *Gastroesophageal Reflux Disease: Pathogenesis, Diagnosis, Therapy.* Mount Kisco, NY, Futura Publishing Co., Inc., 1985.

Definition of a Mechanically Incompetent Cardia

In man, the anti-reflux mechanism consists of a valvular cardia and the propulsive pump-like function of the body of the esophagus. Failure of one of these components can usually be compensated for by the other. Failure of both components inevitably leads to abnormal esophageal exposure to gastric juice. In one-half of the patients with documented increased esophageal acid exposure, the cause is a mechanical failure of the anti-reflux mechanism. Gastric pathology accounts for the remaining half.[1]

Mechanical failure of the valvular component of the anti-reflux mechanism is diagnosed by measuring inadequate mechanical characteristics of the cardia on manometry. The key factor in the competency of the cardia is the distal esophageal sphincter pressure, but the efficiency of the sphincter pressure can be nullified by an abnormal location (Figure 1) or an abnormally short overall resting length of the sphincter (Figure 2). Based on our experience correlating esophageal manometry with 24-hour esophageal pH monitoring, we have defined a mechanically incompetent cardia as having an average sphincter pressure of 5 mm of mercury or less, an average length of sphincter exposed to the positive pressure environment of the abdomen of 1.4 cm or less, and/or a sphincter with an average overall resting length of 2.4 cm. or less.[2-4] Patients with a low sphincter pressure or those with a normal pressure but a short length of sphincter exposed to the abdominal pressure are unable to protect against fluctuations of abdominal pressure caused by daily activities or changes in position (Figure 1). Similarly, patients with a low sphincter pressure or those with a normal pressure but a short overall sphincter length are unable to protect against challenges of intragastric pressure independent of intra-abdominal pressure. The patient who has one, two, or all three of these abnormalities has a mechanically defective cardia as a basis for experiencing the symptoms and complications associated with the regurgitation of gastric contents into the esophagus. Such patients are less apt to receive benefits from medical therapy because their problem is a mechanical deficiency. They have a pathophysiologic defect that a surgical anti-reflux procedure is designed to correct.

Mechanical failures of the esophageal pump component of the anti-reflux mechanism are due to motility disorders, the presence of a hiatal hernia, or myogenic abnormalities. Each of these abnormalities produce inefficiency in the propulsive pumping action of the body of the esophagus. Consequently, physiologic reflux episodes are unable to be cleared out of the esophagus effectively and result in prolonged mucosal acid exposure even in patients with a normal

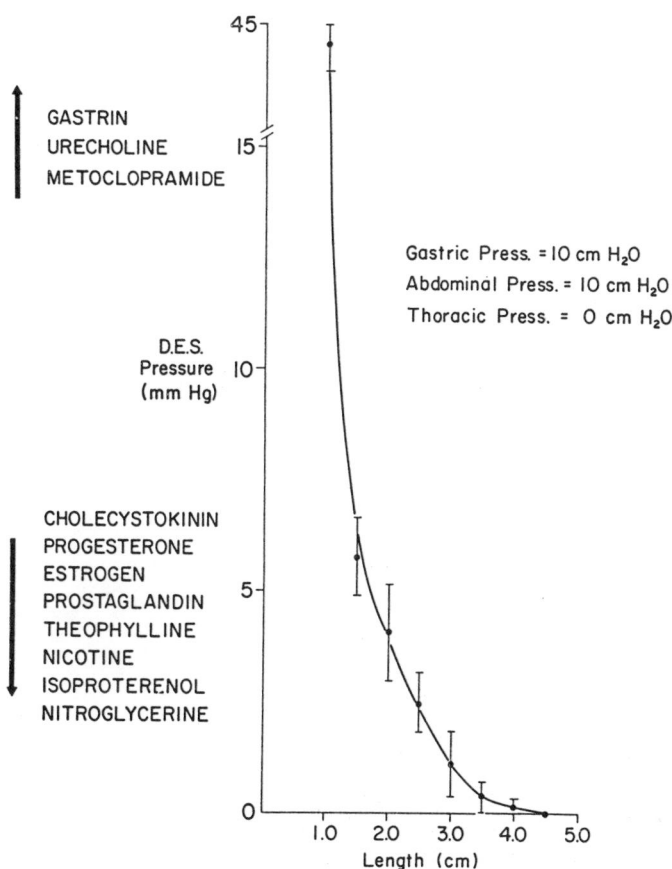

Figure 1: *The relationship of distal esophageal sphincter (DES) pressure and length of sphincter exposed to the positive pressure environment of the abdomen to competency of the cardia. The plotted line represents the pressure necessary for a given length to obtain competence. Patients with 1.5–2 cm of abdominal sphincter require at least 7–5 mmHg of sphincter pressure to remain competent. If abdominal length is less than 1 cm, competency is difficult to achieve irrespective of the level of sphincter pressure. The effect of drugs and hormones on DES pressure are indicated.*

valvular component of the anti-reflux mechanism.[1,5] Studies have indicated that surgery can improve the efficiency of the esophageal pump by reducing a hiatal hernia but provide no benefit to the other causes of pump failure.[6]

Habitual swallowing as an effort of the esophageal pump to compensate for a defective valvular component of the anti-reflux mechanism can lead to an excessive amount of air being pumped into

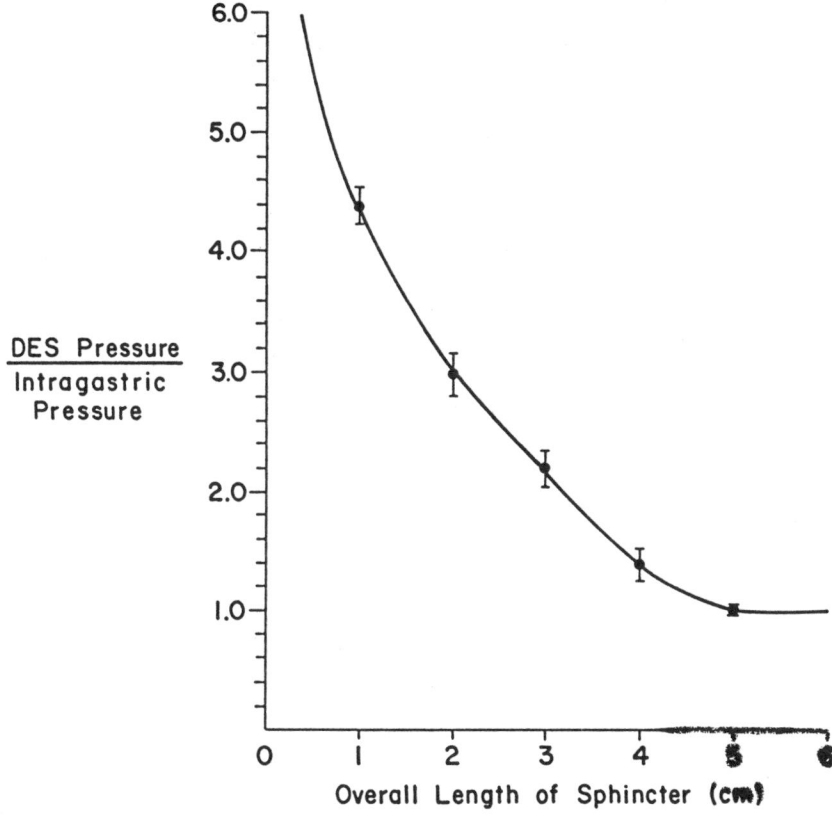

Figure 2: *The relationship of the ratio of distal esophageal sphincter (DES) pressure/intragastric pressure and overall length of sphincter to competency of the cardia. The plotted line represents the pressure ratio necessary to maintain competence for a given overall sphincter length. As the sphincter length shortens, a greater ratio is required for competency. For example, a sphincter length of 2 cm requires a ratio of 3, whereas a sphincter length of 4 cm requires a ratio of 1.5.*

the stomach. This results in gastric dilatation and repetitive belching with further reflux of gastric contents into the esophagus.[5] Surgical correction of the defective valvular component will usually remove the need for the esophageal pump to compensate and alleviate the symptoms of gastric distension. Other causes of habitual swallowing that can lead to excessive air intake are attempts to compensate for a decreased saliva production, or the loss of secondary peristalsis. A surgical anti-reflux procedure has no benefit in these situations.

Competency of the cardia against increases in gastric pressure or gastric dilatation is based, as mentioned before, on the overall sphincter length and the ratio of sphincter to intragastric pressure (Figure 2).

Gastroesophageal reflux can occur whenever an increase in gastric pressure exceeds the sphincter pressure that is necessary to provide competency for the overall length of sphincter present. Similarly, reflux of gastric contents can occur whenever gastric distension results in shortening of the overall length of the sphincter, like the shortening of the neck of a balloon on inflation, to the point where the sphincter length drops below that which is necessary for the sphincter pressure present to maintain competency. Thus, an individual who has a short overall sphincter length on a resting esophageal motility study is at a disadvantage in protecting against reflux caused by normal gastric pressure and dilatation. In an individual with a normal overall sphincter length, it is possible for primary gastric pathology to be the cause of increased esophageal exposure to gastric juice by promoting the reflux of gastric contents into the esophagus through a mechanically competent cardia. The first situation is a form of a mechanically incompetent cardia and can be corrected by an anti-reflux procedure. The second situation may require gastric surgery to correct and is due to: (a) a persistent gastric reservoir secondary to delayed gastric emptying caused by diabetes, neuromuscular disorders, viral infection, vagotomy, pyloric dysfunction, or duodenal dysmotility; (b) increased intragastric pressure secondary to outlet obstruction or the loss of active relaxation following vagotomy; or (c) distension of the stomach secondary to gluttony or the aerophagia caused by habitual swallowing.[5]

Patient Selection and Indication for Anti-reflux Surgery

Prior to any rational therapy for gastroesophageal reflux, a precise diagnosis as to the cause for abnormal acid exposure of the esophagus is necessary. An anti-reflux procedure should be considered only for those patients with a mechanically incompetent cardia. Other causes for abnormal esophageal acid exposure should be searched for if the cardia is manometrically normal. The clinical indications for an anti-reflux operation in patients with a mechanically incompetent cardia are the presence of a complication of reflux, namely persistent endoscopic esophagitis, esophageal stricture, Barrett's columnar lined esophagus, or radiographic evidence of repetitive aspiration pneumonia.

The development of esophagitis as a complication of gastroesophageal reflux appears to be related to the composition of the refluxed material and the pattern in which it is exposed to the esophageal mucosa.[7,8] Thus, it is possible to have a mechanical failure of the cardia and not develop esophagitis. In our experience, this occurs in about 50% of symptomatic patients.[9] Patients with esophagitis and a mechanically incompetent cardia commonly receive little long-term benefit from medical therapy and will usually require a surgical anti-reflux procedure to correct the condition. If severe endoscopic esophagitis is present, surgery should be performed rather quickly, since in these patients strictures can develop while receiving medical therapy.[10] If 24-hour esophageal pH monitoring is normal in a patient with unequivocal endoscopic esophagitis, then the possibilities of alkaline, drug induced, or retention esophagitis should be considered.

A benign esophageal stricture secondary to reflux esophagitis in a patient with a mechanically incompetent cardia represents a failure of medical management and is an indication for surgical therapy. Prior to surgery a malignant etiology of the stricture should be excluded. This can be difficult, and the roentgenographic barium swallow can be misleading. To make this differentiation, several biopsies and brushing from within the lumen of the stricture should be obtained. Occasionally, a rigid scope may be required to get an adequate biopsy. When a malignant etiology has been excluded, the stricture is progressively dilated up to a No. 60 bougie French prior to surgery. When fully dilated, esophageal manometry and 24-hour pH monitoring are performed. Manometry is used to determine the adequacy of peristalsis in the distal esophagus, and the ability of the distal esophageal sphincter to relax on deglutition. If either of these measurements are deficient, caution should be exercised in performing an anti-reflux procedure and serious consideration given to a colon interposition. If 24-hour esophageal pH monitoring is normal, the cardia is either competent, indicating that the stricture is probably secondary to drug ingestion and dilation may be all that is needed, or pure alkaline reflux is present.

Barrett's esophagus is a columnar-lined esophagus acquired as a complication of persistent reflux esophagitis. It is almost always associated with a severe mechanical defect of the cardia.[11] A patient with a Barrett's esophagus is at risk of developing a stricture, hemorrhage from esophageal ulcer, and adenocarcinoma. It is now established that control of the reflux by an anti-reflux procedure can avert the complications of bleeding ulceration and stricture, and probably does protect against the development of adenocarcinoma by causing a reduction in the degree of dysphagia.[12] The presence of a Barrett's esophagus is an indication for multiple mucosal biopsy. If marked mucosal atypia or carcinoma in situ is found, an esophageal resection should be considered. If these changes are not found, an anti-reflux procedure should be performed.

Patients with roentgenographic evidence of previous recurrent pneumonias and a history of episodes of nocturnal choking, waking up with gastric contents in their mouth, or soilage of their bed pillow, may be suffering from repetitive pulmonary aspiration secondary to gastroesophageal reflux. The chest roentgenogram often shows a large hiatal hernia and signs of pleural thickening, bronchiectasis, and pulmonary fibrosis. In such patients 24-hour pH monitoring should be done to confirm the presence of increased esophageal acid exposure. If present, esophageal manometry should be performed, and if a mechanical defect of the cardia is found, an anti-reflux procedure is indicated. Usually, these patients have a nonspecific motility abnormality of the esophageal body which tends to propel the refluxed material toward the pharynx.[13,14] Other esophageal pathology that can cause this clinical presentation are achalasia, a hiatal hernia with a narrow diaphragmatic hiatus which interferes with the flow of esophageal contents into the distal stomach leading to its regurgitation back into the esophagus from the supra diaphragmatic portion of the stomach, and an esophageal or pharyngeal diverticulum. The former is often associated with a nonspecific motility disorder.

The indication for anti-reflux surgery in the absence of complications of reflux is the patient's unwillingness to put up with the symptoms of heartburn or regurgitation that persist despite the best medical therapy. In this situation, it is important to objectively demonstrate the presence of abnormal reflux with 24-hour pH monitoring.[19] If reflux is objectively shown but the complications of reflux are not present, the patient should be placed on medical therapy. If the symptoms persist over 4 to 6 months and there is a mechanical defect of the cardia on esophageal manometry, an anti-reflux repair should be done. If there are normal mechanical components of the cardia, a gastric or esophageal cause for the increase in esophageal acid exposure should be searched out. If the 24-hour esophageal pH monitoring test is normal, a cause for the symptoms other than reflux should be investigated.

Chronic atypical symptoms of reflux that indicate the need for operative therapy are pulmonary symptoms such as chronic cough, hoarseness or wheezing;[13,14] and chest pain from a reflux-induced esophageal irritation or spasm.[15] Generally, these atypical symptoms overshadow any gastroesophageal complaints and focus the physician's attention on the lung or heart. The tip-off that the pulmonary symptoms may be related to reflux is the history of recurrent pneumonias, the presence of chronic interstitial pulmonary fibrosis on the chest x-ray, adult onset of asthma, or a chronic cough that eludes all efforts to uncover its etiology. Chest pain indistinguishable from coronary artery disease can be caused by reflux. These patients are usually thought to have coronary artery disease, but have normal coronary arteries on arteriography or have had a previous coronary artery bypass procedure without relief of their chest pain.

The relationship of the pulmonary or cardiac symptoms to reflux episodes can be clarified with 24-hour esophageal pH monitoring by correlating the timing of the onset of the symptom with a reflux episode. If the symptoms occur during or immediately after a reflux episode and the patient has a mechanically defective cardia without the complication of reflux, medical therapy should be tried. This should consist of reducing the number of reflux episodes by elevating the head of the bed and prescribing cimetidine to alkalinize the pH of the refluxed gastric juice.[16] Urecholine can be added to increase esophageal clearance of the refluxed material.[16] If this therapy fails, an anti-reflux procedure can be helpful in controlling or abolishing the symptoms. If normal mechanical components of the cardia are found, the presence of a motility disorder in the body of the esophagus should be investigated. Attempts to induce esophageal spasm and precipitate an episode of chest pain may be helpful.[17]

A third indication for an anti-reflux procedure is the symptom of dysphagia, regurgitation or chest pain on eating. These symptoms are usually related to the presence of a large paraesophageal hernia, intrathoracic stomach, or a small hiatal hernia with a Schatzski ring or a narrow diaphragmatic hiatus.[18] Heartburn can be associated with a paraesophageal hernia but is uncommon in the latter two conditions. It is absent in patients with an intrathoracic stomach because saliva pools within the stomach and neutralizes the gastric acid. These patients are easily identified with an upper gastrointestinal roentgenographic barium examination. A sliding hiatal hernia with Schatzski ring or a narrow diaphragmatic hiatus can cause dysphagia and chest pain during eating secondary to contraction of the portion of the esophagus immediately above the Schatzski ring or distension of that portion of the stomach above the diaphragmatic opening. Occasionally, the contents in the herniated portion of the stomach can be regurgitated back into the esophagus and, in some patients, up into the pharynx. These patients have little or no heartburn since only swallowed food is regurgitated. Between meals, the cardia may be competent and reflux of gastric contents does not occur. They are best identified with the cine- or video-esophagram using thick barium or a barium-coated hamburger. The surgical repair of these abnormalities includes an anti-reflux procedure because of the associated incompetency of the cardia initially or the potentiality of destroying the competency of the cardia during their repair.

Prior to a surgical anti-reflux repair, the patient should be evaluated for complaints of epigastric pain, nausea, vomiting, and loss of appetite. In the past, we tended to accept these symptoms as part of the reflux syndrome, but now realize that they can be due to duodenogastric reflux which occurs independently or in association with gastroesophageal reflux. It is seen commonly in patients who have had previous upper gastrointestinal surgery, although this is not absolutely necessary.[19] In such patients, the correction of only the incompetent cardia will result in a disgruntled individual who continues to complain of nausea and epigastric pain on eating. In these patients, 24-hour pH monitoring of the stomach for the percent of time the pH is below 3 is being evaluated as a method of documenting the duodenogastric reflux.[20] The diagnosis can also be documented with a Tc-Hida scan if excessive reflux of bile from the duodenum into the stomach can be demonstrated.[21] When diagnosed, the use of sucralfate may relieve the symptoms. If surgery is necessary to control gastroesophageal reflux and severe duodenogastric reflux is present, consideration should also be given to performing a bile diversion procedure as well. When diagnosed after an anti-reflux repair, the administration of sucralfate may give relief of postoperative nausea and epigastric pain.

Prior to an anti-reflux repair, it is also important to evaluate the propulsive force of the body of the esophagus to determine if it has sufficient power to propel a bolus of food through a newly reconstructed valve. This can be done by esophageal manometry or better, with the radioisotopic studies of esophageal transit time.

The Surgeon's Approach to Anti-reflux Surgery

There are three important points to be remembered by the surgeon when performing an anti-reflux operation. First, the performance of esophageal surgery for gastroesophageal reflux requires a shift in surgical thinking. The primary goal of an anti-reflux procedure is to re-establish the competency of the cardia by improving its function. To accomplish this, it is paramount that the surgeon understands the physiology of the cardia and how its function can be improved by surgical reconstruction. Consequently, anti-reflux surgery is different from the simple extirpation of a diseased organ whose function is of no concern since it will be destroyed with its removal.

Rather, anti-reflux surgery is designed to improve the function of an organ that will remain in the patient and provide complete and permanent relief of all symptoms and complications of gastroesophageal reflux secondary to an incompetent cardia. Ideally, the reconstructed cardia should permit the patient to swallow normally, belch to relieve gaseous distension, or vomit when it is necessary to do so. The end result should restore the patient to a normal full life, with no further need for medical, postural, or dietary therapy. The more anti-reflux surgery can achieve these goals safely and dependably, the wider the indications for the operation should become.

The persistence of nausea, heartburn, regurgitation, dysphagia, chest pain, or epigastric pain after an anti-reflux procedure represents a clinically poor result due to either an incorrect initial diagnosis or technical failure. The problem with using symptoms as an indicator of success is that oftentimes a patient who has undergone surgery because of a desire to achieve freedom from his symptoms, will not readily admit to the presence of postoperative symptoms. Thus, using only the lack of postoperative symptoms as an indication of operative success is inadequate. Similarly, the report of a normal barium swallow is not a dependable criterion of success since the symptoms of reflux or its complications may be present in a patient who has no radiological evidence of a hiatal hernia or regurgitation of barium from the stomach into the esophagus. Rather, the success of a procedure depends on: (a) the relief from symptoms, (b) the objective evidence on 24-hour esophageal pH monitoring that reflux has been reduced to physiological levels, and (c) evidence on esophageal manometry that the mechanical defect of the cardia has been corrected.

A second important point is that the surgeon needs to become familiar with the use of diagnostic tools to objectively assess the patient's symptoms. Approximately 10% of the patients referred to me with a previously failed anti-reflux procedure were incorrectly diagnosed prior to their initial surgery. The error in diagnosis is usually due to an incomplete investigation of the patient's symptoms prior to surgery, a failure to objectively document increased esophageal acid exposure when it was thought to be present, or the failure to determine the correct cause for the increased exposure when it was known to be present. Only when increased esophageal acid exposure has been shown to be due to reflux of gastric contents through an incompetent cardia can the surgeon properly consider the use of an anti-reflux procedure. Too often the words diagnosis and indication are confused. If a patient has a symptomatic indication for anti-reflux surgery, we often assume that the diagnosis of gastroesophageal reflux secondary to a mechanically defective cardia is objectively supportable. This is not always so; this lazy thinking must be curbed if we expect to improve the results of surgical therapy.

A problem develops in this regard since surgeons find themselves inept concerning diagnostic instrumentation because they have shunned familiarization with the use of these tools during their training. Consequently, the gastroenterologist now does most of the esophagoscopy and esophageal function testing and as a result, the use of these procedures is no longer under the direction of surgeons. This situation has come about through a shift in the emphasis of surgical education from disease-oriented to procedure-oriented training programs. Only a few programs provide an opportunity for the trainee to gain experience in all aspects of esophageal disease, from endoscopy and laboratory diagnosis through medical and surgical management. Today, most programs direct their attention solely to the surgical procedure, and graduates of such programs have difficulty using the existing technology to diagnose the presence of reflux disease or evaluate the results of surgical therapy. In general, if a surgeon understands the physiology of the cardia and the principles necessary for its reconstruction, and he appropriately selects his patients by preoperative testing, he will collect a group of very gratified patients, relieved of their symptoms, and endeared to him for life. Such a reward makes the time and effort exerted in understanding and applying the science of surgery to gastroesophageal reflux meaningful.

The third point to be remembered in anti-reflux surgery is that a poor surgical result can be attributed to the surgeon who makes his own modification in technique without knowing what effect it will have on the organ's function. Only recently have we begun to appreciate that when an operation is designed to improve organ function, surgical technique becomes paramount and changes in technique can have a profound effect on postoperative function. No change in technique should be made indiscriminately; changes should be accepted and applied only after their effect on function has been carefully evaluated.

Surgical Principles for the Reconstruction of the Anti-reflux Mechanism

As emphasized, it is necessary for the surgeon to understand the physiology of the foregut when performing an anti-reflux procedure. Regardless of the type of anti-reflux repair used, there are five principles that must be kept in mind when surgically constructing a competent and permanent anti-reflux mechanism.

First, maintain or increase the overall length of the distal esophageal sphincter to at least 3 cm and restore its pressure to a level three times resting gastric pressure (15–25 mmHg). As previously discussed, mechanical incompetency of the cardia can result from either a reduction in the distal esophageal sphincter pressure or its overall length. The probability of gastroesophageal reflux secondary to increases in intragastric pressure, independent of intra-abdominal pressure, is 90% for a cardia with an overall sphincter length of less than 2 cm and a ratio of resting gastric to sphincter pressure of less than 3 (Figure 2). Therefore, the overall sphincter length and the sphincter pressure must be corrected if initially abnormal in order to restore competency. Pre- and postoperative esophageal manometry measurements have shown that the overall sphincter length and the resting sphincter pressure can be surgically augmented over preoperative values, and that the change in the latter is a function of the extent of the gastric wrap around the distal esophagus (Figure 3).

Second, place an adequate length of the distal esophageal sphincter in the positive pressure environment of the abdomen by a method that assures its response to changes in intra-abdominal pressure. As previously discussed, the degree of competency provided by a seg-

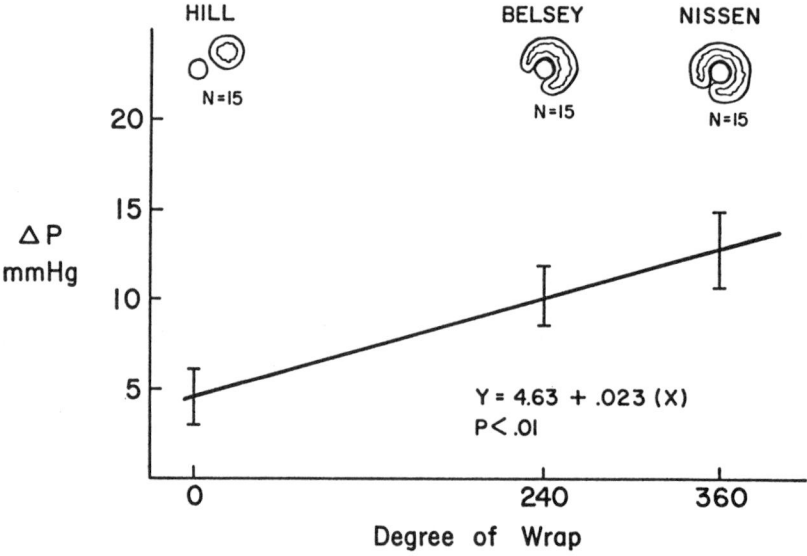

Figure 3: *The relationship between the augmentation of sphincter pressure over preoperative pressure (ΔP) and the degree of gastric fundic wrap.*

ment of intra-abdominal sphincter to challenges in intra-abdominal pressure in the absence of intrinsic sphincter tone is a function of its length (Figure 4). Its efficiency is augmented by the presence of intrinsic sphincter pressure in that the greater the pressure, the shorter the abdominal length required to maintain competency. To function mechanically, however, a minimum of 1.5 cm of abdominal sphincter must be present. The probability of gastroesophageal reflux secondary to challenges of intra-abdominal pressure is 90% if the length of sphincter exposed to the abdomen is less than 1 cm, irrespective of its resting pressure. Since the abdominal sphincter length rarely exceeds 3 cm, a minimum intrinsic pressure of 7 mmHg is also required for competency. The permanent restoration of 1.5−2 cm of abdominal esophagus in a patient with a sphincter pressure greater than 10 mmHg will maintain the competency of the cardia over various challenges of intra-abdominal pressure. Figure 5 shows that all three of the popular anti-reflux procedures increased the length of sphincter exposed to abdominal pressure by an average of 1 cm. However, this did not consistently occur, and in some patients the operations actually resulted in a reduction of the length of abdominal sphincter. If the operation results in less than 1 cm of sphincter

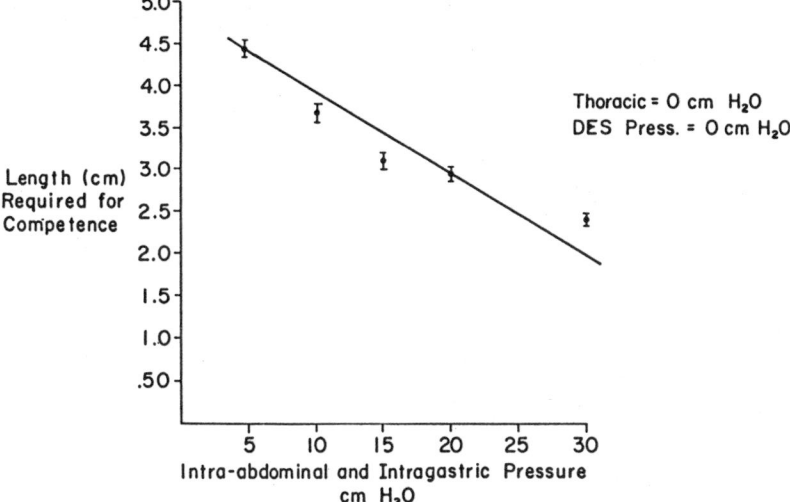

Figure 4: *The mechanical efficiency of the intra-abdominal length of sphincter required to counteract reflux due to increases in intragastric pressure caused by increases in intra-abdominal pressure. The greater the challenge of intra-abdominal pressure, the less abdominal sphincter length required to maintain competency.*

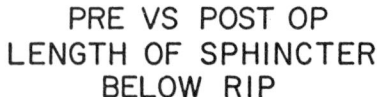

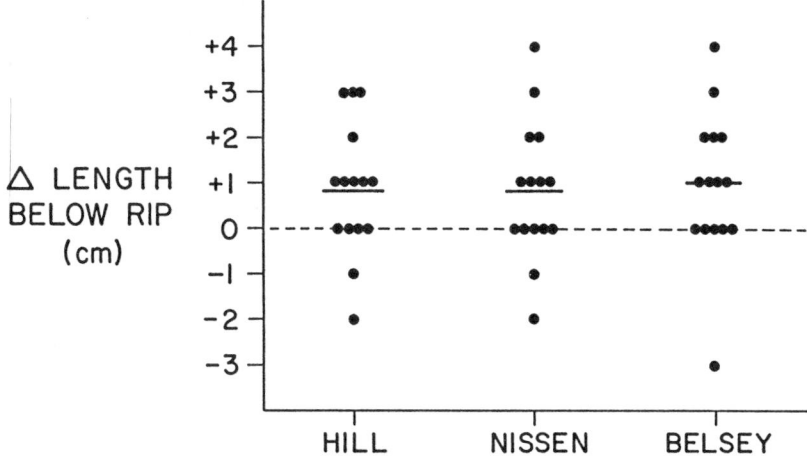

Figure 5: *The change over preoperative values in abdominal sphincter length expected after the three major anti-reflux procedures. Over the average, all the procedures increased the length by 1 cm. However, in some patients the procedure actually decreased the length. (RIP = respiratory inversion point).*

exposed to abdominal pressure, incompetency of the cardia results regardless of the amount that the sphincter pressure was increased by the procedure.

Increasing the length of sphincter exposed to abdominal pressure will improve competency of the cardia if it can be acted upon by challenges of intra-abdominal pressure. Thus, the creation of a conduit that will assure the transmission of intra-abdominal pressure changes around the abdominal portion of the sphincter is a necessary aspect of the surgical repair. The fundoplication in the Nissen and Belsey repair serves this purpose (Figure 6). In the absence of a fundic wrap, as in the Hill procedure, the development of peri-esophageal adhesions can prevent the transmission of intra-abdominal pressure to the abdominal esophagus. This will allow for postural-induced pressure changes in the abdominal cavity to be transmitted unequally to the stomach and the abdominal portion of the sphincter and result in a reflux episode.

Third, assure that the reconstructed cardia relaxes on deglutition. To facilitate normal swallowing after an operative repair, the distal

HILL BELSEY NISSEN

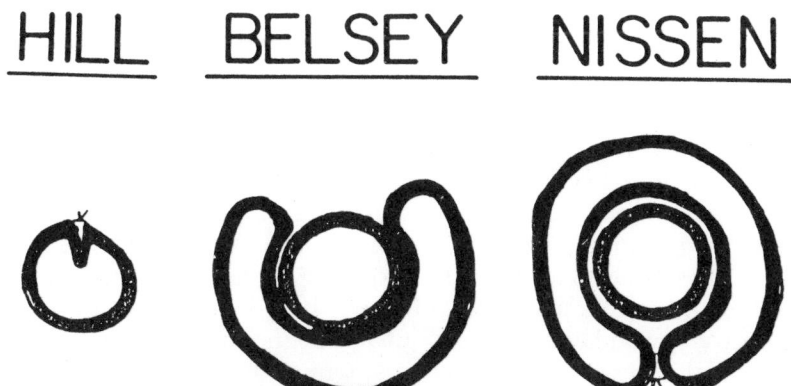

Figure 6: *Schematic cross-section of the cardia after the three major repairs, illustrating how the Belsey and Nissen repair create a conduit that assures the transmission of intra-abdominal pressure changes around the abdominal portion of the sphincter.*

esophageal sphincter must be able to relax. On deglutition, a vagal-mediated relaxation of the distal esophageal sphincter and fundus of the stomach occurs. The relaxation lasts for approximately 10 seconds and is followed by rapid recovery to its former tonicity. To ensure relaxation of the cardia, only the fundus of the stomach should be used since it is known to relax in concert with the sphincter.[22] It is paramount that the innervation of the cardia be protected since inadvertent vagal damage will result in failure of relaxation.

Fourth, be sure the resistance of the reconstructed cardia does not exceed the peristaltic power of the body of the esophagus. The diameter of a 360° wrap should be adequate to allow a No. 60 French bougie to pass into the stomach with ease to ensure that the relaxed cardia will have an adequate lumen size with minimal resistance to be overcome by the esophageal peristalsis. This is not necessary when constructing a partial wrap. The choice between a total 360° or a partial 240° wrap is influenced by the strength of the peristaltic contractions in the body of the esophagus. The esophagi having normal motility and strong peristaltic contractions do well with a 360° wrap. Where peristalsis is absent or of low magnitude, the Belsey two-thirds wrap is the procedure of choice.

Fifth, the crura of the diaphragm should be approximated to assure that the fundoplication will remain within the abdomen. Failure to do so results in the operative conversion of a sliding hiatal hernia into a para-esophageal hernia with all the complications associated with that condition.[23]

Technique of the Nissen Fundoplication

Through personal experience during the last ten years, I have settled on the following operative technique for the transabdominal and transthoracic Nissen fundoplication. Several of the patients have submitted themselves voluntarily to postoperative studies consisting of esophageal manometry, 24-hour esophageal pH monitoring, and a thorough questioning about their esophageal symptoms. Comparison of these studies to the patient's preoperative studies and similar studies obtained from normal volunteers have helped me to evaluate objectively what has been accomplished by the surgical repair. I have selected the Nissen operation because it initially gave the best results in a randomized study of the three available operations. I have continued to follow these and subsequent patients who have had the Nissen operation and made modifications in the operative technique only when the results of the postoperative studies indicated that I was not achieving the stated goals. The current technique represents only minor refinement over the method initially published by Dr. Nissen and, if performed as I have described, will give excellent results to surgeons endowed with average skill.

The Nissen fundoplication, as initially described, consists of wrapping the fundus of the stomach 360° around the lower esophagus for a distance of 4–5 cm. I have modified the originally described procedure only by limiting the length of the wrap to 1.5 cm. When done transthoracically, the fundic wrap lies over the anterior and lateral surfaces of the esophagus with the sutures posterior. When done transabdominally, the fundic wrap lies over the posterior, left lateral, and anterior surfaces of the esophagus, with the sutures on the right anterolateral surface, in line with the insertion of the gastrohepatic ligament along the lesser curve of the stomach. The modification I have made resulted out of my experience in redoing previously failed Nissen operations. Since these patients made up a sizable portion of my referral practice, I took a special interest in determining why they failed. In some patients who complained of recurrent heartburn and regurgitation, traces of a previous fundoplication were completely absent. This was due, I believe, to the breakage or pulling out of the fundic sutures and indicated the need to use stronger sutures placed in a more durable manner. Other patients had marked dysphagia even though a No. 60 French dilator could be passed, in some with force and others with ease, into the stomach. In these patients the fundic wrap was either too tight or too long. From these clinical observations, along with observations made from a model of the cardia, it became evident that the gastric wrap should be only 1.5–2 cm in length and held in place with permanently reinforced sutures. A technique was developed that used one permanent 2–0 Proline horizontal mattress suture reinforced with four 1.5 by 0.5 cm Teflon pledgets placed in a manner to be described subsequently. It is important that Teflon pledgets are cut to exact size. This keeps the wrap a standard length and gives reproducible results. With experience the technique has settled into what is described below and if followed exactly will give gratification to the work of the surgeon and dramatic symptomatic relief to the patient while preserving his eating enjoyment.

The Transabdominal Approach

The transabdominal Nissen fundoplication is performed through an upper mid-line abdominal incision extending from the lower end of the sternum laterally around the xiphoid process and down to the umbilicus. Paramount in performing the procedure is to have excellent exposure of the esophageal hiatus. In our experience, this requires a specialized upper abdominal retractor. We have taken a Weinberg retractor and welded it to a Balfour handle. This retractor is placed under the liver down to the esophageal hiatus. The patient is placed in a reverse Trendelenburg position and the retractor is lifted cephalad in a 45° angle and secured to an overhead bar attached to the table (Figure 7). This elevates the anterior chest wall and lifts the liver out of the way, providing excellent exposure to the area of the esophageal hiatus. Without this exposure, careful dissection of the hiatus is difficult, time consuming, and dangerous. A Balfour retractor is used to open the incision laterally and the exposure obtained with the combination of the two retractors makes the operation a pleasure to perform.

The first step of the procedure is to dissect out the esophageal hiatus by dividing the gastrohepatic ligament in the area where it is thin and usually transparent. Care should be taken not to damage the anterior hepatic branch of the vagus nerve. The temptation to divide this nerve should be resisted, even though it appears initially that it will compromise the exposure. The upper portion of the gastrohepatic ligament should be palpated between the thumb and index finger to prevent transecting an aberrant hepatic artery coming directly from the celiac axis. If a large artery is identified, it should be spared and the operation performed by working around the isolated artery. Cephalad to the hepatic branch of the anterior vagus nerve, the gastrohepatic ligament is divided and the incision carried superiorly over the

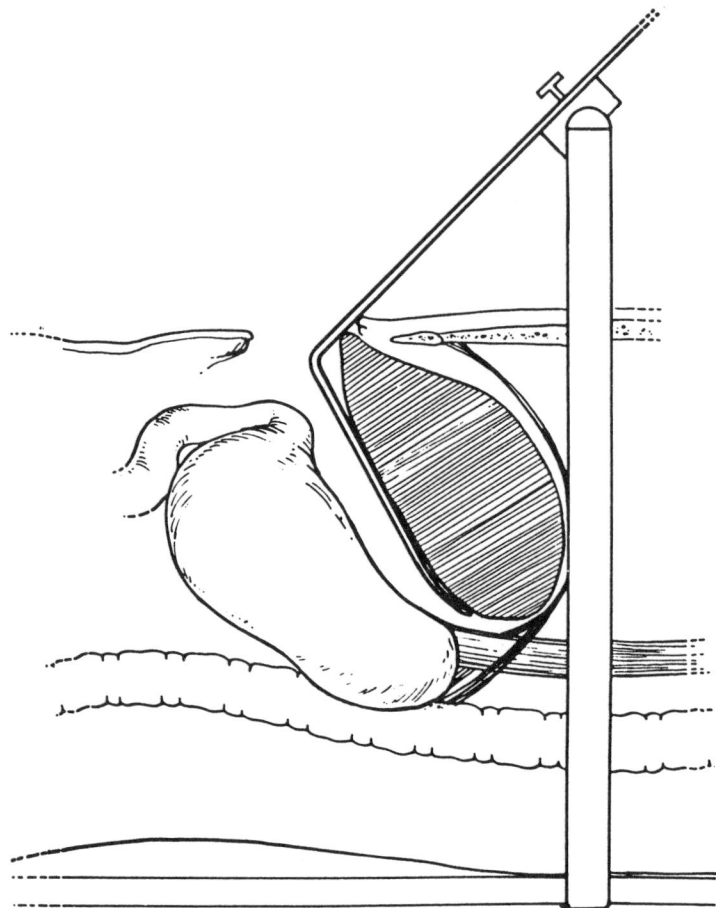

Figure 7: *Position of a modified Weinberg retractor to provide continuous exposure of the esophageal hiatus.*

anterior surface of the esophagus, dividing the reflection of the parietal peritoneum of the diaphragm onto the esophagus and stomach. This incision should not be made up on the diaphragm as this will engender bleeding from the phrenic veins, but rather, within the esophageal hiatus, taking care not to damage the anterior vagal trunk. The incision is continued down the left lateral surface of the esophagus until the left crus of the esophageal hiatus is identified.

The loose areolar tissue over the superior surface of the esophagus is removed. The esophagus is dissected circumferentially within the posterior mediastinum using the thumb and index finger of the surgeon's right hand. This is done by blunt finger dissection over the anterior surface of the aorta encircling both the right vagal trunk and esophagus. When a large hiatal hernia is present, it is helpful to perform this finger dissection high within the posterior mediastinum. This will allow for an easier dissection around the esophagus and aids in reducing the hiatal hernia. When encircled, the right or posterior vagus is identified and a soft rubber drain is passed around the esophagus, excluding the posterior vagal trunk. While retracting on the rubber drain, the loose fibrous tissue, posterior to the esophagus and cephalad to the branches of the left gastric artery, is divided to clearly identify the right and left crus of the esophageal hiatus. The decussation of the right and left crus over the anterior surface of the aorta represents the inferior extent of the dissection (Figure 8).

The second step of the procedure is to mobilize the fundus of the stomach by dividing the short gastric vessels, starting at the point where the veins begin to drain superiorly toward the spleen, rather than inferiorly toward the right gastroepiploic vein. This is about one-third the distance down the greater curvature from the cardioesophageal junction (Figure 9). It should be remembered that the gastric epiploic mesentery is out along the greater curvature to both the anterior and posterior surface of the stomach. In each of these mesentery leaves are branches of the short gastric vessels. It is helpful to

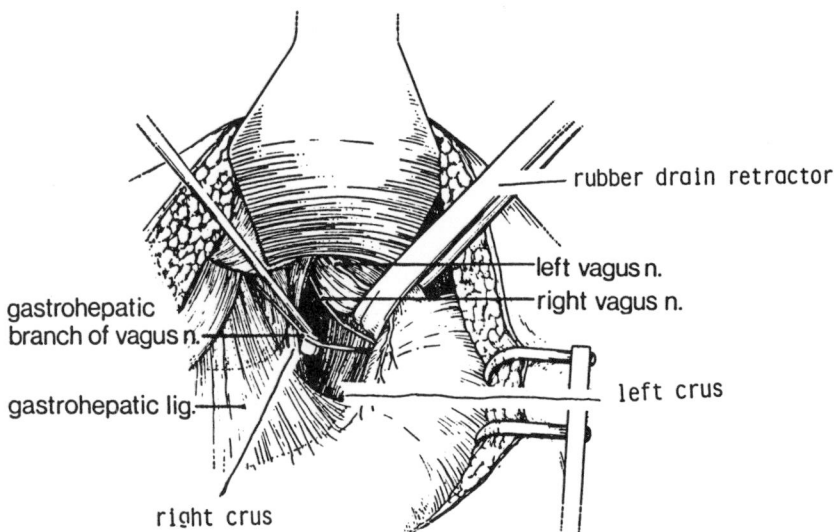

Figure 8: *Completed hiatal dissection done through the transabdominal approach showing the vagal nerves, position of the rubber drain around the esophagus, and the right and left crus.*

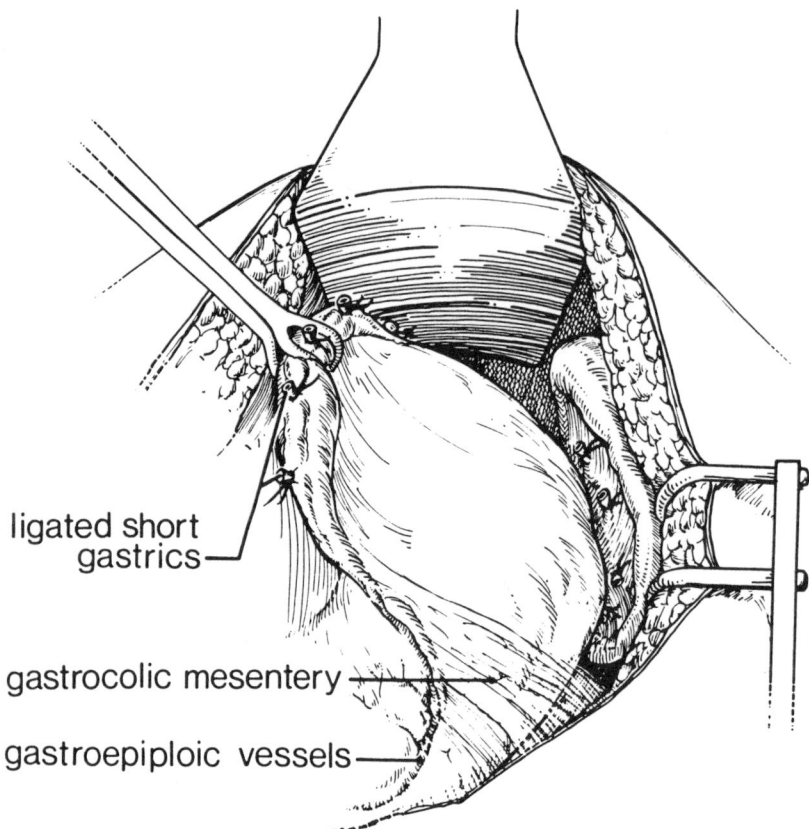

ligated short
gastrics

gastrocolic mesentery

gastroepiploic vessels

Figure 9: *The mobilized gastric fundus after division of the short gastric vessels can take a retroperitoneal course, tethering the fundus of the stomach posterior.*

divide the vessels in the anterior reflection of the mesentery first, and then those in the posterior leaf, to avoid crimping the gastric wall when both leaves are taken together with bulk ties. Occasionally, at the most superior aspect of the greater curvature, one will find that the short gastric vessels take a retroperitoneal course, tethering the fundus of the stomach to the posterior abdominal wall. One can appreciate how these vessels, if not divided, force the surgeon to construct the fundoplication with a portion of the body of the stomach rather than the fundus. Excellent exposure is required to free a tethered gastric fundus; if the retractor described initially is used, few problems in exposure are encountered.

The third stage of the operation is to close the esophageal hiatus.

To do so, the esophagus is retracted to the left with a specially designed esophageal retractor, and the right and left limbs of the crura are approximated with interrupted 0-silk sutures, starting inferiorly where they decussate over the aorta. The sutures are placed at 1 cm intervals, advancing the esophageal body anteriorly as the hiatus is closed. Usually six sutures are required to complete the closure (Figure 10). Care is taken not to place the uppermost sutures on the right side in the fascia of the diaphragm as this will result in a constriction of the hiatus and dysphagia. All sutures should be placed within the muscle of the crura and tied with a tension that causes tissue approximation without strangulation. When complete, the hiatus should freely admit a fingertip adjacent to the esophagus. It is better to err in making the closure of the hiatus too loose rather than too tight. The purpose of the crural closure is only to maintain the repair within the abdomen.

The fourth step of the operation is to construct the fundic wrap. A No. 60 French bougie is passed by the anesthesiologist into the stomach to display the gastroesophageal junction. The pad of areolar tissue, which lies on the anterior surface of the gastroesophageal junction, is removed to allow proper identification of the junction and encourage the fusion of the fundic wrap to the esophagus. Care should be taken while removing the fat pad not to injure the anterior vagus nerve. The bleeding that occurs during removal can be con-

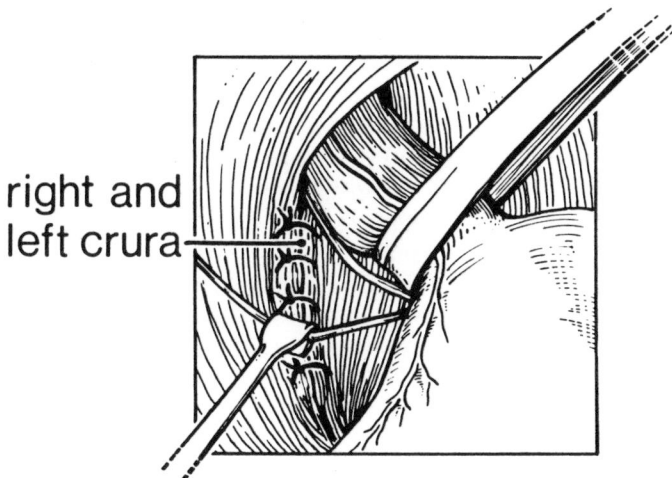

right and left crura

Figure 10: *The closed esophageal hiatus. Notice that the esophageal body has been displaced anteriorly by the approximation of the right and left crura.*

trolled by placing a lap pad on the esophagus and squeezing it around the bougie for a few moments. Any remaining bleeding points can be ligated or bovied. To attempt to clamp and tie all the small vessels during the removal of the fat pad is both time consuming and potentially damaging to the anterior vagus. Failure to control the bleeding can result in a postoperative hematoma within the fundic wrap and dysphagia.

The freed posterior wall of the fundus is pulled between the right vagal trunk and the posterior wall of the esophagus containing the No. 60 French bougie. The anterior wall of the fundus is pulled across the anterior wall of the esophagus. This results in wrapping the distal esophagus with the stomach by enveloping it within the fundus. The needles at both ends of a 2.0 Proline suture are passed through a 1.5 × 0.5 cm Teflon pledget 1 cm apart, and then through the left lip of the fundic wrap, again 1 cm apart. Both ends of the suture are passed through a second pledget sandwiching the lip of the stomach between the two pledgets. One of the limbs of the suture is then passed through the anterior wall of the esophagus at the gastroesophageal junction, incorporating the tissue down to, but not through, the muscularis mucosa. The second limb is similarly passed through the anterior wall of the esophagus 1 cm cephalad to the first stitch. Both ends of the suture are passed through a third Teflon pledget, again 1 cm apart and then through the right lateral lip of the fundic wrap. Both ends of the suture are then passed through the fourth and final Teflon pledget. The completed horizontal mattress stitch, or U-stitch as we term it, sandwiches the stomach between the first and second pledget, the esophagus between the second and third pledget, and the stomach again between the third and fourth pledget (Figure 11).

A single tie is then placed in the suture approximating the two lips of the fundic wrap around the esophagus containing the No. 60 French bougie. The ability for Proline suture to slide through tissue without sawing allows for this test approximation of the fundic wrap without causing tissue damage or hematoma formation. When drawn together, the fundic wrap should be large enough to accept the insertion of the surgeon's index finger alongside the esophagus containing the No. 60 French bougie. If the surgeon is unable to insert his finger or feels tight bands over his finger, the wrap is too tight and the left end of the horizontal U-stitch must be replaced more laterally and inferiorly on the anterior wall of the fundus. This enlarges the internal diameter of the wrap. If there is excessive space, the wrap is too floppy and the left end of the U-stitch must be replaced more medially and superiorly on the anterior wall of the fundus. This reduces the internal diameter of the wrap. When the wrap is proper size, the bougie is removed and the limbs of the U-stitch are tied securely (Figure 11).

Since only one U-stitch suture is used to hold the wrap, it is important that it is made of permanent material and that the Teflon pledgets are used to reinforce its pressure on the tissue. The use of Teflon pledgets has not resulted in the development of postoperative infection or wall erosion. This is probably due to the compression of one pledget against the other, excluding the lumen of the esophagus and stomach (Figure 12). The placement of the fundic wrap between the esophagus and right vagal trunk posteriorly and passing the U-stitch through the anterior wall of the esophagus holds the fundic wrap around the gastroesophageal junction and prevents the development of a slipped Nissen.

Figure 12 is a transverse section of the stomach and distal esophagus at the level of the fundoplication. It illustrates the position of the four pledgets and the placement of the U-stitch. The completed

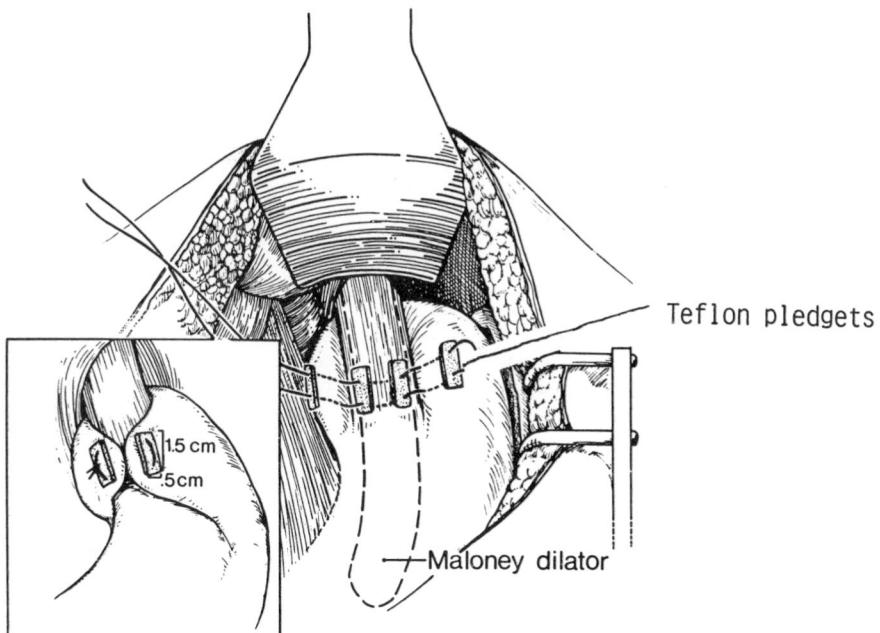

Figure 11: *Construction of the fundoplication by the transabdominal approach illustrating the placement of the horizontal mattress stitch and the positions of the pledgets. The wrap is formed over a No. 60 French bougie with enough space left over to allow the passage of an index finger through the wrap adjacent to the bougie. Insert shows the amplified fundoplication.*

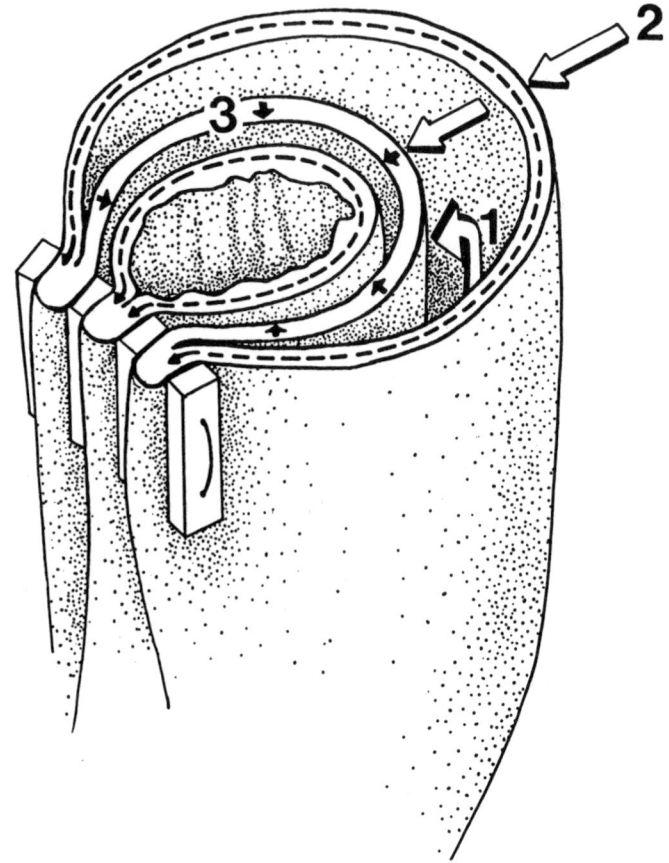

Figure 12: *Schematic cross-section of a Nissen fundoplication done with 1.5 × 0.5 cm pledgets illustrating how (a) intragastric, (b) intra-abdominal pressure, and (c) gastric fundic muscle tone are transmitted to the sphincter.*

fundoplication has an external length of only 1.5 cm and a circumference of slightly less than 360° wrap. Both factors reduce the resistance to the passage of food through the cardia. The illustration also shows how (a) intragastric pressure, (b) intra-abdominal pressure, and (c) gastric muscle tone is applied to the distal esophageal sphincter.

The Transthoracic Approach

The indications for a transthoracic approach for an anti-reflux procedure are: (a) The patient who has had a previous hiatal hernia repair. With this approach a peripheral circumferential incision in the diaphragm can be made for simultaneous exposure of the upper abdomen and safe dissection of the previous repair from both the abdominal and thoracic sides of the diaphragm. (b) The patient who requires a concomitant esophageal myotomy for achalasia or diffuse spasm. (c) The patient who has an esophageal stricture. In this situation the thoracic approach is preferred in order to obtain maximum mobilization of the esophagus to place the repair without tension below the diaphragm. (d) The patient with a sliding hiatal hernia that does not drop below the diaphragm during a roentgenographic barium study in the upright position. This can indicate esophageal shortening and again, a thoracic approach is preferred for maximum mobilization of the esophagus. (e) The patient who has associated pulmonary pathology. In this situation, the nature of the pulmonary pathology can be evaluated and the proper pulmonary surgery in addition to the anti-reflux repair can be performed. (f) The patient who is overly obese. In this situation, the abdominal procedure is difficult because of poor exposure, whereas the thoracic approach gives better exposure and allows a more precise repair.

The hiatus is approached transthoracically through a left posterior lateral thoracotomy incision in the sixth intercostal space, i.e., over the upper border of the seventh rib. For patients who have a previously failed anti-reflux repair and are undergoing a second procedure, I prefer to use the seventh intercostal space, i.e., above the superior border of the eighth rib. This allows better exposure of the abdomen through the diaphragm incision. When necessary, the diaphragm is incised circumferentially 2–3 cm from the chest wall for a distance of approximately 10–15 cm. An adequate fringe of diaphragm must be preserved along the chest wall to allow for reapproximation of the muscle. This diaphragm incision also provides excellent exposure of the left upper abdomen for a concomitant surgical procedure on the stomach or performing a left colon interposition for re-establishing gastrointestinal continuity following resection of the distal esophagus. If further abdominal exposure is necessary, the thoracic incision can be extended across the costal margin and diagonally across the rectus muscle to the abdominal midline. The operation is made easier if the anesthetic is delivered through a double lumen endotracheal tube and the left lung is selectively deflated.

The first step in the operation is to mobilize the esophagus from the level of the diaphragm to the aortic arch. Care is taken not to injure the vagal nerves. There are two vessels that arise from the proximal descending thoracic aorta and pass over the left lateral surface of the esophagus to the left main stem bronchus. They are the left superior and inferior bronchial arteries. These are ligated individually and represent the cephalad extension of the esophageal mobilization. In addition to these arteries, there are two or three direct esophageal branches coming directly from the distal descending thoracic aorta to the lower third of the esophagus. They are also ligated and divided. One need not worry about ischemic necrosis of the esophagus with this degree of dissection. In our experience, this has not occurred in over 700 anti-reflux procedures in which the esophagus has been so mobilized. There is sufficient blood supply through the intrinsic arterial plexus of the esophagus, fed by the inferior thyroid artery in the neck and branches of the right brachial artery in the thorax, to maintain the integrity and prevent ischemic necrosis of the muscle. This degree of mobilization is absolutely necessary in order to place the reconstructed cardia into the abdomen without undue tension. Failure to adequately mobilize the esophagus is one of the major causes for subsequent breakdown of a transthoracic repair and return of symptoms.

The second step of the operation is freeing the cardia from the diaphragm and is the most difficult portion of the transthoracic procedure. To accomplish this, it is not necessary to make an incision through the central tendon of the diaphragm or to enlarge the hiatus by dividing the crura. With experience, this portion of the operation can be completed through the hiatus. The dissection is started by gaining access into the abdominal cavity through the phrenoesophageal membrane. It can be difficult to find the right tissue plane since the properitoneal fat tends to protrude through the incision once the membrane has been divided. Persistence and close dissection to the wall of the stomach, away from the gastric vessels, will eventually be rewarded with entry into the free peritoneal space. Entry into the abdominal cavity is easier when a hiatal hernia is present.

The proper stance of the surgeon at the operating table will aid him in the dissection of the hiatus. He should stand adjacent to the patient, facing the head of the table. The left index and middle fingers are placed through the diaphragmatic hiatus into the abdominal cavity with the palm of the hand facing the patient's feet. The surgeon's line of vision is down and backward under his left axilla. With judicial use of the left thumb, index, and middle fingers, the surgeon is able to spread the hiatal tissues and guide the dissection done with a scissors controlled by his right hand. In this position, the left hand is also used to retract the esophagus and protect the vagal trunks. Although the description of this stance sounds somewhat awkward, its use greatly facilitates the most difficult part of the operation. In fact, the stance is quite natural and would be assumed eventually by any surgeon who, on numerous occasions, has experienced the struggle of freeing the cardia from the hiatus.

When all the detachments between the cardia and diaphragmatic hiatus are divided, the fundus and part of the body of the stomach are withdrawn up through the hiatus into the chest. Sometimes this requires detaching the cephalad portion of the dorsal mesentery of the stomach by passing a clamp through the posterior portion of the hiatus and dividing this mesentery just anterior to the aorta. Care should be taken not to injure the left gastric artery or vagal trunks during this maneuver. This portion of the operation is completed by excising the vascular fat pad that lies on the anterior lateral surface of the cardia in a manner similar to that described for the abdominal approach (Figure 13).

The third step of the procedure is the placement of the crura sutures used to close the hiatus. The completely mobilized esophagus and cardia are retracted anteriorly to expose the right and left crura (Figure 14). Usually there is a decussation of muscle fibers from the right crus around the aorta, but occasionally the aorta lies free within the enlarged hiatus. In either situation, the first crural stitch is placed as close as possible to the aorta, taking a generous bite of muscle in each crura. Traction on this first crural suture, and on a Babcock clamp attached to the anterior margin of the hiatus, elevates the right crus toward the surgeon and facilitates the placement of subsequent crural stitches. Occasionally it is necessary to mobilize the pericardium of the diaphragm for better exposure of the fascia and muscle of the right crus. The subsequent crural stitches should incorporate the fascia from the periphery of the central tendon that blends with the muscle fibers of the right crus. On the left, the stitches are placed through the muscle fibers of the crus and the firmly inherent overlying pleura. Approximately six sutures, placed 1 cm apart, are necessary to adequately approximate the crura and reduce the size of the hiatus. If it is felt more sutures are needed, they should be placed at this time since it is easier to remove those not needed than to place additional stitches after completion of the repair. In order to insert the most anterior crural stitch, it is often necessary to push the esophagus posteriorly against the previously placed sutures and place the stitch into the right crus, anterior to the esophagus, pass it posterior to the esophagus, and then through the left crus. The crural sutures are not tied until the reconstruction of the cardia is compete.

The fourth step of the operation is to construct the fundoplication. The fundus of the stomach is brought up into the chest through the hiatus. The wrapping of the fundus around the distal esophagus is performed in a manner similar to that described for the abdominal

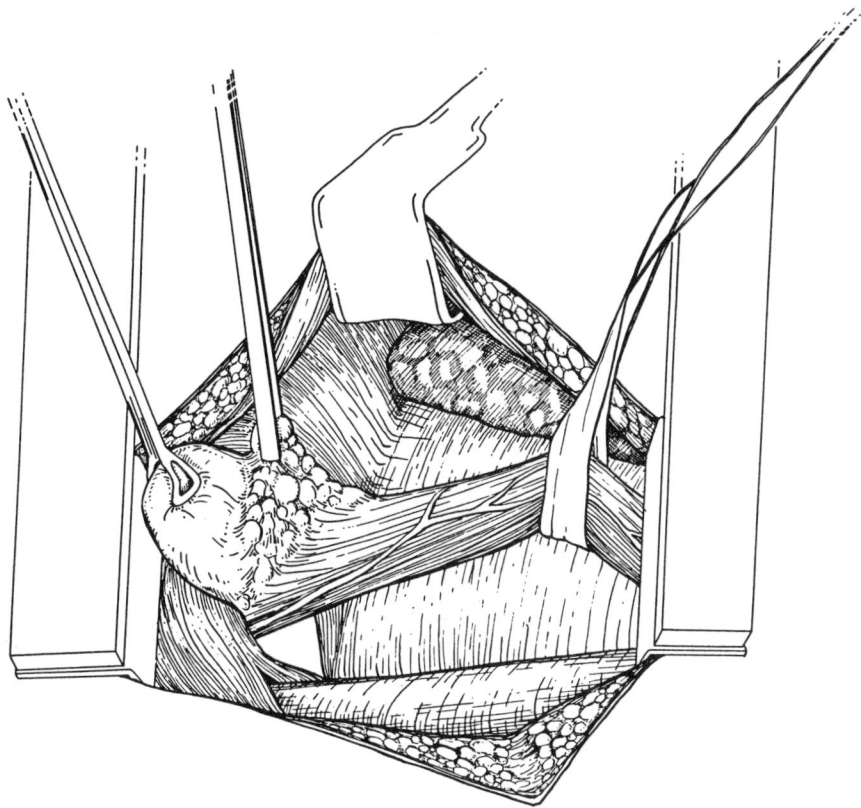

Figure 13: *A left posterolateral thoracotomy approach to the esophageal hiatus showing complete mobilization of the esophagus and freeing of the cardia from the diaphragmatic hiatus, the fundus of the stomach is drawn through the hiatus into the chest with a Babcock clamp. The forceps is on the vascular fat pad at the cardioesophageal junction.*

approach except that the fundus is anterolateral instead of posterolateral, and the hold suture posterior instead of anterior. As in the abdominal approach, the distal esophagus is invaginated into the stomach by pulling the lips of the fundus around posteriorly (Figure 15). The technique used to secure the wrap is similar to that described in the transabdominal approach. The needles of a double armed 2.0 Proline suture are passed through a 1.5 × 0.5 cm Teflon pledget 1 cm apart and then through the right lateral lip of the fundic wrap, again 1 cm apart. This is the inferior lip of the wrap as seen by the surgeon when operating through a left lateral thoracotomy incision. Both ends of the suture are passed through a second Teflon pledget, sand-

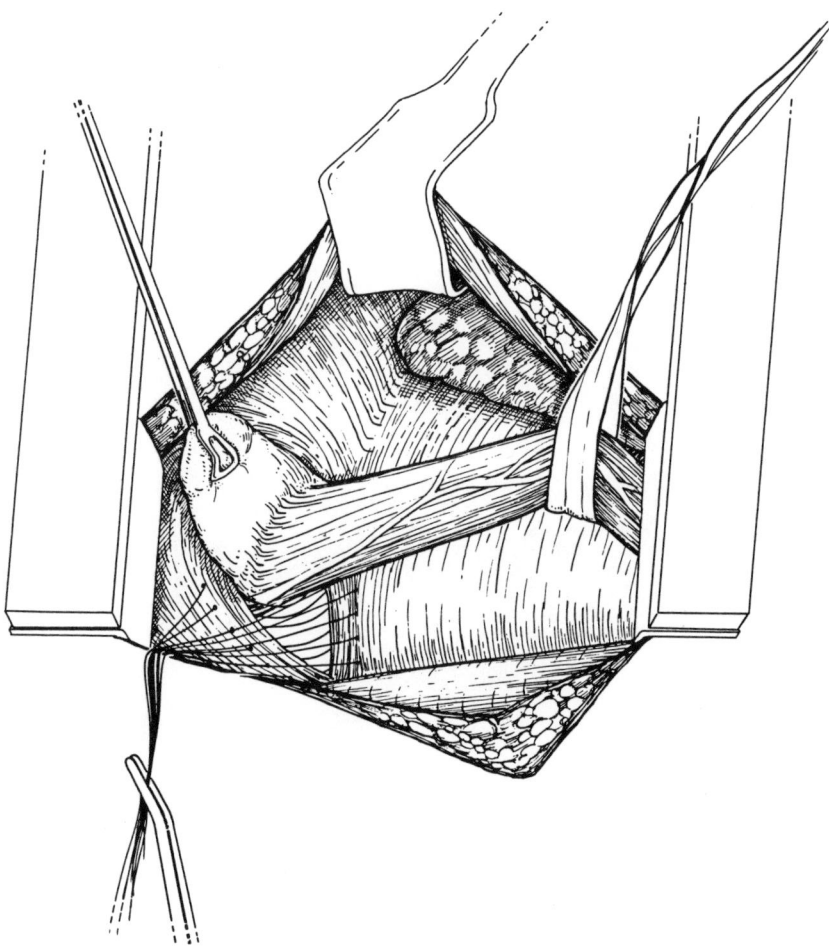

Figure 14: *A transthoracic repair through a left lateroposterior thoracotomy showing the vascular fat pad removed, and the anterior retraction of the esophagus to illustrate the placement of the crural sutures posteriorly. The sutures are tied after the fundoplication is completed.*

wiching the lip of the stomach between the two pledgets. A No. 60 French bougie is passed by the anesthesiologist into the stomach, as in the abdominal procedure, for accurate sizing of the wrap and proper identification of a posterior border of the gastroesophageal junction (Figure 16). One of the limbs of the stitch is then passed through the posterior wall of the esophagus at the level of the gastroesophageal junction, incorporating tissue down to, but not through, the muscu-

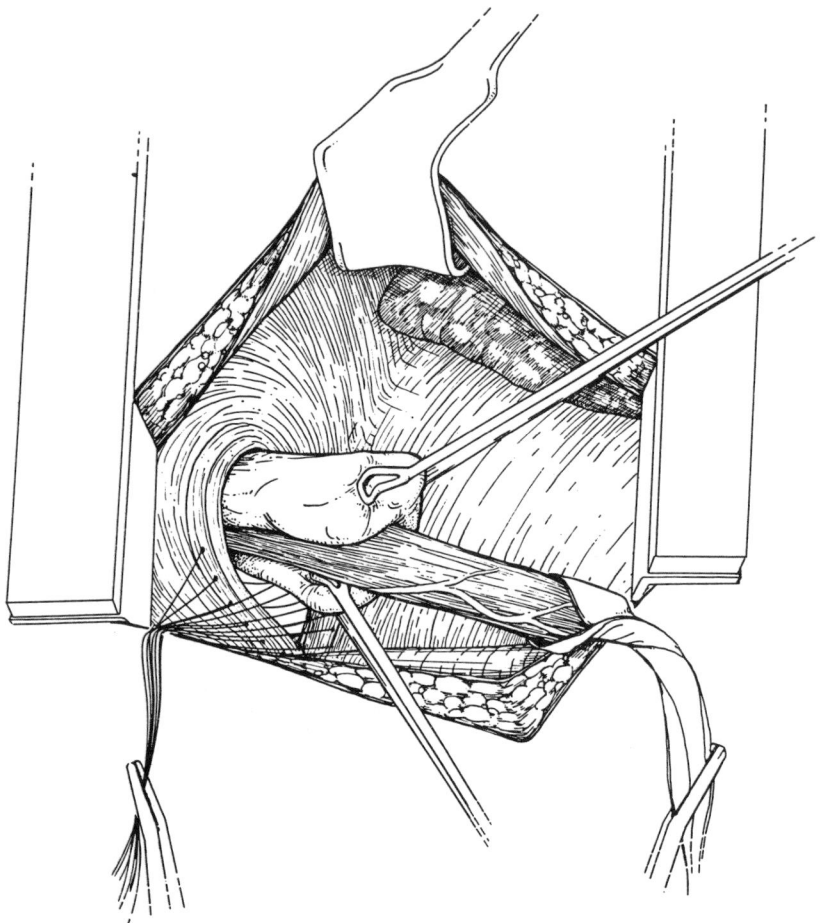

Figure 15: *Construction of a Nissen 360° gastric fundic wrap showing the fundus of the stomach brought up through the hiatus anterior to the esophagus.*

laris muscosa. The second limb is similarly passed through the posterior wall of the esophagus 1 cm cephalad to the first stitch. Both ends of the suture are passed through a third Teflon pledget, again 1 cm apart and then through the left lateral lip of the fundic wrap. This is the superior lip of the wrap as seen by the surgeon when operating through a left lateral thoracotomy incision. Both ends of the suture are then passed through the fourth and final Teflon pledget (Figure 17). A single tie is used initially to approximate the two lips

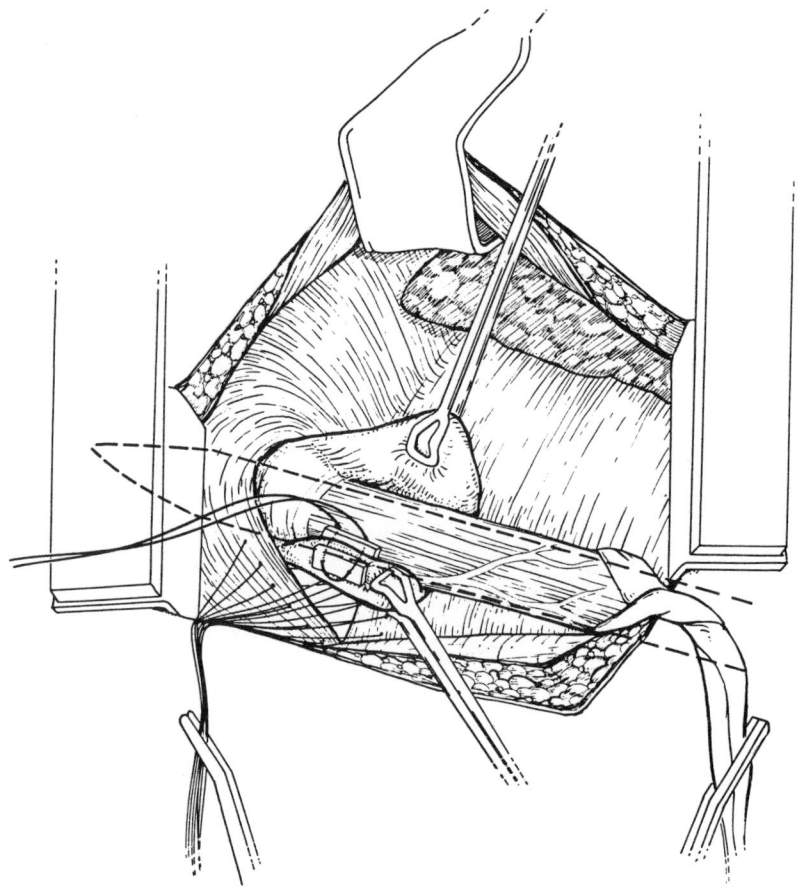

Figure 16: *Continued construction of a transthoracic Nissen fundoplication showing the placement of the horizontal mattress stitch and the position of the Teflon pledgets in the right lateral lip of the fundic wrap. The esophagus and stomach have been rotated to the right for easier placement of this stitch. A No. 60 French bougie is passed into the stomach to allow accurate sizing of the wrap and identification of the posterior border of gastroesophageal junction.*

of the fundoplication around the esophagus containing the No. 60 French bougie. Again, as with the abdominal repair, the wrap, when drawn together, should be large enough to accept the insertion of the surgeon's index finger between the stomach and the esophagus containing the No. 60 French dilator (Figure 18). If unable to do so, or if the wrap is too loose, the size of the wrap must be adjusted, as discussed in the abdominal approach. If the size of the wrap is correct,

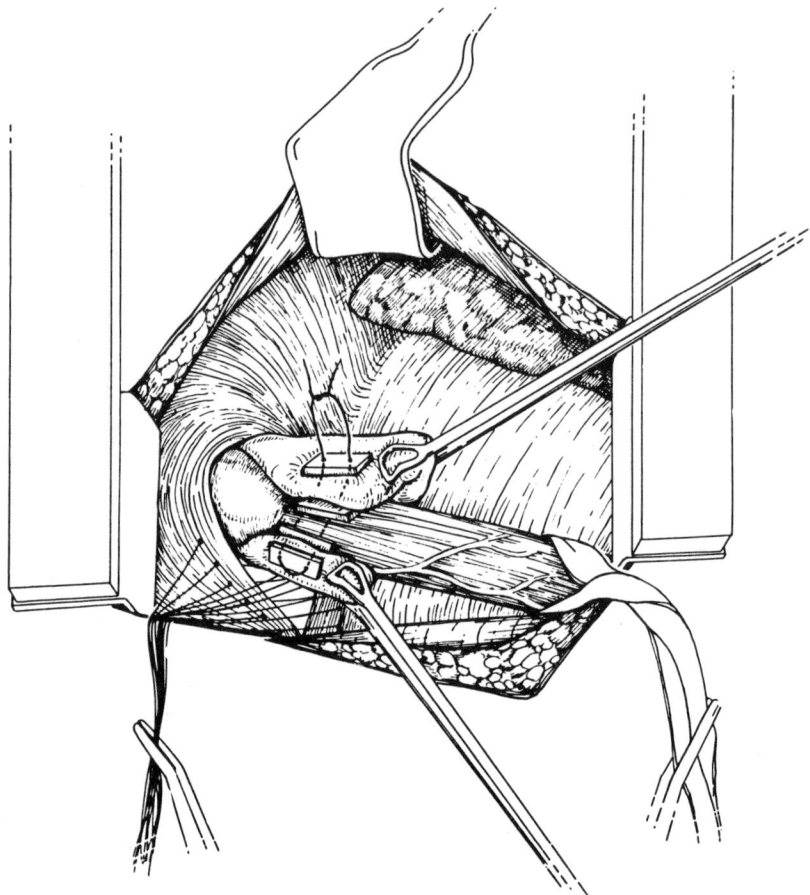

Figure 17: *Continued construction of a transthoracic Nissen fundoplication showing the placement of the horizontal mattress stitch and the position of the four Teflon pledgets. See text for complete description. Again, the stomach and esophagus have been rotated to the right for easier placement of the holding stitch.*

the stitch is tied sandwiching the stomach and esophagus together (Figure 19).

When complete, the fundoplication is placed into the abdomen by compressing the fundic ball with the hand and manually maneuvering it through the hiatus. Resistance to placing the repair into the abdomen can result from the shoelace obstruction of the previously placed crural sutures. Opening the crural sutures, like loosening the shoelaces of the shoe, relieves the obstruction and aids in placing

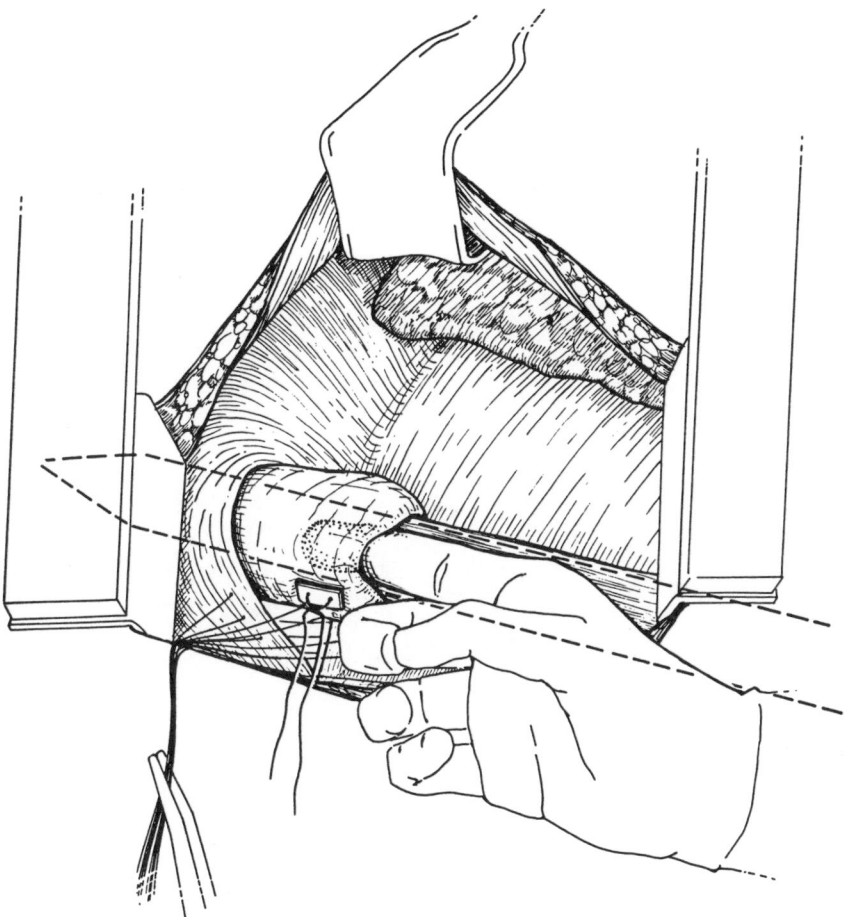

Figure 18: *Continued construction of a transthoracic Nissen fundoplication showing the sizing of the diameter of the wrap by the insertion of the tip of the surgeon's index finger between the gastric wrap and the esophagus containing the No. 60 French dilator. The stomach and esophagus have rotated back to their normal position with the U-stitch located posteriorly.*

the reconstructed cardia into the abdomen. Once in the abdomen, the fundoplication should remain there, and a gentle up-and-down motion on the diaphgram should not encourage it to emerge back through the esophageal hiatus into the chest. If the repair remains in the abdomen unaided, the previously placed crural sutures are tied (Figure 20).

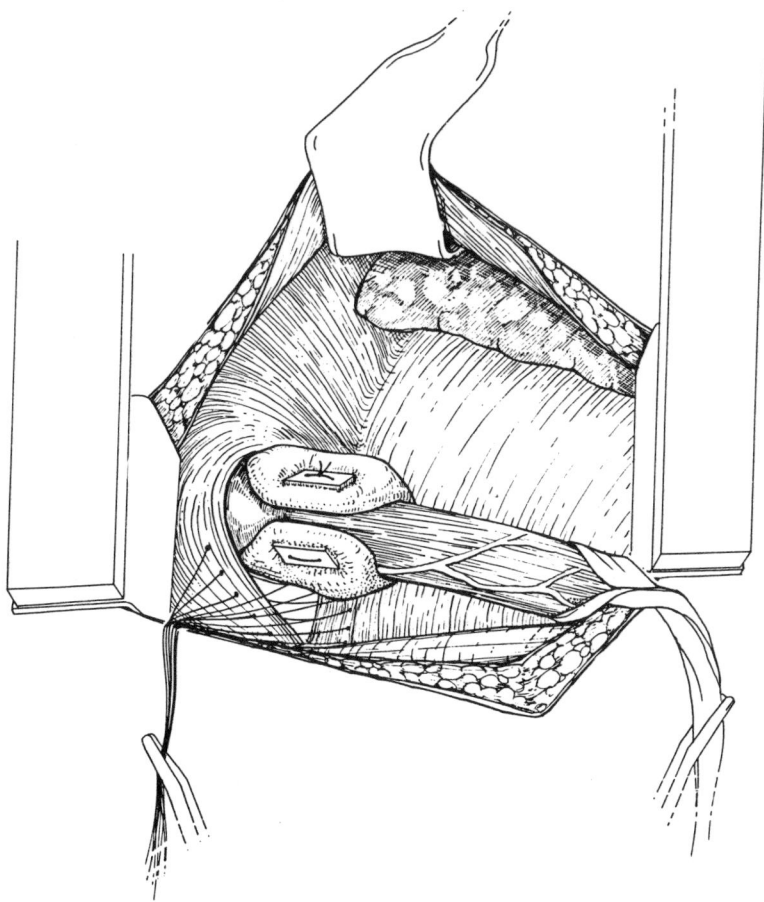

Figure 19: *Continued construction of a transthoracic Nissen fundoplication showing the position of the Teflon pledgets after tying the horizontal mattress suture. Again, the stomach and esophagus have been rotated to the right to demonstrate the holding suture.*

If the fundoplication tends to ride up through the hiatus, tension on the repair is too great and is usually due to inadequate mobilization of the esophagus. If there has been complete mobilization and the fundoplication still tends to ride up through the hiatus, then the branches of the left vagus nerve to the left pulmonary plexus can be divided in an effort to reduce the tension and allow for easier placement of the reconstructed cardia in the abdomen. If the tendency to ride up through the hiatus still exists after this maneuver, a Colles'

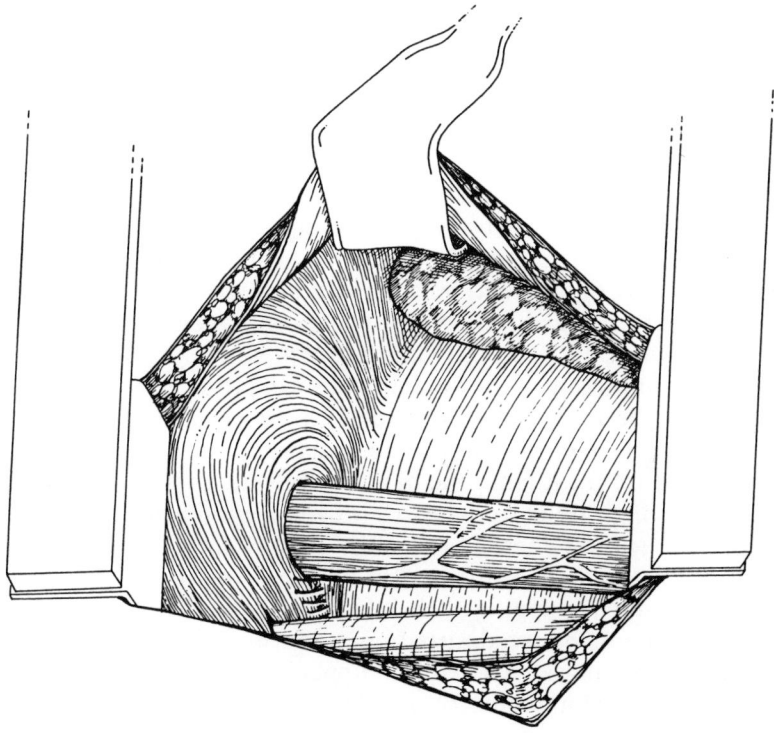

Figure 20: *The completed transthoracic repair after reducing the fundoplication into the abdomen and approximating the right and left crura by tying the previously placed crural sutures.*

gastroplasty or a resection of the cardia using a short left colon interposition to re-establish gastrointestinal continuity is done. This becomes a serious consideration in only two out of every 100 uncomplicated repairs.

When performing the repair, it is important that the vagi are protected and not injured. This will insure the relaxation of the gastric fundic wrap in concert with the distal esophageal sphincter on deglutition. At the completion of the procedure, a nasal gastric tube should be able to be passed, without guidance from the surgeon, directly into the stomach to assure that there has been no angulation of the distal esophagus. A chest tube for drainage of the pleural cavity is properly placed and the chest incision closed.

Postoperative Management

After either the abdominal or thoracic repair, the patient is kept on nasogastric suction for approximately five days to prevent distension of the stomach during the healing period. Gastric distension prior to complete healing can cause a breakdown of the repair. A barium swallow is obtained on the seventh postoperative day to demonstrate the unobstructed passage of barium into the stomach prior to starting a solid oral diet. Initially, a slight dysphagia may be experienced by the patient, but this will disappear as the traumatic edema resolves. Occasionally, dysphagia may persist for a longer period of time and is usually due to the presence of an intramural hematoma at the site of the fundoplication. If present, the hematoma will usually be absorbed within four to six weeks and the dysphagia will subside. One of the immediate benefits of an anti-reflux procedure is that from the time the patient recovers from anesthesia, he notes and enjoys relief from heartburn and regurgitation. Before discharge, the patient should be counseled that until the habit of air swallowing is broken, he may experience increased flatus and gastric distension due to trapping of the air in the stomach.

Our patients are readmitted one year after the operation for a critical symptomatic evaluation, upper gastrointestinal contrast study, esophageal manometry, and 24-hour esophageal pH monitoring. These studies assure us that we have accomplished our goals of: (a) correcting the patient's symptoms without contributing to dysphagia; (b) establishing an anatomical and functional repair of the cardia by increasing the distal esophageal sphincter pressure without interfering with its ability to relax, increasing the overall length of the sphincter if inadequate preoperatively, and increasing the length of the sphincter exposure to the positive pressure environment of the abdomen; and (c) the cessation of gastroesophageal reflux documented by 24-hour esophageal pH monitoring.

References

1. Joelsson BE, DeMeester TR, Skinner DB, LaFontaine E, Waters PF O'Sullivan GC: The role of the esophageal body in the antireflux mechanism. *Surgery* 1982; 92 (2):417-424.
2. DeMeester TR, Wernly JA, Bryant GH, Little AG, Skinner DB: Clinical and in vitro analysis of gastroesophageal competence: A study of the principles of antireflux surgery. *Am J Surg* 1979; 137:39.

3. O'Sullivan GC, DeMeester TR, Joelsson BE, et al: The interaction of the lower esophageal sphincter pressure and length of sphincter in the abdomen as determinants of gastroesophageal competence. *Am J Surg* 1982; 143:40−47.

4. Wernly JA, DeMeester TR, Bryant GH, Wang CI, Smith RB, Skinner DB: Intraabdominal pressure and manometric data of the distal esophageal sphincter. *Arch Surg* 1980; 115:534−539.

5. DeMeester TR: Pathophysiology of gastro-oesophageal reflux. In: Watson A, Celestin, LR, eds. *Disorders of the Oesophagus Advances and Controversies*. Pitman. 1984: 73−93.

6. DeMeester TR, LaFontaine E, Joelsson BE, et al: The relationship of hiatal hernia to the function of the body of the esophagus and the gastroesophageal junction. *J Thorac Cardiovasc Surg* 1981; 82:547−558.

7. Kranendonk SE: Reflux oesophagitis: An experimental study in rats. *En Volgens Besluit Van Het College Van Dekanen*, June, 1980.

8. DeMeester TR, Johnson LF, Joseph GJ, et al: Patterns of gastroesophageal reflux in health and disease. *Ann Surg* 1976; 184:459−470.

9. DeMeester TR, Wang CI, Wernly JA, et al: Technique, indications and clinical use of 24-hour esophageal pH monitoring. *J Thorac Cardiovasc Surg* 1980; 79:656−667.

10. Behar J, Sheahan GG, Biancani P: Medical and surgical management of reflux esophagitis. *N Engl J Med* 1975; 293(6):263−268.

11. Iascone C, DeMeester TR, Little AG, et al: Barrett's esophagus: Functional assessment, proposed pathogenesis and surgical therapy. *Arch Surg* 1983; 118(5):543−549.

12. Skinner DB, Walther BC, Ridell RI, et al: Barrett's esophagus: Comparison of benign and malignant cases. *Ann Surg* 1983; 198(4):554.

13. Pellegrini CA, DeMeester TR, Johnson LF: Gastroesophageal reflux and pulmonary aspiration: Incidence, functional abnormality and results of surgical therapy. *Surgery* 1979; 86:110−119.

14. DeMeester TR, Iascone C, Courtney JV, et al: Prospective evaluation of patients with chronic respiratory symptoms for the presence of occult esophageal disease. *J Thorac Cardiovasc Surg* (in press).

15. DeMeester TR, Cimochowski GE, O'Drobinak J: Esophageal function in patients with angina-type chest pain and normal coronary angiograms. *Ann Surg* 1982; 196(4):488−498.

16. Johnson LF, DeMeester TR: Evaluation of elevation of the head of the bed, bethanechol, and anatacid foam tablets on gastroesophageal reflux. *Dig Dis Sci* 1981; 26:673−680.

17. Benjamin SB, Richter JE, Cordova CM, et al: Prospective manometric evaluation with pharmacologic provocation of patients with suspected esophageal motility dysfunction. *Gastroenterology* 1983; 84:393−401.

18. Walther BS, Courtney JV, DeMeester TR, et al: The effect of paraesophageal hernia on sphincter function. *Am J Surg* 1984; 147:111−116.

19. O'Sullivan GC, DeMeester TR, Smith RB, et al: Twenty-four hour pH monitoring of esophageal funcion: Its use in evaluation in symptomatic patients after truncal vagotomy and gastric resection or drainage. *Arch Surg* 1981; 116:581−590.

20. Little AG, DeMeester TR, Skinner DB: Combined gastric and esophageal 24-hour pH monitoring in patients with gastroesophageal reflux. *Surg Forum* 1979; XXX:351−353.

21. Tolin RD, Malmud LS, Stelzer F, et al: Enterogastric reflux in normal subjects and patients with Bilroth II gastroenterostomy: Measurement of enterogastric reflux. *Gastroenterology* 1979; 77:1027–1033.
22. Lind JF, Duthie HL, Schlegel JF, et al: Motility of the gastric fundus. *Am J Physiol* 1961; 201:197–202.
23. Richardson JD, Larson GM, Polk HC: Intrathoracic fundoplication for shortened esophagus. Treacherous solution to a challenging problem. *Am J Surg* 1982; 143:29–35.

16

Complications of Gastroesophageal Reflux

Charles F. Barish, M.D., and
Wallace C. Wu, M.B., B.S.

Chapter Contents

From Castell DO, Wu WC, Ott DJ (eds): *Gastroesophageal Reflux Disease: Pathogenesis, Diagnosis, Therapy.* Mount Kisco, NY, Futura Publishing Co., Inc., 1985.

The complications of gastroesophageal reflux disease include esophagitis, esophageal ulcers and bleeding, esophageal strictures, Barrett's esophagus, and pulmonary disease. This chapter primarily reviews esophageal strictures and reflux-related pulmonary disease. Esophagitis, esophageal ulcers and bleeding, and Barrett's esophagus are discussed more briefly. A thorough review of Barrett's esophagus is contained in Chapter 17.

Esophageal Strictures

Introduction

A lower esophageal stricture is believed to result from fibrosis when damage from chronic, long-standing gastroesophageal reflux extends below the mucosa.[1] Which patients with reflux are destined to develop a stricture is not known, nor is the pathogenesis of stricture formation well understood. Although peptic strictures can occur at any age and in patients without prior heartburn, those affected are generally older and usually have a long history of heartburn. Factors predisposing to stricture formation include reflux while supine, gastric intubation, peptic ulcer disease, gastric hypersecretory states, such as the Zollinger–Ellison syndrome, post-gastrectomy conditions, scleroderma, and treated achalasia.[2] In the latter two circumstances, loss of esophageal peristalsis with subsequent prolonged acid exposure is a significant contributing factor. Up to 11% of patients with reflux disease have been reported to develop strictures.[3]

Manometric studies in patients with strictures have shown decreased lower esophageal sphincter pressures. In one study, 25 patients with benign peptic stricture all had lower esophageal sphincter pressures below 8 mmHg with a mean value of 4.9 ± 0.5 ($\pm$ SE) mmHg compared with 19.2 ± 1.3 mmHg in normal subjects.[3] In addition, many patients with stricture have been shown to have nonspecific esophageal motor disorders, such as simultaneous or repetitive contractions. Impaired peristalsis may contribute to esophagitis and stricture due to delayed esophageal acid clearing. Whether the manometric abnormalities in such patients contribute to stricture formation or are an effect of long-term gastroesophageal reflux is not clear. Nevertheless, such abnormal manometric findings in patients with gastroesophageal reflux might alert physicians to patients having a greater risk for stricture development.

Presentation

Dysphagia is usually the presenting complaint in patients with peptic strictures. Typically, heartburn from gastroesophageal reflux subsides with the onset of dysphagia. Initially, dysphagia is mostly for solids, but it can develop for liquids as well as with progressive narrowing of the stricture. Prolongation of eating, pain from food impaction, and regurgitation become prominent complaints.[4] Patients will frequently adjust their diet and may not present to their doctors until the stricture is far advanced. Occasionally, there will be no history of reflux symptoms.

Evaluation

The first step in evaluating any patient with dysphagia is a barium esophagram, which will usually demonstrate the presence and location of a stricture. To best evaluate the stricture radiographically, the esophagus should be well distended with barium. Time should be allowed to observe passage of barium into the stomach; the length and nature of the stricture can then be evaluated further by allowing barium to reflux into the esophagus from below. A stricture can also be assessed by having the patient swallow a marshmallow or piece of bread impregnated with barium.

A proper performed barium esophagram can accurately detect esophageal strictures with a sensitivity approximately that of endoscopy.[5] In fact, the radiographic method is probably the best way to determine the caliber of a stricture, and initially may be the only way to evaluate tight strictures that do not allow passage of an endoscope. Radiographically, benign strictures typically have smooth margins with a tapered appearance. There may be dilatation of the esophagus above a long-standing stricture. Active esophagitis often produces irregularity of the stricture margins; however, eccentric and irregular narrowing radiographically suggests malignancy.

Patients with dysphagia should have endoscopy after their radiologic study to evaluate further the extent of luminal narrowing and the gross appearance of the mucosa.[2] A benign stricture is usually smooth although mucosal ulceration may be present, while a malignant stricture appears more irregular, friable, and necrotic. Since the endoscopic appearance of a stricture can be misleading, esophageal biopsy and cytology must be done to exclude malignancy. Biopsies should be obtained, if possible, from the narrowest portion of the stricture. It would also be ideal to obtain biopsies from all four quadrants of the stricture as well as samples from passing the forceps through the stricture. Cytologic material is obtained by brushing the lumen of the stricture. If suspicion for malignancy is high and the initial pathologic material not diagnostic, repeat biopsy of the stricture can be done after esophageal dilatation.

Endoscopic biopsy should also be used in patients with peptic stricture to exclude Barrett's esophagus. Although such strictures are not necessarily associated with Barrett's esophagus, epithelial changes diagnostic of this disorder have been described in up to 44% of patients with chronic peptic stricture.[6] In another study, benign strictures were identified radiographically in 61% of patients with Barrett's esophagus.[7]

All strictures should be examined from below if the endoscope passes through the narrowed area. Sometimes an initial dilatation can be achieved by passage of the endoscope, while at other times the endoscope will pass freely through the narrowed area seen on the barium study. The latter may result if the diameter of the endoscope is smaller than the stricture lumen (particularly with use of the smaller caliber endoscopes), the narrowed area is stretched by the endoscope due to an elastic component, or the narrowed area is due to muscle spasm, in which case the mucosa usually appears normal. Untreated achalasia may simulate peptic stricture radiographically; however, the endoscope usually passes into the stomach with only slight pressure in this circumstance.

Treatment

Esophageal Dilatation and Medical Management

Most peptic strictures can be treated successfully using forceful dilatation. There are several different dilators available. The most commonly used mercury-filled dilators (bougies) are the Maloney and Hurst types. The Maloney dilator has a tapered end that more easily negotiates the lumen of longer strictures, while Hurst dilators have a blunted end that can exert more direct force.[8] Strictures having a very narrow or tortuous lumen are best dilated by first locating the lumen with a guide wire or the end of a swallowed string.[9] The Eder–Peustow metal dilator is inserted over a spring-tipped guide wire that is placed into the stomach either endoscopically or fluoroscopically.[10,11] Olive-shaped metal dilators of increasing size are screwed onto a flexible metal staff and are passed until the force required for easy passage is considered to be excessive. The risk of complications is reduced by fluoroscopic monitoring.

Other esophageal dilators include the tapered solid "neoplex" dilators, which are also inserted over a guide wire.[12] Although somewhat rigid, these dilators are flexible enough to follow the curve of the pharynx and allow for uniform, gentle dilatation of the stricture, rather than on abrupt stretching that might result in rupture of the esophagus. A Gruntzig balloon catheter passed over a fluoroscopically placed torqueable guide wire has also been used in esophageal dilatation.[13] This technique might be useful for initial dilatation of strictures that do not permit the passage of the Eder–Peustow spring-tipped guide wire. After balloon dilatation of the stricture to a maximum diameter of 9 mm, more conventional methods of esophageal dilatation can be used.

Generally, most patients having esophageal dilatation need only mild sedation, such as with meperidine or diazepam. Many patients require no medication, especially if they are accustomed to esophageal dilatation. Topical anesthesia in the pharynx may also be used. With the patient usually sitting, esophageal dilators of increasing size are passed through the stricture using gentle pressure. Fluoroscopic monitoring during the procedure can be helpful, particularly if the stricture is tortuous or the esophagus significantly dilated. In fact, fluoroscopy may be the only way to assure passage of the dilator through the stricture. Esophageal dilatation should be continued in one or more sessions with progressively larger dilators until at least a 45 French dilator passes easily (1 French [F] = 0.32 mm diameter). The patient is then seen at frequent intervals to test the luminal patency with the appropriate dilators or to redilate if necessary. Gradually, dilatation intervals can be lengthened depending on the patient's response or recurrence of dysphagia. Some patients can be trained to dilate themselves at home. Patients should follow a rigid anti-reflux medical regimen to avoid further damage to the esophagus and to discourage further stricture formation.

Conservative treatment of patients with peptic strictures using esophageal dilatation and a medical anti-reflux regimen has shown good success. An earlier study of 133 patients with peptic strictures describes a good response in 70%,[14] while another report of 90 patients with peptic strictures describes good results in 79%.[15] In another study of 68 patients with peptic strictures, 88% had a good response to conservative management.[16] Successful management by bougienage alone is described in 84.5% of 103 patients with benign esophageal stricture followed for 6 to 87 months in another recent report.[17] Nearly half of the patients in this report, however, required further dilatations during the first year after the initial series of dilatations, and two-thirds of these needed dilatations in subsequent years.

Esophageal dilatation for peptic stricture is associated with less morbidity and mortality than is surgery, and is usually the recommended initial treatment in elderly patients, particularly if they have cardiopulmonary disease. Nevertheless, esophageal dilatation is not without risk. The major complications include perforation, bleeding, aspiration, myocardial infarction, cardiac arrhythmias, respiratory arrest, and allergic reaction to sedative or anesthetic medications.[18] The cardiopulmonary complications seem to be more associated with the use of intravenous sedation or pharyngeal anesthesia. Depending on the method of esophageal dilatation, the complication rates ranged from 0.4 to 1.8%.[18] Mercury bougie dilatation is associated with bleeding more than perforation, while metal olives have a greater risk of esophageal perforation. The reported perforation rate for Eder–Peustow dilatation is about 0.6% compared with 0.4% for mercury bougienage.[18]

Complications are less likely if prior radiologic studies of the esophagus are reviewed, fluoroscopic monitoring is available during the procedure, sedation and anesthesia are used cautiously, resuscitative equipment is readily at hand, and x-ray examination with a water-soluble contrast medium is done in suspected perforation. Although it is generally felt that esophageal perforation should be treated surgically with primary closure and drainage, conservative management with fasting, nasoesophageal suction, and antibiotics has been described in confined perforations.[16]

Surgical Management

Surgical management of peptic strictures is indicated when esophageal dilatation is unsuccessful, or when a patient is unwilling to have repeated dilatations. It may be particularly desirable in younger patients with peptic stricture and severe gastroesophageal reflux. Several surgical techniques have been used with variable success. Historically, one of the first procedures was resection of the esophageal stricture with interposition of a segment of colon, small bowel, or stomach.[19] Due to significant morbidity, mortality, and high recurrence rate of strictures, these interposition procedures were abandoned for simpler operations. The Thal procedure includes incision of the stricture anteriorly and application of a gastric fundic patch in an attempt to open the stricture and guard against gastro-esophageal reflux by creation of a valve mechanism.[20] It is necessary, however, to add a fundoplication to the Thal procedure because reflux is usually not adequately controlled.

More recent operations with good results have replaced those mentioned above.[21] The surgical approach has been partly governed by determining the extent and severity of the stricture in the operating room.[22] Intraoperative dilatation of severe strictures has been done antegrade with conventional bougies or retrograde through a gastrotomy with cylindrical bougies of gradually increasing size. Such intraoperative dilatation combined with an adequate anti-reflux procedure, such as Nissen fundoplication, has produced excellent results in most patients followed for several years. Restoration of normal esophageal mucosa and an adequate esophageal lumen have been noted.[22] The use of anti-reflux surgery alone without intraoperative dilatation may also be successful, since post-operative resolution of strictures and return of esophageal mucosa to normal has been reported.[23] The currently recommended surgical management of peptic stricture should, therefore, include an effective anti-reflux procedure possibly combined with intraoperative dilatation.

Esophageal Ulcers and Bleeding

Overview

Esophagitis is a relatively common complication of gastroesophageal reflux. Endoscopically, patients with esophagitis have friable mucosa and linear erosions, sometimes with superficial or deep ulcerations. While superficial ulcerations are not uncommon, only a small percentage of these progress to deep ulceration involving the muscular layers of the esophagus.[1,24] Esophagitis generally responds to anti-reflux management. Deep ulcers may be more difficult to treat, requiring, at times, prolonged cimetidine therapy[25] or surgery. Symptoms associated with deep esophageal ulceration include constant severe pain radiating to the back and not related to meals or body position,[24] dysphagia, weight loss, or bleeding. Melena or hematemesis may be a presenting complaint, and massive bleeding may require surgical treatment.[26] Chronic occult esophageal bleeding can also occur in reflux patients, and may result in the development of iron deficiency anemia. This latter presentation is often related to an unsuspected esophageal ulcer.[26]

Deeper esophageal ulcers are generally associated with a Barrett's esophagus. Indeed, a deep, punched-out ulcer above the gastroesophageal junction is often associated with a Barrett's esophagus. These deep ulcers tend to occur in the columnar epithelium and can have the appearance of benign gastric ulcers.[26] Other potential problems include ulcer perforation and an increased risk of malignancy.[25] Barrett's esophagus is discussed more extensively in Chapter 17.

Pulmonary Manifestations

Introduction

Although a causal relationship between esophageal reflux and pulmonary disease is difficult to establish, it has been shown to exist in selected patients. Gastroesophageal reflux may even be one of the most common non-infectious causes of chronic or recurrent laryngeal, tracheobronchial, and pulmonary disease. Although most patients will experience co-existing gastroesophageal symptoms, they are not always present or may be overlooked. For this reason, gastroesophageal reflux may not be suspected as the etiology for the pulmonary disease. It has been stated that up to 10% of patients with gastroesophageal reflux have tracheobronchial aspiration syndrome.[27] Respiratory problems sometimes attributable to gastroesophageal reflux include chronic asthma (especially with nocturnal wheezing or cough), bronchiectasis, laryngitis, hoarseness, bronchitis, aspiration pneumonia, atelectasis, and hemoptysis. Pulmonary fibrosis and cor pulmonale have also been reported, as have seizures secondary to hypoxia after aspiration. The respiratory symptoms are usually recurring and nonseasonal.

Unfortunately, documentation of pulmonary aspiration of gastric contents has been difficult. Radionuclide scintiscanning may be used to demonstrate pulmonary aspiration following placement of technetium-99m sulphur colloid in the stomach. One study[28] of six adults with suspected nocturnal aspiration showed positive scintiscans of the lung in three who also had prolonged espisodes of gastroesophageal reflux during overnight pH monitoring. Conversely, another study[29] showed that none of ten asthmatics with gastroesophageal reflux had documentation of aspiration. Similarly, Pope's laboratory was unable to document aspiration in any of twelve subjects with subjective histories.[1] In seven children tested in another study, only two had evidence of radionuclide aspiration.[30] These reports suggest one or more of the following conclusions: (a) the radioisotope technique is relatively insensitive, (b) aspiration occurs in only a small number of asthmatics with reflux, or (c) reflux occurs so infrequently that it is difficult to detect. It appears, therefore, that the role of radionuclide scintiscanning in evaluating patients with suspected esophagopulmonary aspiration has yet to be established. Despite this uncertainty, a positive scintiscan is still reliable documentation of reflux-related aspiration.

Another possibility explaining the rarity of demonstrating actual aspiration in some patients with asthma and gastroesophageal reflux is the observation that they may have a neurally mediated reflex mechanism producing their symptoms. Studies in 15 asthmatics[31] with clinical gastroesophageal reflux who underwent intraesophageal acid provocation testing showed increased pulmonary flow resistance when symptoms of acid reflux occurred. Treatment with antacids reversed the pulmonary changes, suggesting relief of bronchospasm. The explanation may be related to stimulation of esophageal receptors that trigger vagally mediated bronchoconstriction. This concept is supported by experimentation in dogs with esophagitis showing that intraesophageal acid infusion caused a fall in respiratory conductance that did not occur after bilateral vagotomy.[32] Consequently, aspiration may not be necessary to explain respiratory symptoms in patients with gastroesophageal reflux.

Reflux-induced Respiratory Disorders in Children

Much of the information on pulmonary complications of gastroesophageal reflux has been reported in children. Gastroesophageal reflux is a frequent cause of recurring emesis in infants, usually improving during the first year. Serious reflux in infants and young children, however, can result in apnea or failure to thrive from esophagitis, stricture, anemia secondary to esophageal bleeding, and pulmonary disease. In some children, the pulmonary disorder may be the only manifestation of reflux. Children with recurrent pulmonary infections or intractable asthma should be evaluated for gastroesophageal reflux since repeated episodes of aspiration may lead to chronic pulmonary disease with fibrosis.

Several patterns of nocturnal asthma related to reflux have been described in children.[33] Affected children often eat bedtime snacks, large or late suppers, or take large volumes of liquids with their evening meal or at bedtime. The asthmatic attacks seem to occur regularly at night after an otherwise well child has gone to bed. They commonly occur 1 to 2 hours after lying down and are frequently preceded by bouts of paroxysmal coughing and wheezing. Attacks have also been described between midnight and four A.M. and in the morning while the child is dressing.

Investigations of children with pulmonary manifestations of gastroesophageal reflux have been reported. Foglia et al[34] compared the sensitivity of various tests for detecting gastroesophageal reflux in 42 children ages 7 weeks to 19 years old (median 3.8 years). Thirty-four of them had bouts of recurring pneumonia, 17 had moderate to severe asthma or recurrent atelectasis, and nine had no gastrointestinal symptoms. The children underwent several studies before treatment, including radiographic examination, esophageal manometry, esophageal pH testing,and endoscopy. The radiographic study showed barium reflux in 81%, esophageal manometry revealed decreased lower esophageal sphincter pressure (less than 15 mmHg) or motility problems in 72%, endoscopy demonstrated esophagitis in 72%, a 1-hour pH test showed reflux in 74%, and 24-hour pH monitoring showed reflux in 92% of patients tested. The cine-esophagram was felt to be the simplest screening test, while 24-hour pH monitoring was considered the most sensitive. A normal control group was not included in the report.

Christie et al[35] evaluated 15 patients with recurrent acute respiratory symptoms for gastroesophageal reflux. Eight of 15 tested had reflux during barium esophagram while all of 10 tested had positive acid reflux tests and decreased lower esophageal sphincter pressure on manometry. The acid reflux test was performed by instillation of 300 ml/1.7 m^2 of 0.1 N HCl into the stomach by nasogastric tube and measurement of pH in the esophagus by a probe 3 cm above the gastroesophageal junction. The test was considered positive if two episodes of acid reflux, defined as a decrease in esophageal pH to less than four and lasting more than 15 seconds, occurred within a 20-minute period.[36] In those patients not having spontaneous reflux within 10 minutes, provocative maneuvers were done to promote reflux. The authors concluded that the acid reflux test was the more sensitive measure of gastroesophageal reflux, and that an incompetent lower esophageal sphincter may be the cause of abnormal reflux.

Thirty children, aged one to 18 years, with either chronic asthma or at least two episodes of pneumonia in one year were evaluated in another study.[37] Using acid reflux tests, esophageal manometry, endoscopy with biopsy, and barium esophagrams, 63% of the children had gastroesophageal reflux based on two or more positive tests. In these patients, 17 had a history of nocturnal cough within 1–3 hours after retiring. The cough occurred alone or preceded wheezing. Many of the patients had a history of vomiting during infancy. The conclusions of this study were that the acid reflux test was indispensable in the evaluation of children with suspected reflux-related pulmonary disease and that esophageal manometry and the barium esophagram were also useful.

Danus et al[38] studied 43 children, 4 months to 5 years of age, with recurrent obstructive bronchitis (repeated attacks of dyspnea, wheezing, rales, rhonchi, and fever), but no prominent gastrointestinal symptoms, by barium esophagram and manometry. Radiographic examination showed gastroesophageal reflux in 26 patients, who also had a mean lower esophageal sphincter pressure of 6.3 mmHg (normal 21.9 mmHg). The other 17 patients without barium reflux had a mean lower sphincter pressure of 10 mmHg. Ten of 14 patients with radiographic and manometric evidence of reflux had disappearance of their pulmonary symptoms after appropriate treatment. Five of six patients without barium reflux, but with a hypotensive sphincter, also had good results with such management.

Jolley et al[39] evaluated 27 infants with respiratory symptoms and gastroesophageal reflux documented by clinical history and extended esophageal pH monitoring. These infants were compared with 14 controls with reflux but no respiratory symptoms. The children with respiratory symptoms were treated for reflux and followed for at least a year. They were classified as having reflux-related respiratory disease (17 patients) if their pulmonary symptoms ceased, reflux-unrelated disease (seven) if the pulmonary symptoms persisted, or indeterminate (three) if neither reflux symptoms nor pulmonary symptoms improved. Findings on 18- to 24-hour pH recordings in the distal esophagus seemed to indicate that the duration of reflux during sleep and more than 2 hours post-prandially provided the best separation between the groups. In the children with reflux-related symptoms, 94% and 74% had a mean duration of reflux during sleep greater than 4 minutes and 6 minutes respectively. In the control group of 14 children with reflux but no respiratory symptoms, only 50% and 7% had a mean duration of reflux greater than 4 minutes and 6 minutes, respectively. None of the seven patients with reflux-unrelated symptoms nor the six asymptomatic controls had a mean duration over 4 minutes. One of the three patients in the intermediate group had a mean duration of reflux of over 4 minutes.

Presumably, acid reflux should closely precede respiratory distress if it is the cause of the respiratory symptoms. This study suggested such a relationship in only 41% of patients who had resolution of their respiratory symptoms with anti-reflux therapy. Thus, the mean duration of acid reflux during sleep might provide a good indicator of reflux-induced respirtory symptoms even when a direct relationship is not observed during pH monitoring.

It has been suggested that sudden infant death syndrome might be related to laryngeal sensitivity to refluxing gastric contents, resulting in apnea, laryngospasm, and respiratory arrest.[34] Gross aspiration would not be necessary in these instances, and is, in fact, difficult to document in those infants who have died from the syndrome. A report[36] of 14 infants with symptomatic gastroesophageal reflux that also had respiratory distress, apnea, and chronic pulmonary disease since birth describes the results of simultaneous recordings of esophageal pH, heart rate, impedance pneumography, and nasal air flow. All the infants had reflux on a barium esophagram, all but one had a positive pH reflux test, and all had radiographic changes compatible with bronchopulmonary dysplasia. In five infants, gastroesophageal reflux preceded apnea, and the tracings recorded what appeared to be laryngospasm. Apnea was also induced by the infusion of dilute acid into the esophagus, but not by similar infusion of water or formula. Thus, apnea may have resulted from an exaggerated response to stimulation of chemoreceptors near the pharynx sensitized by refluxing gastric contents. Eight infants had cessation of apnea and improvement in their pulmonary disease after intensive medical therapy, while the six who failed medical management had a good response to surgical control of gastroesophageal reflux.

Spitzer et al[40] studied 15 otherwise healthy infants with awake apnea, described as a sudden startled or staring expression, rigid posturing followed by hypotonia, absence of tonic–clonic movements, and occurrence within an hour of feeding. The symptoms were often precipitated by sudden flexing of the legs during diaper changing or by moving from a lying to sitting position. All 15 infants were compared with a control group of infants using 24-hour pH monitoring, nasal thermistor measurement of air flow, impedance pneumography, and heart rate. All 15 had significant gastroesophageal reflux by pH probe, and 13 had documented episodes of airway obstruction in association with reflux. No such episodes occurred in the control group. Ten infants had their apnea successfully managed at home using reflux precautions, three had reflux prevented by the use of bethanechol, and two required Nissen fundoplication.

In a study of 19 children with chronic allergic steroid-dependent asthma, Shapiro and Christie[41] suggested that gastroesophageal reflux should probably be considered more a potential cause of chronic pulmonary disease in children who are not atopic. The children studied were classified as atopic based on family history, skin testing, serum IgE concentrations, and chronic wheezing exacerbated by extrinsic factors. Eight of the 19 children had a lower esophageal sphincter pressure of less than 12 mmHg, and nine had a positive acid reflux test. Barium esophagram, however, showed reflux in only two. The children were treated for three weeks with a medical anti-reflux regimen but there was no significant change in their asthma symptoms or pulmonary function tests. All patients were taking theophylline preparations. Since theophylline may decrease lower esophageal sphincter pressure, the LES pressures were remeasured in seven patients after stopping the medication for 12–18 hours. In five of the patients, initially low sphincter pressures returned to normal. It was suggested that children with an atopic history and pulmonary symptoms may have gastroesophageal reflux that is either unrelated to the pulmonary problems or that is a result of medication that lowers the LES pressure. The 3 weeks of anti-reflux therapy may have been, however, too short to provide a fair evaluation in this study.

Management

Medical managment of children with gastroesophageal reflux includes elevation of the head of the bed, small evening meals with less than 4 ounces of fluid, and no food for at least 3 hours before going to bed.[33] Patients with pyrosis or esophagitis are also treated with antacids, 10–30 ml 1 and 3 hours post-prandially and at bedtime. Infants are treated with thickened feedings (flour added to their milk and thickened smaller meals) and upright positioning for 30 to 60 minutes after feeding. Orenstein and Whitington[42] described good success with prone, head-elevated positioning in a simple cloth harness. If children still remain symptomatic, bethanechol has been used successfully.[43,44] The use of H_2 blockers in young children has not been adequately studied. Anti-reflux surgery should be considered in severely symptomatic patients refractory to medical therapy.

The choice between medical and surgical management in patients with reflux-related pulmonary disease remains controversial. Davis[27] studied 18 children with severe recurrent pneumonitis or bronchitis, comparing nine patients treated surgically and nine treated medically. Over a period of four years or more, the postoperative patients continued to do well, while the medically managed patients continued to have bronchopulmonary problems. Larger series of randomized patients using more current modes of medical therapy will be needed, however, to clarify this issue.

Reflux-induced Respiratory Disorders in Adults

Reflux-related respiratory disease in adults has also been a subject of considerable interest. Kjellen et al[45] compared 22 exogenous asthmatics with a known precipitating allergan to 75 endogenous asthmatics without an atopic history using esophageal manometry, intraesophageal acid perfusion testing, and spirometry. Both groups had frequent esophageal abnormalities such as a motility disorder, decreased lower esophageal sphincter pressure, or a positive acid perfusion test. Surprisingly, the incidence of esophageal disorders was 95% in the exogenous group compared with 58% in the endogenous group. The asthmatic patients with objective esophageal disease were noted to have more pyrosis, heartburn, chest pain, wheezing, and nonproductive coughing. These findings do not clearly support or refute the theory that gastroesophageal reflux is a cause of asthma in adults. Gastroesophageal reflux may be a secondary phenomenon in asthmatic patients attributable to changes in intrathoracic and intraabdominal pressure induced by the asthma. Along with the theophylline-containing drugs affecting the lower esophageal sphincter pressure, a complicated relationship between reflux and asthma may exist.

Mays[46] described 28 adults with severe asthma, 20 of whom had onset of their asthma in adulthood. Compared with a control group, the asthmatics had a significantly higher incidence of gastroesophageal reflux. Past history, allergy skin testing, sinus x-rays, and pulmonary and gastrointestinal evaluations were obtained. If the history and laboratory data did not clearly establish whether the asthma was endogenous or exogenous, further importance was given to age of onset, the time of day that symptoms occurred, and previous response to therapy. Those who had adult onset, had smoked, had predominantly nocturnal episodes of coughing and wheezing, and who were more resistant to conventional therapy, were more likely to be classified as having endogenous asthma. The non-allergenic asthmatics over 30 years old had a stronger association with gastroesophageal reflux than other patients. It was proposed that patients with pre-existing asthma may become worse after the development of gastroesophageal reflux.

Pellegrini et al[47] studied 100 patients with abnormal gastroesophageal reflux documented by 24-hour esophageal pH monitoring, including 48 patients with a history of possible aspiration. After more careful evaluation during 24-hour pH monitoring, only 17% of the 48 had reflux-induced respiratory symptoms documented by a drop in esophageal pH occurring simultaneously with pyrosis and coughing or wheezing. Only one patient had a history of more than mild heartburn. Eleven percent had coughing or wheezing before reflux occurred, while another 19% were considered potential aspirators because they did have reflux but did not develop pulmonary symptoms. Interestingly, 75% of the documented aspirators had abnormal esophageal manometry with delayed clearance of acid in the supine position. The potential aspirators had rapid esophageal clearance of refluxed acid by normal peristalsis. Also, the patients with respiratory symptoms preceding reflux, who therefore were presumed to have a primary pulmonary disorder, had higher esophageal pressures and normal motility. This would infer that the incidence of aspiration is less than suspected by history and occurs more in patients with esophageal motility disorders that interfere with esophageal clearing. Identification of the primary problem can serve to clarify the best approach to therapy.

Another study of 30 asthmatics[48] with variable reflux symptoms reinforces the importance of a subjective and objective association between respiratory symptoms and gastroesophageal reflux. In 18 of these patients, nocturnal asthma was associated with pyrosis. Intra-esophageal infusion of 0.1 N HC1 produced a significant decrease in pulmonary function in 10 of these 18 patients, and antacid relief of pyrosis resulted in improved pulmonary function tests. The 12 patients who had no historical association between their pyrosis and asthma did not have a change in pulmonary function with acid infusion.

In summary, gastroesophageal reflux may cause pulmonary symptoms in only a subset of patients initially suspected. Although a careful history may help to identify these patients, esophageal symptoms may be minimal or absent. For this reason, patients with suspected reflux-related respiratory symptoms and those with chronic pulmonary disease of unknown etiology should be considered for gastrointestinal evaluation. A suggested approach is shown in the flow diagram found in Figure 1.

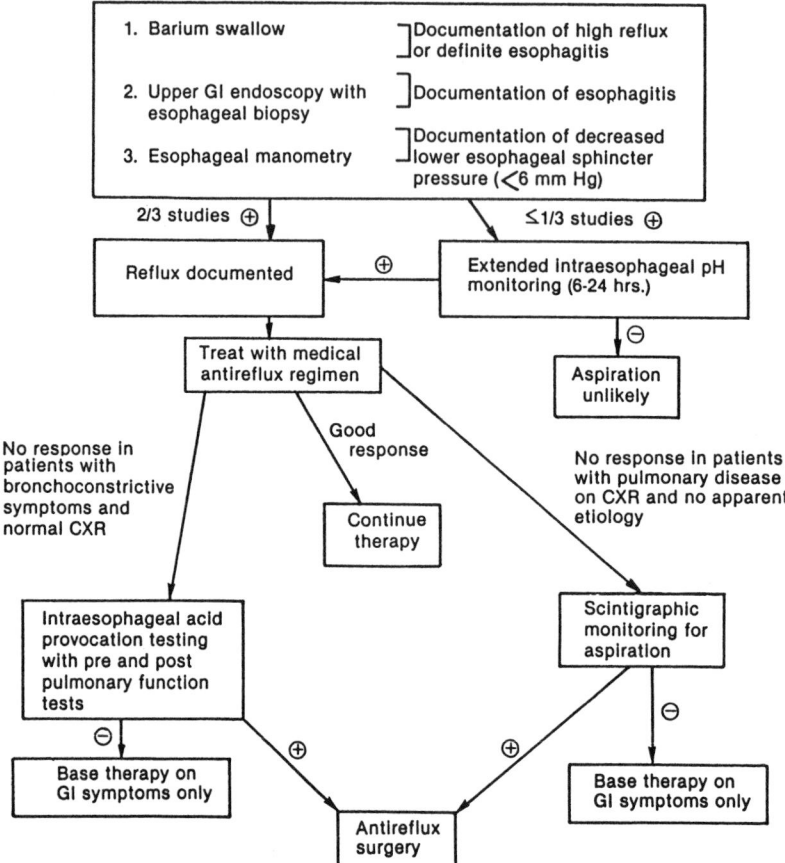

Figure 1: *Suggested approach to patients with suspected reflux-induced respiratory disease. Patients who are positive for gastroesophageal reflux in at least two of the initial three studies are treated with a medical anti-reflux regimen. If none, or only one, of the initial studies are positive, intraesophageal pH monitoring is performed before treatment with a medical anti-reflux regimen. Patients with documented gastroesophageal reflux refractory to medical management undergo intraesophageal acid provocation testing or scintigraphic aspiration monitoring to document whether pulmonary symptoms are related to reflux before being subjected to surgery.*

Management

Treatment of reflux-induced pulmonary disease in adults has received much attention. A report of 18 patients[49] diagnosed as having asthma and gastroesophageal reflux by esophagram, endoscopy, pH monitoring, intraesophageal acid infusion, and pulmonary function tests describes the results of a 6-week double-blind crossover study with cimetidine. The cimetidine resulted in significant improvement of both reflux and nocturnal asthma symptoms, as well as a statistical improvement in the evening peak flow values compared with placebo. The cimetidine presumably helps by decreasing both gastric acid production and volume of gastric juice. Although H_2 receptors may be present in the lung, their role in the regulation of bronchoconstriction is unclear, and no studies have shown any significant bronchodilator effect attributable to cimetidine. Another study[50] consisted of a randomized trial of medical and surgical therapy for gastroesophageal reflux in adults with endogenous asthma. Twenty-seven patients were treated for 6 months with cimetidine, 26 with anti-reflux surgery, and 28 with placebo for 6 months. During that time, 20 (74%) patients treated with cimetidine, 20 (77%) treated surgically, and 10 (36%) from the placebo group had improvement in their pulmonary symptoms. In another study, 28 adult asthmatics with known reflux were treated with intensive anti-reflux medical therapy; there was notable improvement with none requiring surgery.[51]

Most of the earlier reports of patients with pulmonary disease and associated gastroesophageal reflux described the results of anti-reflux surgery. For example, 24 (89%) of 27 patients with asthma treated by anti-reflux surgery in one study[52] were completely relieved of their symptoms. Others have also shown good results in treating pulmonary disease with anti-reflux surgery.[53-57]

Generally, patients with suspected reflux-related respiratory symptoms should be initially managed with a medical anti-reflux regimen as discussed in Chapter 14. Any respiratory medications being used therapeutically in patients should be weaned slowly while response to treatment of reflux is closely followed. If respiratory symptoms persist after an adequately enforced trial of medical therapy, anti-reflux surgery should be considered.

References

1. Pope CE: Gastroesophageal reflux disease (reflux esophagitis). In: Sleisenger MH, Fordtran JS, eds. *Gastrointestinal Disease—Pathophysiology, Diagnosis, Management.* 3rd ed. Philadelphia: W.B. Saunders Co. 1983:449–476.

2. Bennett JR: Oesophageal strictures. *Clin Gastroenterol* 1978; 7:555–569.

3. Ahtaridis G, Snape WJ, Cohen S: Clinical and manometric findings in benign peptic strictures of the esophagus. *Dig Dis Sci* 1979; 24:858–861.

4. Vantrappen G, Hellemans J, Geboes K: Etiology and non-surgical treatment of organic esophageal stenosis. In: Vantrappen G, Hellemans J, eds. *Diseases of the Esophagus.* New York: Springer-Verlag. 1974:795–806.

5. Ott DJ, Gelfand DW, Lane TG, Wu WC: Radiologic detection and spectrum of appearances of peptic esophageal strictures. *J Clin Gastroenterol* 1982; 4:11–15.

6. Spechler SJ, Sperber H, Doos WG, Schimmel EM: The prevalence of Barrett's esophagus in patients with chronic peptic esophageal strictures. *Dig Dis Sci* 1983; 28:769–774.

7. Skinner DB, Walther BC, Riddle RH, Schmidt H, Iascone C, DeMeester TR: Barrett's esophagus—comparison of benign and malignant cases. *Ann Surg* 1983; 198:554–566.

8. Johnson RB, Lukash WM: Medical management of esophageal strictures. *Hosp Med* 1972; 808:64–70.

9. Pagliero KM: Facilitating oesophageal bougienage. *Lancet* 1973; 1:467.

10. Moskowitz SA, Burbige EJ: Esophageal dilatation with Eder–Peustow dilators under direct visual control. *Am J Proct Gastroenterol Colon Rectal Surg* 1982; 33–7:14–15.

11. Price JC, Stanciu C, Bennett JR: A safer method of dilating oesophageal strictures. *Lancet* 1981; 1:1141–1142.

12. Celestin LR, Campbell WB: A new and safe system for oesophageal dilatation. *Lancet* 1981; 1:74–75.

13. London RL, Trotman BW, Dimarino AJ, Oleaga JA, Freiman DB, Ring EJ, Rosato EF: Dilatation of severe esophageal strictures by an inflatable balloon catheter. *Gastroenterology* 1981; 80:173–175.

14. Benedict EB: Peptic stenosis of the esophagus—a study of 233 patients treated with bougienage, surgery, or both. *Am J Dig Dis* 1966; 11:761–770.

15. Lanza FL, Graham DY: Bougienage is effective therapy for most benign esophageal strictures. *JAMA* 1978; 240:844–847.

16. Wesdorp ICE, Bartelsman JFWM, Hartog Jager FCA, Huibregtse K, Tytgat GN; Results of conservative treatment of benign esophageal strictures: A follow-up study in 100 patients. *Gastroenterology* 1982; 82:487–493.

17. Patterson DJ, Graham DY, Smith JL, Schwartz JT, Alpert E, Lanza FL, Cain GD: Natural history of benign esophageal stricture treated by dilatation. *Gastroenterology* 1983; 85:346–350.

18. Mandelstam P, Sugawa C, Silvis SE, Nebel OT, Rogers BHG: Complications associated with esophagogastroduodenoscopy and with esophageal dilatation. *Gastroint Endo* 1976; 23:16–19.

19. Orringer MB, Kirsh MM, Sloan H: Esophageal reconstruction for benign disease—technical considerations. *J Thor Cardiovasc Surg* 1977; 73:807–812.

20. Thal AP, Hatafuku T, Kurtzman R: New operation for distal esophageal stricture. *Arch Surg* 1965; 90:464–472.

21. Hill LD, Gelfand M, Bauermeister D: Simplified management of reflux esophagitis with stricture. *Ann Surg* 1979; 1972:638–651.

22. Herrington JL, Wright RS, Edwards WH, Sawyers JL: Conservative surgical treatment of reflux esophagitis and esophageal stricture. *Ann Surg* 1975; 181:552–566.

23. Larrain A, Csendes A, Pope CE: Surgical correction of reflux: an effective therapy for esophageal strictures. *Gastroenterology* 1975; 69:578–583.

24. Mangla JC: Barrett's esophagus: An old entity rediscovered. *J Clin Gastroenterol* 1981; 3:347–356.

25. Kothari T, Mangla JC, Kalra TMS: Barrett's ulcer and treatment with cimetidine. *Arch Intern Med* 1980; 140:475–477.

26. Sjogren RW, Johnson LF: Barrett's esophagus: A review. *Am J Med* 1983; 74:313–321.

27. Davis MV: Relationship between pulmonary disease, hiatal hernia, and gastroesophageal reflux. *NY St J Med* 1972; 72:935–938.

28. Chernow B, Johnson LF, Janowitz WR, Castell DO: Pulmonary aspiration as a consequence of gastroesophageal reflux—a diagnostic approach. *Dig Dis Sci* 1979; 24:839–844.

29. Ghaed N, Stein MR: Assessment of a technique for scintigraphic monitoring of pulmonary aspiration of gastric contents in asthmatics with gastroesophageal reflux. *Ann Allergy* 1979; 42:306–308.

30. Reich SB, Earley WC, Ravin TH, Goodman M, Spector S, Stein MR: Evaluation of gastropulmonary aspiration by a radioactive technique: Concise communication. *J Nucl Med* 1977; 18:1079–1081.

31. Mansfield LE, Stein MR: Gastroesophageal reflux and asthma: A possible reflex mechanism. *Ann Allergy* 1978; 41:224–226.

32. Mansfield LE, Hameister HH, Spaulding HS, Smith NJ, Glab N: The role of the vagus nerve in airway narrowing caused by intraesophageal hydrochloric acid provocation and esophageal distention. *Ann Allergy* 1981; 47:431–434.

33. Dees SC: The role of gastroesophageal reflux in nocturnal asthma in children. *NCMJ* 1974; 35:230–233.

34. Foglia RP, Fonkalsrud EW, Ament ME, Byrne WJ, Berquist W, Siegel SC, Katz RM, Rachelefsky GS: Gastroesophageal fundoplication for the management of chronic pulmonary disease in children. *Am J Surg* 1980; 140:72–79.

35. Christie DL, O'Grady LR, Mack DV: Incompetent lower esophageal sphincter and gastroesophageal reflux in recurrent acute pulmonary disease of infancy and childhood. *J Pediatr* 1978; 93:23–27.

36. Herbst JJ, Minton SD, Books LS: Gastroesophageal reflux causing respiratory distress and apnea in newborn infants. *J Pediatr* 1979; 95:763–768.

37. Euler AR, Byrne WJ, Ament ME, Fonkalsrud EW, Strobel CT, Siegel SC, Katz RM, Rachelefsky GS: Recurrent pulmonary disease in children: A complication of gastroesophageal reflux. *Pediatrics* 1979; 63:47–51.

38. Danus O, Casar C, Larrain A, Pope CE: Esophageal reflux—an unrecognized cause of recurrent obstructive bronchitis in children. *J Pediatr* 1976; 89:220–224.

39. Jolley SG, Herbst JJ, Johnson DG, Matlak ME, Book LS: Esophageal pH monitoring during sleep identifies children with respiratory symptoms from gastroesophageal reflux. *Gastroenterology* 1981; 80:1501–1506.

40. Spitzer AR, Boyle JT, Tuchman DN, Fox WW: Awake apnea associated with gastroesophageal reflux: A specific clinical syndrome. *J Pediatr* 1984; 104:200–205.
41. Shapiro GG, Christie DL: Gastroesophageal reflux in steroid-dependent asthmatic youths. *Pediatrics* 1979; 63:207–212.
42. Orenstein SR, Whitington PF: Positioning for prevention of infant gastroesophageal reflux. *J Pediatr* 1983; 103:534–537.
43. Euler AR: Use of bethanechol for the treatment of gastroesophageal reflux. *J Pediatr* 1980; 96:321–324.
44. Strickland AD, Chang JHT: Results of treatment of gastroesophageal reflux with bethanechol. *J Pediatr* 1983; 103:311–315.
45. Kjellen G, Brundin A, Tibbling L, Wranne B: Oesophageal function in asthmatics. *Eur J Respir Dis* 1981; 62:87–94.
46. Mays EE: Intrinsic asthma in adults—association with gastroesophageal reflux. *JAMA* 1976; 236:2626–2628.
47. Pellegrini CA, DeMeester TR, Johnson LF, Skinner DB: Gastroesophageal reflux and pulmonary aspiration: Incidence, functional abnormality, and results of surgical therapy. *Surgery* 1979; 86:110–119.
48. Spaulding HS, Mansfield LE, Selner J: Further investigaions of the association between gastroesophageal reflux and bronchoconstriction. *J All Clin Immunol* 1979; 63:218 (abstract).
49. Goodall RJR, Earis JE, Cooper DN, Bernstein A, Temple JG: Relationship between asthma and gastro-oesophageal reflux. *Thorax* 1981; 36:116–121.
50. Larrain A, Carrasco J, Gallesguillos J, Pope CE: Reflux treatment improves lung function in patients with intrinsic asthma. *Gastroenterology* 1981; 80:1204 (abstract).
51. Mays EE, Dubois JJ, Hamilton GB: Pulmonary fibrosis associated with tracheobronchial aspiration—a study of the frequency of hiatal hernia and gastroesophageal reflux in interstitial pulmonary fibrosis of obscure etiology. *Chest* 1976; 69:512–515.
52. Urschel HC, Paulson DL: Gastroesophageal reflux and hiatal hernia—complications and therapy. *J Thorac Cardiovasc Surg* 1967; 53:21–32.
53. Davis MV: Evolving concepts regarding hiatal hernia and gastroesophageal reflux. *Ann Thor Surg* 1969; 7:120–133.
54. Babb RR, Notarangelo J, Smith VM: Wheezing: A clue to gastroesophageal reflux. *Am J Gastroenterol* 1970; 53:230–233.
55. Kennedy JH: "Silent" gastroesophageal reflux: An important but little known cause of pulmonary complications. *Dis Chest* 1962; 42:42–45.
56. Overholt RH, Ashraf MM: Esophageal reflux as trigger in asthma. *NY St J Med* 1966; 66:3030–3032.
57. Overholt RH, Voorhees RJ: Esophageal reflux as a trigger in asthma. *Dis Chest* 1966; 49:464–466.

17

Barrett's Esophagus—
A Special Problem

*Gregory L. Eastwood, M.D., and
Canan Avunduk Bonnice, M.D., Ph.D.*

Chapter Contents

From Castell DO, Wu WC, Ott DJ (eds): *Gastroesophageal Reflux Disease: Pathogenesis, Diagnosis, Therapy.* Mount Kisco, NY, Futura Publishing Co., Inc., 1985.

Barrett's esophagus is a condition in which a portion of the normal stratified squamous epithelium of the esophagus is replaced by a columnar glandular metaplastic epithelium (Figure 1). The identification of Barrett's esophagus is more than a histological curiosity; it has special clinical relevance because patients with Barrett's esophagus have a higher risk of developing esophageal adenocarcinoma.

Historical Perspective

In 1950, N.R. Barrett, a British surgeon, described chronic ulcers of the lower esophagus in association with an epithelium that was not squamous but rather columnar.[1] In that paper he called attention to Tilestone's description in 1906 of peptic ulcers occurring in the lower esophagus.[2] Tilestone had reviewed the literature and claimed that there had been 44 examples of such ulcers published. The histology of these ulcers was identical to chronic gastric ulcer and the

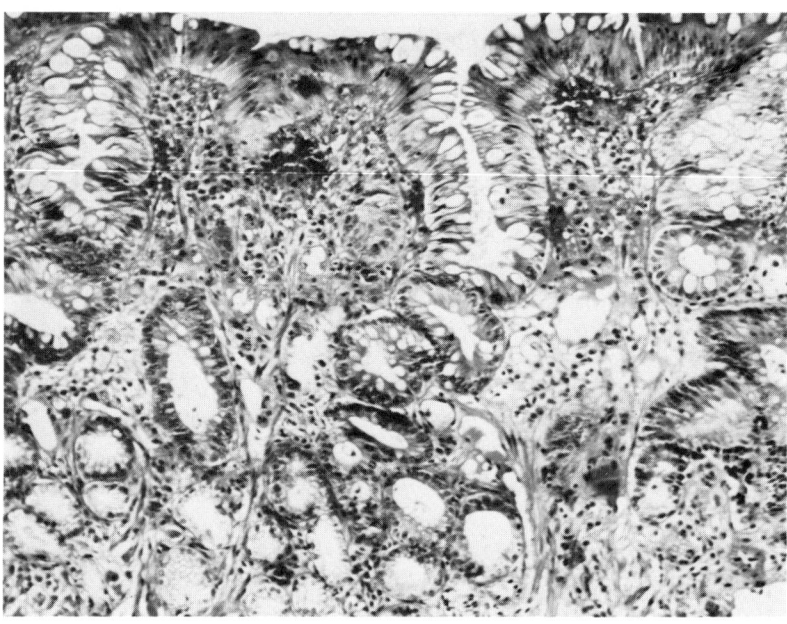

Figure 1: *Photomicrograph of Barrett's epithelium. Intestinal-type goblet cells are interspersed between the columnar cells lining the glands and covering the mucosal surface. Parietal and chief cells are absent. This particular example would conform to the specialized columnar type of Paull et al[15] or to the intestinal metaplastic type of Mangla.[16]*

adjacent mucosa was gastric in appearance. Tilestone assumed the "gastric" mucosa was ectopic because it lined the lower esophagus. Barrett extended this concept further. He proposed that the ulcers were gastric ulcers in mediastinal extensions of the stomach and the patients in fact had congenital short esophagi.

Others also had described peptic ulcers of the esophagus within columnar epithelium before Barrett. In 1937, Lyall presented eight cases of peptic ulceration of the esophagus, one of which was surrounded by intact "heterotopic gastric mucosa."[3] This mucosa resembled normal gastric mucosa with wide, short glands and few parietal cells. In 1943, Allison et al reported 10 cases of peptic ulcer of the lower esophagus associated with shortening of the esophagus and "gastric" mucosa in and below an esophageal stricture.[4] They postulated that the stomach was pulled up either due to a congenitally short esophagus or due to shortening of the esophagus from extensive ulceration and fibrosis. This resulted in herniation of the stomach above the hiatus.

In 1953, after Barrett's paper had been published, Allison and Johnstone used the term "Barrett's ulcer" to describe peptic ulcerations in the columnar-lined lower esophagus.[5] They noted that this columnar-lined lower esophagus had no peritoneal covering, contained the musculature of the lower esophagus, included islands of squamous epithelium within it, and had typical esophageal submucosal mucous glands. Further, it had the same blood supply as the esophagus. Therefore, they argued, these ulcers were in fact in the esophagus and not in the mediastinal extension of the stomach.

Barrett in 1957, revised his views and suggested that this entity be referred to as the lower esophagus lined by columnar epithelium.[6] However, since his first description in 1950, the columnar-lined lower esophagus and related conditions have been referred to as Barrett's epithelium, esophagus, and ulcers.

Histology of the Normal Esophagus

The esophagus is a muscular tube about 25 cm long. It is lined by stratified, nonkeratinized squamous epithelium (Figure 2). Papillae of lamina propria project upward into the epithelium to a distance not more than 65% of the total epithelial thickness.[7] The epithelium of the esophagus undergoes constant renewal.[8] The area within the epithelium in which new cells are formed, the so-called proliferative zone, is the basal layer of polygonal epithelial cells. This layer is applied to the basement membrane overlying the lamina propria in

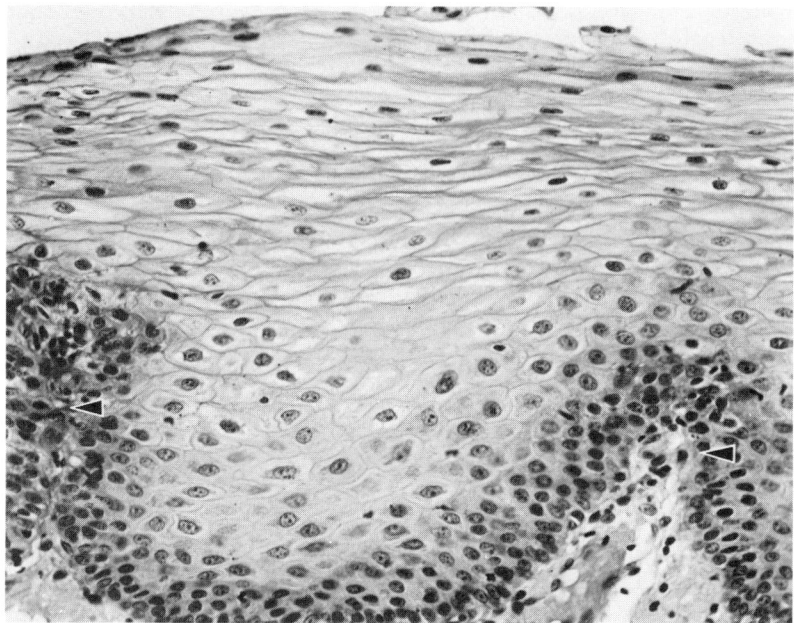

Figure 2: *Photomicrograph of normal human esophageal stratified squamous epithelium. Papillae of lamina propria project into the epithelium (arrows).*

the interpapillary region as well as over the papillary projections. As cells migrate toward the esophageal lumen, they become more squamous in appearance. After a week or more, the cells reach the surface of the epithelium and are sloughed into the esophageal lumen.[9,10] At the junction of the esophagus and the stomach, at about the level of the diaphragm and corresponding to the lower esophageal sphincter (see below), the epithelium changes abruptly from stratified squamous to columnar-glandular in the stomach, forming an irregular junctional line called the Z-line.

The lamina propria is thin and usually contains superficial esophageal glands. In the lower esophagus these glands are called cardiac glands. Below the lamina propria is a thin layer of muscle, the muscularis mucosae.

Beneath the muscularis mucosae is the submucosa, which contains the deeper esophageal mucous glands. Several glands drain into a common duct lined by stratified columnar epithelium, which passes through the muscularis mucosae into the esophageal lumen. The ramified lymphatic plexus within the loose connective tissue network of the submucosa accounts for the early and extensive spread of esophageal carcinoma.

The main muscle coat of the esophagus, the muscularis propria, is well developed with inner circular and outer longitudinal layers. The lower 2–4 cm of the muscularis propria constitute a zone of higher pressure than either the intragastric or intraesophageal pressure and is called the lower esophageal sphincter (LES). Histologically the LES cannot be distinguished from adjacent esophageal or gastric muscle. The esophagus has no serosal layer, which also facilitates the spread of esophageal carcinoma within the mediastinum.

Histology of Barrett's Esophagus

A variety of cell types and histological patterns has been associated with Barrett's esophagus. Barrett, in his original 1950 paper,[1] was convinced that the columnar epithelium was gastric in type, but he did not elaborate on its histology. Later, in 1957,[6] he described the columnar epithelium as containing shallow tubular glands resembling normal deep esophageal glands. Scattered parietal cells were present only in the lower esophagus adjacent to the stomach. At any level within the segment of columnar epithelium were patches of normal appearing squamous epithelium.

Hershfield et al described their biopsies of Barrett's epithelium as having the typical appearance of gastric mucosa.[11] They found chief cells containing pepsinogen granules and parietal cells that secreted hydrochloric acid in response to histamine stimulation. Abrams and Heath noted at least two different epithelia composing Barrett's esophagus in the patient they studied.[12] At 30 cm from the teeth, a villous pattern resembling small intestinal mucosa was identified. Between 30 and 33 cm, the appearance was similar to gastric fundic mucosa. Here, the surface epithelium was composed of simple mucous-secreting cells; the glands beneath contained mucous neck, parietal, and argentaffin cells. Trier obtained biopsies of Barrett's epithelium occurring distal to mid-esophageal stricture in five patients and examined them by light and electron microscopy.[13] He found three epithelial cell types. The most abundant was a columnar cell that had numerous apical microvilli and contained many glycoprotein granules. In addition, there were many mucous-secreting goblet cells and a few argentaffin cells, both similar in appearance to those seen normally in intestinal epithelium. No gastric parietal or chief cells were observed in any of the biopsies. Finally, Schreiber et al even identified Paneth cells within Barrett's epithelium.[14] Paneth cells normally are found at the base of the crypts in the small intestine.

The foregoing would indicate that there was no agreement as to whether Barrett's epithelium is gastric or intestinal in nature, or perhaps an entirely separate histological type with some characteristics of both gastric and intestinal epithelium. An attempt to reconcile these conflicting observations was presented by Paull et al.[15] They carefully examined 112 suction biopsies from various levels above the LES in 11 patients with Barrett's epithelium. They found three distinctly different types of epithelium: (a) a specialized columnar epithelium with a villiform surface, mucous glands, and periodic acid-Schiff (PAS) and alcian blue staining intestinal-type goblet cells, but no parietal or chief cells; (b) a gastric junctional type epithelium with cardiac-like mucous glands and no parietal or chief cells; and (c) a gastric–fundic type epithelium that did contain parietal and chief cells. In a single patient, a tiny island of squamous epithelium was found within a segment of specialized columnar-type epithelium. Not all three epithelial types were identified in all patients, but when present, the specialized columnar epithelium always was the most proximal, the gastric fundic type most distal, and the junctional epithelium was interposed between gastric fundic and specialized columnar or normal squamous epithelium.

The findings of Paull et al were elaborated further by Mangla.[16] He obtained endoscopic biopsies in patients with Barrett's epithelium every 2–4 cm starting at the LES and proceeding toward the upper esophagus. He noted five mucosal types: (a) simple epithelium consisting of columnar cells with basally oriented nuclei and small intracytoplasmic PAS positive granules; (b) gastric–fundic type epithelium with sparse and shortened fundic glands that contained parietal and chief cells; (c) intestinal metaplastic-type epithelium with crypt-like glands and villi lined by intestinal type columnar cells and goblet cells; (d) junctional-type epithelium with normal gastric surface mucous cells and mucous glands without goblet cells, parietal cells, or chief cells; and (e) antral-type epithelium with no parietal or chief cells. Argentaffin cells were present in the first four types. No zonation of these epithelial types was observed when they coexisted. Biopsies from the same area sometimes contained an admixture of two or three types of epithelia.

In all the above studies, either suction or endoscopic biopsies were used to describe cells, glands, and architectural types of epithelium found in Barrett's esophagus. The findings have been inconsistent from one study to another. The enigma of Barrett's epithelium may have been resolved by Thompson et al.[17] They examined eight en bloc esophagogastrectomy specimens obtained from patients presenting with adenocarcinoma within Barrett's esophagus. When the epithelial patterns from the entire specimens were considered, Barrett's epithelium could not be described as zonal or of only three or five types. Rather, it was found to be a complex mosaic of various cell, gland, and villous architectural types, showing variable degrees of atrophy and maturation toward intestinal and gastric epithelium. With the exception of a slight tendency for gastric–fundic type epithelium to occur distally, no zonation was observed. Ulcerations and residual squamous islands were universally present and occurred at all levels. A villiform surface lined by goblet and absorptive cells was found in all cases. Surface mucous, goblet, absorptive, mucous neck, mucous gland, and neuroendocrine cells were found in all cases and at all levels above the gastroesophageal junction. Paneth, chief, and parietal cells were found in half of the cases. Chief and parietal cells were seen more frequently distally, but also occurred in the mid and upper portions of the Barrett's epithelium.

Whether Barrett's epithelium containing adenocarcinoma is typical of Barrett's epithelium that does not contain adenocarcinoma is conjectural. Unfortunately, en bloc segments of esophagus with Barrett's epithelium from patients who do not have cancer are not commonly available, except perhaps at autopsy. Nevertheless, the observations of Thompson et al indicate that Barrett's epithelium bears a resemblance to that of atrophic small intestinal and gastric mucosa, but is a metaplastic epithelium with characteristics that allow it to be differentiated from normal intestinal and gastric epithelium.

Pathogenesis of Barrett's Epophagus

Over the years there has been some controversy as to whether Barrett's esophagus is a congenital or an acquired lesion. The congenital theory is based on the observation that during the 3–34 mm stage of embryogenesis, the esophagus is lined by stratified columnar epithelium as it develops from the foregut.[18] The columnar epithelium becomes ciliated at the 40 mm stage and lines the entire esophagus up to the 130 mm stage. Then, stratified squamous epithelium gradually replaces the columnar epithelium, appearing first in the middle third of the esophagus and progressing in both directions. This re-epithelization is completed in the lower esophagus first and in the upper esophagus last. Patches of ciliated columnar epithelium may persist in the upper esophagus at birth and later in life.[18] Although conversion to squamous epithelium normally is completed before birth, an arrest in the developmental process may result in a columnar-lined lower esophagus. Columnar-lined lower esophagus has been reported in a neonate,[19] in children,[20] and in an adult.[21]

Despite this evidence, the case for the congenital theory has been weakened by the following observations. This embryonic esophageal epithelium does not contain goblet cells, which commonly are seen in Barrett's esophagus. Other cell types that may be present in Barrett's esophagus, such as parietal, chief, and Paneth cells, also have not been found in the embryonic columnar epithelium.[18]

Today, the theory that Barrett's esophagus is an acquired lesion is generally accepted. Over the last 25 years, much clinical and experimental evidence has been collected to support this theory.

Virtually all patients with Barrett's esophagus have gastroesophageal reflux and many have severe erosive lesions in the stratified squamous portion of the esophagus.[22,23] It is assumed that the chronic exposure of the lower esophagus to acid, pepsin, and bile results in inflammation and destruction of the squamous epithelium, leading to its replacement by a columnar epithelium that is perhaps more resistant to injury. This concept is supported by reports of patients with reflux esophagitis in whom successive esophageal mucosal biopsies have documented the development and progressive ascent of Barrett's epithelium up the esophagus over several years.[24,25]

In other patients who had undergone partial esophagogastrectomy with reanastomosis and pyloroplasty, Barrett's epithelium was seen to develop in 6–10 years.[26] Similarly, Barrett's epithelium developed in a patient 16 years after a Heller esophagomyotomy for achalasia.[27] In all these cases, gastroesophageal reflux was present due to the removal of the LES or compromise of the gastric reservoir function.

Other factors may be important in the genesis of Barrett's esophagus. These include bile reflux into the esophagus after total gastrectomy with esophagojejunal anastomosis,[28] delayed esophageal clearance after repair of esophageal atresia in children [29] or in patients with scleroderma,[30] and mid-esophageal stricture secondary to lye ingestion which may have retarded esophageal clearance after episodes of reflux.[31] However, in all these instances chronic prolonged exposure of the squamous epithelium to acid, pepsin, and/or bile seems to be the underlying prerequisite to its placement by columnar epithelium.

Bremner et al succeeded in experimentally producing a columnar lining of the lower esophagus in dogs.[32] In one group of dogs, they removed the squamous epithelium and submucosal glands of the lower esophagus, but left the LES intact. In these animals, the distal esophagus was re-epithelized rapidly by squamous epithelium. A second group of dogs underwent surgical removal of the esophageal mucosa and a myotomy of the LES with creation of a hiatus hernia. In these dogs, the distal esophagus re-epithelized almost equally by columnar epithelium from below and squamous epithelium from above. In the third group, the dogs underwent the same procedures as in the second group but also received histamine to increase gastric acid secretion. In these dogs, where the LES was destroyed and re-epithelization was allowed to occur in the presence of gastroesophageal reflux and increased acid output, the squamous cell regeneration was absent or minimal. Rather, the surgically denuded zone, as well as areas in the more proximal parts of the esophagus which were denuded by reflux esophagitis, became re-epithelized by columnar mucus-producing cells. The authors proposed that the most likely source of the columnar epithelial cells repopulating the distal esophagus was from the gastric columnar epithelium. Some support for this concept comes from the observations of Wong and Finckh.[33] They showed that repeated mechanical injury to the stratified squamous epithelium of the rat forestomach can heal by migration and overgrowth of columnar epithelial cells from adjacent gastric mucosa.

Although the experiments described above, and perhaps common sense, suggest that Barrett's epithelium is derived from adjacent gastric epithelium, other candidates for the cell of origin of Barrett's epithelium have been proposed. These include metaplasia of basal cells from the esophageal squamous epithelium,[28] columnar cells from esophageal cardiac glands,[34] and an undefined primordial stem cell.[35] Because of the diversity of the histologic features of Barrett's epithelium, it is possible that there is more than one site of origin.

Clinical Features of Barrett's Esophagus

Symptoms

Barrett's esophagus itself causes no symptoms. Symptoms that lead to a diagnosis of Barrett's esophagus are related either to gastroesophageal reflux or to a complication, such as a Barrett's ulcer or carcinoma. Patients typically complain of heartburn and regurgitation, which usually have been present for several years. Other symptoms are dysphagia, weight loss, and hematemesis. However, some patients with Barrett's esophagus have had minimal if any symptoms of reflux and present with dysphagia due to adenocarcinoma complicating the disease.

Prevalence

The prevalence of Barrett's esophagus in the general population is unknown simply because the disorder is not always associated with symptoms demanding diagnostic studies. In one study, 140 out of 1,225 patients (11%) with reflux esophagitis examined endoscopically were found to have Barrett's epithelium.[36] However, this was a retrospective study probably weighted toward patients with more severe symptoms. A similar prevalence of 12% was found in an autopsy series.[37]

Barrett's esophagus occurs from early childhood to late adult life. Most patients present at age 45–70 years and there is no sex predominance.

Diagnostic Studies

Barium Swallow X-ray Films

Classically, Barrett's esophagus has been described radiologically as presenting with esophageal stricture or ulcer in association with a hiatus hernia.[38] However, uncomplicated Barrett's esophagus typically does not show any particular abnormality on barium contrast x-ray examination. Fluoroscopy demonstrates normal peristalsis in the body of the esophagus, and gastroesophageal reflux may be evident. In fact, Robbins et al studied 39 patients with histologically proven Barrett's epithelium and found that 72% of them did not fit the classic stereotype of high esophageal stricture of ulcer.[38]

Diagnostic sensitivity may be improved by double-contrast barium studies that may show irregularity, nodularity, and thickening of the mucosa. However, because of the lack of radiographic sensitivity and specificity, the diagnosis of Barrett's esophagus needs to be confirmed by endoscopy and biopsy.

Endoscopy

The normal endoscopic appearance of the squamous epithelial lining of the esophagus is a flat, pinkish-white. If Barrett's epithelium is present, this appearance changes abruptly to a velvety, pinkish-red, and sometimes friable, mucosa at some level above the gastroesophageal junction. The columnar epithelium can be circumferential or appear as islands or fingers of pinkish-red mucosa in the distal esophagus.

To help identify the presence of Barrett's epithelium and define its extent, an iodine-containing solution such as Lugol's solution may be sprayed through the endoscope onto the esophageal mucosa.[39] Iodine will stain the normal glycogen-containing squamous epithelium black, but will not stain the columnar epithelium. It will also not stain neoplastic tissue or severely inflamed squamous epithelium.

Esophagitis may be evident by endoscopy in both the squamous and the columnar epithelium. Ulcers may be present at the squamocolumnar junction or within the columnar-lined esophagus.[23] Adenomatous polyps may be visible. Strictures, when present, typically occur at the junction of the squamous and columnar epithelium.

The definitive diagnosis of Barrett's epithelium is based upon histologic confirmation by multiple biopsies. If strictures are present, it may be necessary to dilate them in order to examine the esophagus adequately and obtain appropriate biopsies. Suspicious areas can be brushed to obtain cytological samples to aid in the diagnosis of adenocarcinoma.[40]

Manometry

Normally, the transition from the pale squamous esophageal epithelium to the darker pink gastric epithelium occurs at the level of the LES, roughly 40 cm from the teeth. If Barrett's epithelium is present, the squamocolumnar junction is situated higher in the esophagus, well above the LES. Because the LES can be identified manometrically, any biopsies taken above the LES are from the esophagus. In some patients, it may be necessary to obtain manometrically guided biopsies to ensure that the columnar epithelium is from the esophagus and not from the stomach, especially in patients who have a short segment of Barrett's epithelium above a hiatus hernia.

Manometric examination of the esophagus in patients with Barrett's epithelium reveals normal or attenuated peristalsis. Most patients have decreased LES pressures, below 10 mmHg.[22] These findings are consistent with the presumed pathogenesis of Barrett's epithelium, namely, chronic gastroesophageal reflux in combination with poor clearing of the esophagus.

Electrical Potential Difference

The mucosal surface of the esophagus is electrically negative with respect to the mediastinal surface, giving a transmural potential difference of about −12 to −15 mV. The transmural potential difference in the stomach has a greater negative value, about −34 to −38 mV. The transition from esophageal to gastric potential difference occurs at the squamocolumnar junction within the LES in normal esophagi and above the LES in patients with Barrett's epithelium where the squamous epithelium changes to columnar epithelium. When ulceration, inflammation, or carcinoma are present, the potential difference may become intermediate between esophageal and gastric, limiting its usefulness. Nevertheless, Orlando et al feel that an abnormal esophageal potential difference is highly specific for the presence of esophageal mucosal disease, and if performed at the time of manometry, may provide additional diagnostic information.[41]

Radioisotope Scanning

Intravenous ^{99m}Tc-pertechnetate is concentrated and secreted by gastric-type mucosa, either in the stomach or in ectopic locations such as Meckel's diverticulum[42] or Barrett's esophagus.[43] Its distribution can be detected by isotope scanning. Because salivary glands also secrete pertechnetate, patients are asked not to swallow during testing. Also, patients are tested while standing to minimize the reflux of gastric juice into the esophagus. The appearance of the isotope above the gastroesophageal junction is considered a positive scan for Barrett's epithelium. The location of the gastroesophageal junction and the presence or absence of a hiatus hernia are verified by a radiograph taken after the patient swallows barium in the upright position. However, because gastric epithelium with parietal cells is found in only about half the cases of Barrett's epithelium[17] and intestinal-type Barrett's epithelium does not concentrate pertechnetate, the diagnosis of Barrett's epithelium may be missed. Occasionally, gastroesophageal reflux or hiatus hernia will give false positive results. Thus, the reliability of this method is uncertain.

Complications

Barrett's esophagus may be complicated by esophagitis, ulceration, stricture, or adenocarcinoma.

Esophagitis

The esophagitis may be superficial or deep and is found both in the squamous and columnar-lined esophagus.

Ulceration

Two types of ulcers have been described in Barrett's esophagus. More commonly, one finds a superficial linear ulcer on the squamous side of the squamocolumnar junction such as is usually seen in reflux esophagitis regardless of whether or not Barrett's epithelium is present. The less common is a deep, circular ulcer resembling a chronic gastric ulcer within the columnar epithelium. This is a true Barrett's ulcer and corresponds to Barrett's original description.[1] Perforation and bleeding of Barrett's ulcers have been reported.[20,44]

Stricture

Strictures are common in Barrett's esophagus, occurring in up to 80% of patients, accounting for the presenting symptom of dysphagia.[22] They usually occur at the squamocolumnar junction.[1,5,6] Thus, the strictures typically are found in the mid or lower esophagus, but may occur in the upper esophagus. Ulcers may develop at the margins or within the stricture.[45]

Adenocarcinoma

The first well documented case of adenocarcinoma occurring in a Barrett's esophagus was reported by Morson and Belcher in 1953.[46] The tumor was found in the upper esophagus. Above the lesion the epithelium was squamous, and below the lesion it was columnar. Similar case reports followed,[47,48] and in 1963 Adler proposed a causal relation between Barrett's epithelium and neoplasia.[23]

Over the years several other lines of evidence have linked Barrett's esophagus with the development of adenocarcinoma. Two studies of epithelial kinetics in Barrett's epithelium have shown a pattern of proliferation resembling that found in other pre-malignant conditions of the gastrointestinal tract, namely, a widened proliferative zone, a decreased generation time, and an increased mitotic index.[49,50] In another study, carcinoembryonic antigen was detected in biopsies from 11 out of 23 patients with Barrett's esophagus, again suggesting a malignant potential in this metaplastic disorder.[51]

Carcinomas in Barrett's epithelium may have a glandular pattern resembling that seen in gastric carcinomas;[52] they may be papillary occurring as single or multiple adenomatous polypoid neoplasms;[53] or they may be diffusely infiltrating with signet ring-type cells.[54]

Theoretically, the malignant change in Barrett's epithelium is the end point of an epithelial response to chronic reflux-induced injury that begins as columnar metaplasia, progresses through dysplasia and carcinoma in situ, and finally becomes invasive carcinoma. If the theory of reflux-induced epithelial transformation is correct, the entire surface of the Barrett's epithelium is at risk for these changes, and there should be a high frequency of multifocal neoplastic disease. When esophagectomy specimens are examined carefully en bloc, in fact this has been observed. Dysplasia ranging from mild to carcinoma in situ has been found not only adjacent to invasive carcinoma but remote from it elsewhere in the columnar epithelium.[17,52,53,55]

Clinically, dysphagia is the predominant presenting complaint of patients with adenocarcinoma associated with Barrett's esophagus (87%).[56] Esophageal stricture (80%) and hiatus hernia (70%) are common. Symptoms of gastroesophageal reflux may be present, but 36% of patients have no history of reflux. The most common site of the cancer is in the distal third of the esophagus. The average age of the patient is 57 years (range 23–88 years), the same as for Barrett's esophagus.[44] The male to female ratio is 5:1.[57] Patients with adenocarcinoma in Barrett's esophagus have a low prevalance of smoking and alcohol abuse, in contrast to patients with squamous cell carcinoma of the esophagus, reflecting possible etiologic differences between the tumors.[55]

The prevalence of adenocarcinoma in Barrett's esophagus is difficult to determine because many patients are investigated for symptoms produced by the tumor itself without a previous diagnosis of Barrett's esophagus. Asymptomatic cases of Barrett's esophagus usually do not come to medical attention. Naef et al performed 6,368 esophagoscopies and identified 1,225 cases of reflux esophagitis, 140 of which (11%) had extensive columnar metaplasia of the distal esophagus.[36] Twelve (9%) of these patients with Barrett's epithelium were found to have adenocarcinoma. In smaller series, the prevalence of adenocarcinoma in Barrett's epithelium varies from 2.5%[58] to 41%.[59] This is particularly impressive since adenocarcinoma of the esophagus is reported to comprise only 2–10% of all esophageal cancers.[60–63]

The recognition that adenocarcinoma in association with Barrett's epithelium may be more common than has been appreciated has led to the concept that most adenocarcinomas of the esophagus may arise from Barrett's epithelium. Other sites of origin for esophageal adenocarcinoma could be from esophageal mucous glands and from adjacent gastric mucosa. Raphael et al reviewed the records of 1,312 patients with the diagnosis of carcinoma of the esophagus or cardia over a 20-year period at the Mayo Clinic.[61] They found 44 patients (3.4%) who were originally considered to have adenocarcinoma of the esophagus. However, when one excludes anaplastic lesions with pseudoglandular formation, tumors apparently arising from the proximal stomach, and a tumor in columnar epithelium, then only 9 adenocarcinomas remain (0.7%) presumably arising from esophageal mucous glands. Further, by the time the adenocarinoma is discovered, it may have grown sufficiently to obliterate all traces of its origin, whether it be from Barrett's epithelium, esophageal mucous glands, or gastric mucosa. In one case of adenocarcinoma of the cardia and lower esophagus, only a small 2 mm fragment of residual Barrett's epithelium was found; this contained both dysplasia and carcinoma in situ.[17] If the tumor had been discovered later, perhaps no residual columnar metaplasia would have been found. Thus, a strong argument can be made to support the idea that most adenocarcinomas of the esophagus in fact arise from Barrett's epithelium.

Treatment

The treatment of Barrett's esophagus consists of the treatment of reflux esophagitis and its complications. In general, an anti-reflux regimen is recommended in conjunction with antacids and a histamine-2 antagonist. Symptomatic improvement and healing of esophagitis and esophageal ulcers have been described after treatment with bethanechol,[64] carbenoxolone, and cimetidine,[65] and antacids and cimetidine.[66] Repeated bougienage of strictures associated with Barrett's esophagus will give temporary relief of dysphagia.

When carcinoma is discovered, either in situ or with invasion of the esophageal wall, the usual treatment is surgical resection.[54,67] The tumors do not appear to be radioresponsive[68] and there is no information on the use of chemotherapy. The prognosis of adenocarcinoma in Barrett's esophagus is similar to the poor prognosis seen with squamous cell carcinoma of the esophagus. However, apparent cure of adenocarcinoma in situ[40] and up to seven years survival after esophageal resection for invasive adenocarcinoma have been reported.[52]

If the extent of Barrett's epithelium bears any relationship to the risk of developing adenocarcinoma, then efforts to reduce the area at risk would be indicated. However, none of the patients treated medically in the studies cited above had regression of columnar epithelium to squamous epithelium.[64–66] One additional study, in abstract form, reported the successful regression of columnar epithelium as well as resolution of severe dysplastic changes in Barrett's epithelium in three patients treated with bethanechol, cimetidine, and antacids.[69] More studies are needed to confirm these important observations.

If reflux symptoms are intractable and there is no healing of esophageal lesions after several weeks of medical treatment, then anti-reflux surgery, such as the Nissen fundoplication, is recommended. If the surgery is successful in eliminating reflux, then esophagitis, ulcers, and strictures resolve and the proximal ascent of the columnar epithelium is arrested.[70] However, the general experience has been that the columnar epithelium persists,[16,25,36] although regression of Barrett's epithelium has been reported in eight patients after Nissen fundoplication.[71,72] In the study by Brand et al[72] successful fundoplication was demonstrated by documenting decreased reflux with esophageal pH probe testing in all four of their patients in whom regression to squamous epithelium was observed by manometrically guided suction biopsies. Acid reflux testing was not done in the other study. As with medical treatment, more patients need to be studied to determine whether anti-reflux surgery indeed is associated with a regression of Barrett's epithelium.

Because Barrett's epithelium is thought to be a metaplastic response to chronic injury caused by gastroesophageal reflux, cessation of the stimulus would be expected to diminish the chance of dysplastic and malignant changes. Unfortunately, adenocarcinoma has been reported to develop in Barrett's epithelium after fundoplication.[36] However, in one of the cases, pH probe testing demonstrated that the fundoplication had been unsuccessful in preventing gastroesophageal reflux. Measurements of pH were not performed in the other patients.[36]

The increased risk of adenocarcinoma in Barrett's esophagus and the multicentric nature of the neoplastic change suggest the need for periodic endoscopic surveillance with multiple biopsies and cytologic examination. The appropriate frequency of surveillance endoscopy in Barrett's esophagus is unknown. Intervals of six months to one year have been recommended.[16,20]

References

1. Barrett NR: Chronic peptic ulcer of the oesophagus and "oesophagitis." *Br J Surg* 1950; 28:175–182.
2. Tilestone W: Peptic ulcer of the esophagus. *Am J Med Sci* 1906; 132:240–265.
3. Lyall A: Chronic peptic ulcer of the oesophagus: A report of eight cases. *Br J Surg* 1937; 24:534–547.
4. Allison PR, Johnstone AS, Boyce GB: Short esophagus with simple peptic ulceration. *J Thorac Surg* 1943; 12:432–457.
5. Allison PR, Johnstone AS: The esophagus lined with gastric mucus membrane. *Thorax* 1953; 8:87–101.
6. Barrett NR: The lower esophagus lined by columnar epithelium. *Surgery* 1957; 41:881–894.
7. Ismail–Beigi F, Horton PF, Pope CE II: Histological consequences of gastroesophageal reflux in man. *Gastroenterology* 1970; 58:163–174.
8. Eastwood GL: Gastrointestinal epithelial renewal. *Gastroenterology* 1977; 72:962–975.
9. Messier B, Leblond CP: Cell proliferation and migration as revealed by radioautography after injection of thymidine-H^3 into male rats and mice. *Am J Anat* 1960; 106:247–285.
10. Bell B, Almy TP, Lipkin M: Cell proliferation kinetics in the gastrointestinal tract of man. III. Cell renewal in esophagus, stomach, and jejunum of a patient with treated pernicious anemia. *J Natl Cancer Inst* 1967; 38:615–623.
11. Hershfield NB, Lind JF, Hildes JA, et al: Secretory function of Barrett's epithelium. *Gut* 1965; 6:535–539.
12. Abrams L, Heath D: Lower esophagus lined with intestinal and gastric epithelia. *Thorax* 1965; 20:66–72.
13. Trier JS: Morphology of the epithelium of the distal esophagus in patients with midesophageal peptic strictures. *Gastroenterology* 1970; 58:444–461.
14. Schreiber DS, Apstein M, Hermos JA: Paneth calls in Barrett's esophagus. *Gastroenterology* 1978; 74:1302–1304.
15. Paull A, Trier JS, Dalton MD, et al: The histologic spectrum of Barrett's esophagus. *N Engl J Med* 1976; 295:476–480.
16. Mangla JC: Barrett's esophagus: An old entity rediscovered. *J Clin Gastroenterol* 1981; 3:347–356.
17. Thompson JJ, Zinsser KR, Enterline HT: Barrett's metaplasia and adeno-

carcinoma of the esophagus and gastroesophageal junction. *Hum Pathol* 1983; 14:42−61.

18. Johns BAE: Developmental changes in the oesophageal epithelium in man. *J Anat* 1952; 86:431−442.

19. Postlethwait RW, Musser AW: Changes in the esophagus in 1000 autopsy specimens. *J Thorac Cardiovasc Surg* 1974; 68:953−956.

20. Borrie J, Goldwater L: Columnar cell lined esophagus: Assessment of etiology and treatment. A 22 year experience. *J Thorac Cardiovasc Surg* 1976; 71:825−834.

21. Raeburn C: Columnar ciliated epithelium in the adult oesophagus. *J Pathol Bacteriol* 1951; 63:157−158.

22. Robbins AH, Hermos JA, Schimmel EM, et al: The columnar lined esophagus. Analysis of 26 cases. *Radiology* 1977; 123:1−7.

23. Adler RH: The lower esophagus lined by columnar epithelium. Its association with hiatal hernia, ulcer, stricture, and tumor. *J Thorac Cardiovasc Surg* 1963; 45:13−34.

24. Goldman MC, Beckman RC: Barrett syndrome: Case report with discussion about concepts of pathogenesis. *Gastroenterology* 1960; 39:104−110.

25. Endo M, Kobayashi S, Kozu T: A case of Barrett epithelization followed up for five years. *Endsocopy* 1974; 6:48−51.

26. Hamilton SR, Yardley JH: Regeneration of cardiac type mucosa and acquisition of Barrett mucosa after esophagogastrectomy. Gastroenterology 1977; 72:669−675.

27. Kortan P, Warren RE, Gardner J, et al: Barrett's esophagus in a patient with surgically treated achalasia. *J Clin Gastroenterol* 1981; 3:357−360.

28. Meyer W, Vollmar F, Bar W: Barrett esophagus following total gastrectomy. A contribution to its pathogenesis. *Endoscopy* 1979; 11:121−126.

29. Winter HS, Madara JL, Stafford RJ, et al: Delayed acid clearance and esophagitis after repair of esophageal atresia. *Gastroenterology* 1981; 80:1317 (abstract).

30. Cameron AJ, Payne WS: Barrett's esophagus occurring as a complication of scleroderma. *Mayo Clin Proc* 1978; 53:612−615.

31. Spechler SJ, Schimmel EM, Dalton JW, et al: Barrett's epithelium complicating lye ingestion with sparing of the distal esophagus. *Gastroenterology* 1981; 81:580−583.

32. Bremner CG, Lynch VP, Ellis FH Jr: Barrett's esophagus: Congenital or acquired. An experimental study of esophageal mucosal regeneration in the dog. *Surgery* 1970; 68:209−216.

33. Wong J, Finckh ES: Heterotopia and ectopia of gastric epithelium produced by mucosal wounding in the rat. *Gastroenterology* 1971; 60:279−287.

34. Adler RH; The esophagus with columnar epithelium. Its clinical significance. *Geriatrics* 1965; 20:109−115.

35. Berenson MM, Herbst JJ, Freston JW: Enzyme and ultrastructural characteristics of esophageal columnar epithelium. *Am J Dig Dis* 1974; 19:895−907.

36. Naef AP, Savary M, Ozzello L: Columnar-lined esophagus: An acquired lesion with malignant predisposition. Report on 140 cases of Barrett's esophagus with 12 adenocarcinomas. *J Thorac Cardiovasc Surg* 1975; 70:826−835.

37. De La Pava S, Pickren JW, Adler RH; Ectopic gastric mucosa of the esophagus—A study on histogenesis. *NY State J Med* 1964; 65:1831–1834.
38. Robbins AH, Vincent ME, Saini M, et al: Revised radiologic concepts of the Barrett esophagus. *Gastrointest Radiol* 1978; 3:377–381.
39. Burbige EJ, Radigan JI: Characteristics of the columnar-cell lined (Barrett's) esophagus. *Gastrointest Endosc* 1979; 25:133–136.
40. Belladonna JA, Hajdu SI, Bains MS, et al: Adenocarcinoma in situ of Barrett's esophagus diagnosed by endoscopic cytology. *N Engl J Med* 1974; 291:895–896.
41. Orlando RC, Rowell DW, Bryson JC, et al: Esophageal potential difference. Measurements in esophageal disease. *Gastroenterology* 1982; 83:1026–1032.
42. Jewett TC Jr, Duszynski DO, Allen JE: The visualization of Meckel's diverticulum with ^{99m}Tc-pertechnetate. *Surgery* 1970; 68:567–570.
43. Berquist TH, Nolan NG, Carlson HC, et al: Diagnosis of Barrett esophagus by pertechnetate scintigraphy. *Mayo Clin Proc* 1973; 48:276–279.
44. Burgess JN, Payne WS, Andersen HA, et al: Barrett's esophagus. *Mayo Clin Proc* 1971; 46:728–734.
45. Berardi RS, Devaiah KA: Barrett's esophagus. *Surg Gynecol Obst* 1983; 156:521–538.
46. Morson BG, Belcher JR: Adenocarcinoma of the esohagus and ectopic gastric mucosa. *Br J Cancer* 1953; 6:127–130.
47. Thomas JV, Hay LJ: Adenocarcinoma of the esophagus. Report of a case of glandular metaplasia of the esophageal mucosa. *Surgery* 1954; 35:635–639.
48. Armstrong RA, Blalock JB, Carrera GM: Adenocarcinoma of the middle third of the esophagus arising from ectopic gastric mucosa. *J Thorac Cardiovasc Surg* 1959; 37:398–403.
49. Herbst JJ, Berenson MM, McCloskey DW, et al: Cell proliferation in esophageal columnar epithelium (Barrett's esophagus). *Gastroenterology* 1978; 75:683–687.
50. Pellish LJ, Hermos JA, Eastwood GL: Cell proliferation in three types of Barrett's epithelium. *Gut* 1980; 21:26–31.
51. Geboes K, Vanstapel MJ, Desmet VJ, et al: Tissue demonstration of carcinoembryonic antigen (CEA) in columnar esophageal epithelium. *Hepato-Gastroenterol* 1981; 28:324–326.
52. Haggit RC, Tryzelaar J, Ellis HF, et al: Adenocarcinoma complicating columnar epithelium-lined (Barrett's) esophagus. *Am J Clin Path* 1978; 70:1–5.
53. McDonald GB, Brand DL, Thorning DR: Multiple adenomatous neoplasms arising in columnar-lined (Barrett's) esophagus. *Gastroenterology* 1977; 72:1317–1321.
54. Berenson MM, Riddell RH, Skinner DB, et al: Malignant transformation of esophageal columnar epithelium. *Cancer* 1978; 41:554–561.
55. Witt TR, Bains MS, Zaman MB, et al: Adenocarcinoma in Barrett's esophagus. *J Thorac Cardiovasc Surg* 1983; 85:337–345.
56. Sjogren RW Jr, Johnson LF: Barrett's esophagus: A review. *Am J Med* 1983; 74:313–321.
57. Poleynard GD, Marty AT, Birnbaum WB, et al: Adenocarcinoma in columnar-lined (Barrett) esophagus—a case report and review of the literature. *Arch Surg* 1977; 112:997–1000.

58. Hawe A, Payne WS, Weiland LH, et al: Adenocarcinoma in the columnar epithelial lined lower (Barrett) oesophagus. *Thorax* 1973; 28:511–514.
59. Dees J, VanBlankenstein M, Frenkel M: Adenocarcinoma involving the esophagus: A report of 13 cases. *Gastroenterology* 1978; 74:1119 (abstract).
60. Hankins JR, Cole FN, Attar S, et al: Adenocarcinoma involving the esophagus. *J Thorac Cardiovasc Surg* 1974; 68:148–158.
61. Raphael HA, Ellis FH, Dockerty MB: Primary adenocarcinoma of the esophagus: 18-year review and review of literature. *Ann Surg* 1966; 164:785–796.
62. Webb JN, Busuttil A: Adenocarcinoma of the oesophagus and of the oesophagogastric junction. *Br J Surg* 1978; 65:475–479.
63. Turnbull ADM, Goodner JT: Primary adenocarcinoma of the esophagus. *Cancer* 1968; 22:915–919.
64. Everhart CW Jr, Humphries TJ: Medical treatment of Barrett's esophagus with bethanechol: Report of three cases with prolonged follow-up. *Gastroenterology* 1978; 74:1003 (abstract).
65. Thompson WG, Barr R: Pharmacotherapy of an ulcer in Barrett's esophagus: Carbenoxolone and cimetidine. *Gastroenterology* 1977; 73:808–810.
66. Wesdorp ICE, Bartelsman J, Schipper MEI, et al: Effect of long-term treatment with cimetidine and antacids in Barrett's esophagus. *Gut* 1981; 22:724–727.
67. Bosch A, Frias Z, Caldwell WL: Adenocarcinoma of the esophagus. *Cancer* 1979; 43:1557–1561.
68. Danoff B, Cooper J, Klein M: Primary adenocarcinoma of the upper oesophagus. *Clin Radiol* 1978; 29:519–522.
69. Patel GK, Clift SA, Schaefer RA, et al: Resolution of severe dysplastic (Ca in situ) changes with regression of columnar epithelium in Barrett's esophagus on medical treatment. *Gastroenterology* 1982; 82:1147 (abstract).
70. Naef AP, Savary M: Conservative operations for peptic esophagitis with stenosis in columnar-lined lower esophagus. *Ann Thorac Surg* 1972; 13:543–551.
71. Bremner CG: The columnar lined (Barrett's) esophagus. *Surg Annu* 1977; 9:103–123.
72. Brand DL, Ylvisaker JT, Gelfand M, et al: Regression of columnar esophageal (Barrett's) epithelium after anti-reflux surgery. *N Engl J Med* 1980; 302:844–848.

Index